PRAISE FOR REBECCA GRANT'S *BIRTH*

Winner of a 2023 Porchlight Business Book Award

"A much-needed perspective on childbirth. . . . I do feel far more informed after reading *Birth,* and I hope that other readers come away feeling the same."

—Porchlight (Editor's Choice)

"A significant and compelling sociological investigation."

—*Kirkus Reviews*

"An enlightening and accessible portrait of maternal health care in America."

—*Publishers Weekly* (starred review)

"As we navigate an endless number of crises, Rebecca Grant's thorough reporting about one such issue—reproductive health in all its facets—is lighting a pathway forward. *Birth* is a testament to Grant's impeccable reporting and storytelling skills, pulling back the curtain on pregnancy in America while also pushing us to understand what the stakes are and what it will take to move forward. *Birth* is the kind of book that should be on the shelves of every obstetrician and gynecologist in a country where giving birth is as dangerous as it has ever been."

—Evette Dionne, author of *Weightless*

"A true feat of intimate, illuminating reporting, *Birth* is a profound examination of the deeply personal and structural forces that shape life-defining choices, experiences, dreams, and futures."

—Rainesford Stauffer, author of *An Ordinary Age* and *All the Gold Stars*

"Grant captures the inherent drama of giving birth with keen insights into the social and political forces that shape pregnancy and motherhood in America. A must-read for anyone who has been born!"

—Atossa Araxia Abrahamian, author of *The Cosmopolites*

BIRTH

Three Mothers, Nine Months, and Pregnancy in America

REBECCA GRANT

AVID READER PRESS

New York London Toronto Sydney New Delhi

Avid Reader Press
An Imprint of Simon & Schuster, LLC
1230 Avenue of the Americas
New York, NY 10020

First Avid Reader Press trade paperback edition April 2024

Interior design by Lexy East

Manufactured in the United States of America

1 3 5 7 9 10 8 6 4 2

Library of Congress Cataloging-in-Publication Data has been applied for.

ISBN 978-1-9821-7042-4
ISBN 978-1-9821-7043-1 (pbk)
ISBN 978-1-9821-7044-8 (ebook)

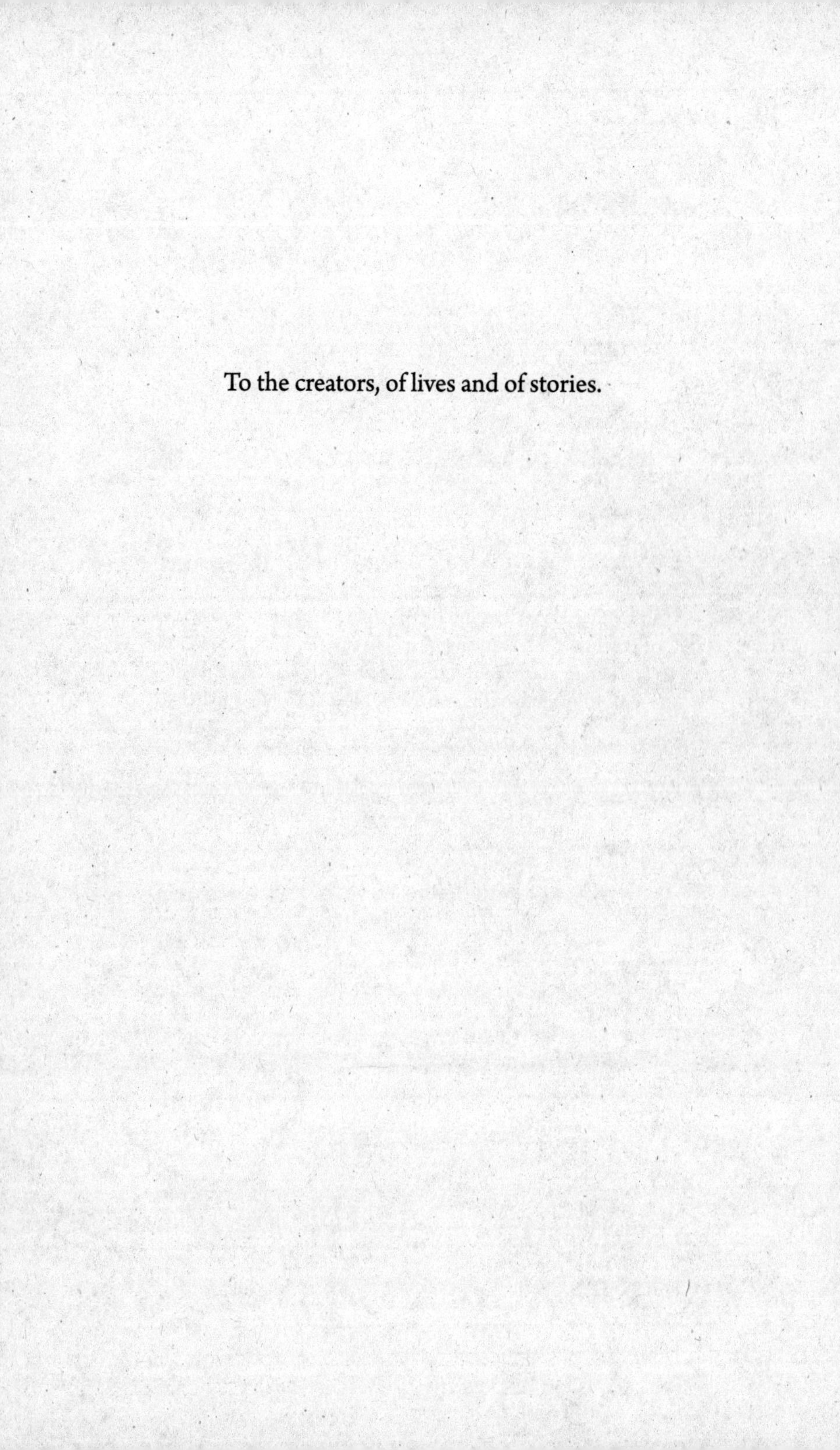

To the creators, of lives and of stories.

CONTENTS

BIRTH

POSTPARTUM

A NOTE ON NAMES AND LANGUAGE

While Jillian, T'Nika, and Alison all chose to use their real first names in this book, part of my embed arrangement with the birth center was that unless a client agreed to be interviewed separately, outside the scope of the appointment, or gave explicit permission, I would not use their real name. Therefore, Andaluz clients, aside from the three protagonists, have each been given a pseudonym. I also used pseudonyms for a handful of people from my sources' lives. These include the names Hallie, Martina, Danielle, Kayla, and Jada.

Throughout the book, I refer both to "women" and to "people" who give birth. Not all people who have uteruses, get pregnant, or give birth identify as women. The use of the term "woman" is not meant to marginalize, diminish, or discount those experiences. Rather, it reflects the gender identity of my three main characters, as well as a majority of the birth center's clients.

We are volcanoes.
When we women offer our experience as our truth,
as human truth, all the maps change.
There are new mountains.
—Ursula K. Le Guin, Bryn Mawr, 1986

FOREWORD

The seed for this book was a very simple question: What is it like, for a woman in our country today, to experience pregnancy and childbirth for the first time?

Having a baby is one of the most physically, mentally, and emotionally significant things a person can do in their life. This is not to say that children are a requirement for a happy or meaningful life or that families aren't made in an infinite variety of ways. It is to say that when someone gets pregnant and has a baby, they are never the same again.

Pregnancy can be a disorienting combination of the momentous and the mundane. The body is in the process of growing a new human. It's an engine of seismic, irreparable transformation, a cleaving into the Before and the After. It can also feel at times like a nine- (or ten-) month slog, an endless parade of physical ailments and discomfort. It's throwing up and taking vitamins and feeling tired and answering the same questions over and over again. It's having one's body taken over and subjected to a steady stream of monitoring and commentary from friends, family, and strangers alike. It's never knowing if a twinge is indigestion or catastrophe. It's being anchored at the center of the universe and swept up in an endlessly repeating cycle, a journey that is both unique and quotidian. There's so much that's unknown, and yet it's happened an infinite number of times before.

There are depths to mine, and yet there is a remarkable lack of narrative resources that convey what it's really like. A lot is left unsaid, or only passed on in whispers.

I hope to change that. While there are thousands of books out there that fall under the category of "pregnancy and childbirth," the vast majority are guides, how-tos, reference manuals, or treatises that espouse specific ways of doing things. There are histories of childbirth; memoirs about motherhood, midwifery, and obstetrical practice; academic and sociological books that examine subjects like cesarean surgeries or medical racism; and journalism about the maternal healthcare system. But few books, if any, have treated the experiences of being pregnant and giving birth as the foundation for reported nonfiction, documenting these experiences in a rigorous, intimate, and unflinching way.

It may be helpful to know at what week a fetus is the size of a papaya or how an epidural works, but it's equally helpful to know how those milestones might make someone feel or the struggles they may face. Stories are the map that's needed. They create a cosmos of all the infinite directions a sperm meeting an egg can go.

This book is rooted in the narratives of three women with similar circumstances and starting points, for whom pregnancy represented a kind of quest—to create a new family, to understand themselves, to assert their values, to question norms, and to venture bravely into the unknown in the hope of securing the future they wanted, grappling with sacrifice and obstacles and encountering moments of epiphany and joy along the way. But where and how someone gives birth—and whether they choose to give birth in the first place—is inseparable from their context. During pregnancy, medical, social, historical, cultural, and spiritual forces interact with the personal, playing across people's bodies and shaping the decisions they make, or can make. That is why the scope of this book expands beyond these three stories, zooming in and out and up and around and back to investigate why things are the way they are—and how to build a better birth system.

There is widespread agreement that maternal healthcare in the US is deeply flawed. Our costs are exponentially higher than peer countries, and yet we have far higher rates of adverse outcomes and persistent racial inequities.

Childbirth is the most common reason for hospitalization in the US and represents a major proportion of hospital-based care. 23 percent of hospital stays are for pregnancy, childbirth, and newborn care—more than any other reason by far. A baby is born roughly every eight seconds in America. That's 3.6 million babies each year, and 98 percent of them are born in a hospital. Within the overarching category of "hospital birth," there is significant variation. There are major teaching hospitals and small community hospitals; public and private hospitals; rural, suburban, and urban hospitals; Catholic and secular hospitals; hospitals designated as "mother" or "baby" friendly; hospitals with nurse-midwifery programs and birth tubs and hospitals with 65 percent cesarean rates. Most births in hospitals are attended by obstetricians or nurse-midwives, although a small percentage, particularly in rural areas, are attended by family medicine doctors. (Osteopaths and naturopaths may attend births as well.)

Each year in the US, $111 billion is spent on maternal and newborn care. One in three babies is born via cesarean surgery. Six of the sixteen most common hospital procedures are for maternal or newborn care, including the most common operating room procedure in the US: the cesarean birth. On average, a vaginal birth costs $23,000 and a cesarean birth costs $43,700. Spontaneous vaginal birth in an American hospital costs five times what it does in Spain, and despite the higher costs, the US ranks lower in health outcomes for mothers and infants than other industrialized countries. Thousands of families go bankrupt each year from having a baby.

For a young, healthy woman encountering the hospital system for the first time, childbirth can be a jarring experience. The pattern is of constant expense, vigilance, and preparation for worst-case scenarios. Interventions intended to improve outcomes for high-risk moms are applied universally to every mother, regardless of their level of risk and preferences. "The modern medical system was built to treat the sickest possible patient," said Dr. Chavi Eve Karkowsky, an OB/GYN and maternal-fetal medicine specialist, in her book *High Risk*—sometimes at the expense of pregnant people who are healthy and low-risk.

In hospitals today, intensive medical management is the norm. That might be fine if it improved outcomes, was cost-effective, or provided what women wanted. But none of those things is true. According to an exhaustive report published by the National Academies of Sciences, Engineering, and Medicine in 2020, "the U.S. maternity care system currently incurs extraordinary costs to produce among the poorest outcomes among high-income nations. . . . [It] is fraught with uneven access and quality, stark inequities, and exorbitant costs."

Around 85 percent of women who labor in hospitals receive continuous electronic fetal monitoring and an intravenous drip. Around one in three pregnant people have their labors induced, while 40 percent report that their maternity care provider tried to induce their labor. 52.4 percent of women said they received Pitocin at some point during their labor. 75 percent get an epidural. 80 percent of people giving birth in hospitals do not eat, and 60 percent do not drink during labor. Most patients are restricted to bed and give birth on their backs. Nurses are typically the most present medical providers during labor, with obstetricians arriving for the actual delivery. Depending on the hospital or practice (or type of insurance), birth may be the first time a woman meets her OB. Far too many American women emerge from birth feeling confused, alienated, discouraged, and traumatized.

This is the birth system that most expectant mothers encounter in America. But what if it could be different?

It was these broader questions and issues that led me to set this book in a birth center. Freestanding birth centers represent a sort of middle ground between the home and the hospital. They do not provide epidurals or opioids for pain relief (relying instead on non-pharmacological measures, such as birth tubs), do not administer Pitocin to induce or augment labor or perform surgery, and use intermittent fetal monitoring, which enables people in labor to move around. Because freestanding birth centers rely on fewer medical interventions, and because they don't have facilities like operating rooms or blood banks on-site for emergencies, they are designed to serve low-risk clients. They are also the domain of a small but mighty category of birth workers: midwives.

Through years of reporting on maternal healthcare, through conducting countless interviews and reading reams of books and research, I—along with many others—have come to see midwives as a critical component of improving maternity care. The benefits of their presence are clear and well-established: fewer cesareans, fewer inductions, significant reductions in severe lacerations and tears, and higher levels of satisfaction, to name a few. Many of the greatest challenges America faces when it comes to maternal healthcare could be mitigated by greater integration of midwifery care into our system, but until somewhat recently, midwives have remained a niche and largely inaccessible option, out-of-hospital birth even more so.

Over the past few years, out-of-hospital, also known as "community," birth has experienced a surge. Between 2004 and 2017, home births increased by 77 percent, while birth center births more than doubled. In 2017, one of every sixty-two births in the US was an out-of-hospital birth. At 1.61 percent, it was the first time in decades that out-of-hospital birth had surpassed the 1 percent mark. Between 2019 and 2020, the percentage of home births increased by 22 percent, marking the highest level since 1990, including significant increases across racial and ethnic lines. Those rises were likely spurred by the outbreak of Covid-19, which led midwives to report significant upticks in the number of families seeking their services. People who may never have considered a birth center or midwives before are becoming more open to the option. Historically, interest in midwifery has followed pendulum swings, but there's reason to think this upswing may be here to stay.

Portland, Oregon, where I live, has a robust midwifery community, and out-of-hospital birth is more common here than in most other parts of the country. In addition, several private insurance carriers and the state's public insurance cover birth center care. As a result, midwifery care is accessed not by only a fervent few, but by a more mainstream subset of the population.

This worked in my favor as the vision for this project took shape. During the summer of 2020, I was on a scouting mission, searching for a birth center where I could immerse and embed as a journalist for nine months, shadowing midwives and following clients as they navigated their pregnancies. Reporters often approach a story with a general sense of the type of source they'd like to find, someone who provides a particular portal or lens to the topic at hand. The women I followed would also need to be willing, and ideally eager and excited, to participate in this project. I needed sources who were on board with opening their lives to a journalist in an intimate and time-consuming way; who would answer endless questions about sex, gassiness, miscarriage, weight gain, nipple chafing, spousal tension, vaginal secretions, and deep-seated anxieties; who were willing to let me nose around their medical records and homes and overhear conversations about hemorrhoids and stool softeners; who might be willing for me to be in the room when they were in various states of undress or even completely naked. And I needed people who thought intensely about their pregnancies and who were as invested in the mission of telling their stories as I was.

I needed the buy-in of midwives as well, so they'd be willing to let me observe them during appointments and introduce me to their clients. In my experience, midwives are passionate about what they do and want more people to know that midwifery is an option. But they also care about their clients' privacy, and the media hasn't always been fair to their profession, so I wasn't sure how easy gaining access would be. When I called the Andaluz Waterbirth Center in Southwest Portland to gauge their interest in the project, my gut said I'd found the right place.

I initially spoke with the birth center's founder, Jennifer Gallardo. I expected to have to make a strong case for why she should let me lurk around for a year, but that didn't turn out to be necessary. After one meeting on her farm, sitting in hammocks as dogs and children ran around, she gave me the green light and left me to my own devices, subject to what individual midwives and clients were comfortable with. As a first step, she recommended I take a tour to see for myself how the birth center worked. That's when I met the birth center's office manager, Jillian, who let me in and showed me around the building. She shared that she had recently graduated from midwifery school, was pregnant with her first child, and was planning a home birth. Right away, I enlisted her as a source. She also connected me directly to about a dozen Andaluz clients, and I met dozens more while sitting in on prenatal and postpartum appointments.

One of those clients was T'Nika, who shared a due date with Jillian. I spent most of our first conversation giggling incessantly. It may not have been the most professional way to conduct an interview, but her mix of wry humor and candid goofiness, along with the creative and surprising ways her mind engaged with pregnancy, provided a captivating perspective—as did her commitment to working for racial justice in maternal healthcare as an aspiring labor and delivery nurse.

My third character, Alison, was something of an outlier. She had toured Andaluz but found another birth center that felt like a better fit because it was more closely aligned with a hospital. She didn't think of herself as a "midwifery" or "birth center" person, but a series of experiences had led her to question the hospital-based birth system and seek out an alternative. Alison approached every decision, every pregnancy milestone, with a great amount of intention and deliberation. She evolved with each passing week of her pregnancy in a way that was compelling to follow.

I had my three main protagonists.

Over the next nine months, the bulk of my reporting unspooled over countless hours of interviews, both in-person and over the phone every week—and sometimes multiple times a week—starting from early in their pregnancies. I talked with each woman about what they were feeling and how they were feeling and why. I asked about their nausea, if they could feel the baby kick, and what they were stressed about. I asked about their childhoods and what they did at work, what they ate for dinner and what type of contraception they had previously used, where they bought maternity pants and how they thought motherhood would change them. I attended their prenatal appointments and read their medical records. I reviewed text messages, photos, videos, journal entries, and emails. I interviewed their partners, midwives, doulas, parents, family members, and friends. I befriended some of their pets, all in the service of documenting in close detail their pregnancy and childbirth journeys. I followed these women through moments of glee, worry, excitement, fear, apprehension, embarrassment, uncertainty, growth, stress, and metamorphosis. Each wrestled with the right time to have a baby and how having a baby would irreparably alter their lives. Each embarked on a journey that offered no guarantees, but that was filled with mystery, courage, promise, and hope.

Jillian, T'Nika, and Alison share certain things in common. They are all older than twenty-seven, making them above the average age for first-time mothers in the US. They are middle-class, cisgender, straight, college educated, and partnered. English is their first language. In many significant ways, their experiences differ from those of, say, teenage mothers, single mothers, immigrant women, and LGBTQ+ parents. They differ from people who have struggled with drug addiction or who are unhoused, and they were all having uncomplicated pregnancies. In these similarities, they reflect the typical profile of people who seek birth center care in the US. Those similarities also created a level foundation upon which to build out each of their narratives. Their three stories are not meant to be symbolic or representational. Instead, they aim to show that, even among women with similar backgrounds, there exists an entire, highly varied spectrum of pregnancy and birth experiences. Observing those experiences in real time provided nuance, detail, honesty, and insight that might otherwise have been lost.

I hope that this book breaks information about pregnancy and birth out of its silo. I hope it helps people, regardless of whether they can or want to have children, understand what this journey can look like. I hope it drives home the point that conversations about pregnancy and birth are inextricable from those about miscarriage and abortion, and that bodily autonomy should never be negotiable. I hope it lets people know that they are not alone, regardless of how their pregnancies unfold or the choices they make. I hope it empowers people with the knowledge that they have agency and choice in their birth experiences.

Finally, I hope this book contributes to broader efforts to evolve our maternal healthcare system into one with the well-being of mothers and infants at its core.

BIRTH

CONCEPTION

There is no greater agony than bearing an untold story inside you.
—Zora Neale Hurston, *Dust Tracks on a Road*

CHAPTER 1
Jillian

Just after 1:00 p.m. on a Thursday in August, Jillian looked at the clock and then around the lobby of the Andaluz Waterbirth Center. No clients were sitting in the muffled quiet of the waiting area, and there weren't any appointments scheduled for another half hour. She cocked an ear toward the hallway behind her, hearing only the faint sound of people chatting in the kitchen. She pushed her chair back from the reception desk, grabbed her water bottle and sweater, and crept down the empty hallway, hoping no one would emerge before she made it to the staircase. The coast was clear as Jillian climbed the wide wooden stairs to the second floor and let herself into the Clara suite, one of the birth center's lesser-used rooms.

The room was decorated in soft yellow and gray, with a bed nestled under a fabric headboard and a framed picture of a beach boardwalk on one wall. Over the wide tub in the bathroom hung a picture of a whale. Jillian sat on the bed and waited, listening for the shuffle of Marilyn's footsteps on the carpet. She was nervous and excited, like a teenager sneaking a beer from her parents' refrigerator. It was unlikely anyone would find them, but the clandestine nature of the meeting added to the thrill.

Jillian had already confirmed her pregnancy with a test and was exhibiting classic early symptoms—aching breasts, nausea, swings in body temperature, and fatigue—but part of her didn't believe it was real yet. When Marilyn suggested they do a little ultrasound tryst, Jillian was relieved. She hoped that by hearing the baby for the first time, by making what was happening internally echo externally, the reality would sink in. She wanted someone to lay their hands on her stomach and say, "Everything looks good," even though it was really too soon to say. At eight weeks, the fetus was only the size of a kidney bean.

After a few moments, Marilyn slipped into the room, a conspiratorial gleam in her eyes. Tall and willowy with a fondness for scarves, she had worked as a midwife at Andaluz for six years. After decades of running her own home birth practice, she had grown tired of being a business owner, weighed down by all the paperwork and administrative work that it entailed, and decided to spend her final years before retirement focused on catching babies.

"Well, isn't this exciting?" she said in a hushed voice. She smiled warmly as she held up a Doppler, a small monitor that used sound waves to detect fetal cardiac activity.

Jillian scooted back on the bed, lay down, and lifted her shirt.

Marilyn smeared gel on the probe and stood to the side, delicately placing it on Jillian's belly. It felt cool and slimy. Both women were quiet. Then, a *whoosh whoosh* sound filled the room—just white noise at first—before an ever-so-slightly more pronounced pulsing began to reverberate.

There it is, she thought.

"Oh my goodness, sweetie," Marilyn said. "Listen to that."

Jillian widened her eyes and grinned, her own heart thumping harder. She held as still and quiet as she could, listening to the sound coming from inside her. With each new vibration, Jillian imagined a tiny ember burning brighter now that it had been exposed to oxygen. She'd listened to fetal heart tones countless times before as a midwifery student, but these were specific pulses. These pulses were hers. Theirs.

Jillian met Marilyn's eyes, glad they were sharing the moment together. They had grown close since Jillian had started apprenticing at the birth center as a midwifery student two years before. She found Marilyn's tender confidence soothing and was glad not to be alone with the secret. Outside of her husband, Chad, and her best friend, Alysa (and now Marilyn), no one knew she was pregnant. A decade before, Jillian had experienced a miscarriage at the end of the first trimester, and this time around, she hoped to pass the twelve-week milestone before making any kind of announcement. However, it was especially difficult to keep a pregnancy under wraps in a workplace that teemed with pregnant women and babies. After forty years as a midwife, Marilyn was like a bloodhound. All it took was one morning when Jillian looked a little ill at the front desk and complained about temperature swings for Marilyn to sniff out her secret.

Pregnancy, at this moment, was not something Jillian had planned. She and Chad had intended to wait a little longer before having a baby because their lives were still getting settled. Jillian had graduated from midwifery school in 2019, but she hadn't yet applied for her midwifery certification or license, and the couple had just moved into a new house. She was still wrapping her mind around the situation and wanted to share the news in her own time and on her own terms.

After listening to the Doppler for a few moments, Jillian wiped the goo off her belly and pulled down her shirt. She and Marilyn walked softly out of the Clara room and back down the stairs before going their separate ways. Marilyn had a full schedule of clients to see that afternoon, and Jillian returned to her position at the front desk, carrying the pulsing little kidney bean with her.

CHAPTER 2
T'Nika

Andaluz was located on a busy road in Southwest Portland. On clear days, the sharp peak of Mount Hood stood out in the distance, framed between a bright purple house and a green one perched on the hillside. The square brick birth center had white columns and frosted windows. It used to be a firehouse and then an insurance company office, and it retained the unglamorous yet dignified look of utilitarian buildings. For over ten years, women had struggled up the brick steps in labor and descended back down them, reassembled into motherhood. But the only hints of what went on within the sturdy walls were a sign out front, three white lockboxes for medical samples, and a certificate in the window that read, "Accredited Birth Center."

T'Nika and her husband, Daniel, parked on the street to avoid the narrow lot that ran in an L-shape along the side and the back of the building. Above the parking lot hung stretched cables for the Portland Aerial Tram, connecting the riverfront to the main campus of Oregon Health and Science University up the hill, where T'Nika had once considered applying for a nursing program. She had driven by the building many times but never noticed the sign hanging from the iron lamppost out front that read, "Andaluz Waterbirth Center," with a photo of a sleeping baby. When she and Daniel pulled up in their car, her first thought was that it seemed like something out of Harry Potter, appearing only now that she knew to look for it.

Now, she stood on the porch and knocked.

The door clicked open, and the couple stepped inside, hit by a gentle gust of air-conditioning. Their eyes immediately went to the mural of a tree on the opposite wall. A brown trunk and branches were painted on a bright blue background, covered with green and yellow paper cutouts of leaves, each with a name and a date written on it—all the babies who had been born at Andaluz, all the way back to 2017. Every few years, the midwives took the leaves down and started filling the tree's branches again.

They walked across the lobby to the reception desk, where a woman who introduced herself as Jillian greeted them. As she checked in T'Nika, she leaned forward and whispered with a smile that she was eight weeks pregnant, too, and their due dates were probably around the same time. *That's cool,* T'Nika thought. It made the birth center seem extra nurturing, like a clubhouse for pregnant people. Jillian said a midwife named Marilyn would be through in a few minutes, but in the meantime she and Daniel could wait on the couches in the lobby.

T'Nika and Daniel surveyed the waiting area. It reminded T'Nika of the birth center where she and her siblings had been born. The walls were painted a soft yellow and lined with photographs and paintings of mothers holding babies and newborns emerging from wombs. Plants were arrayed around the room and the dark wood floors were covered by a plush area rug. Past Jillian's desk and the mural stood a bookcase filled with books about pregnancy and childbirth. (A voracious reader, T'Nika fought the urge to examine the titles for ones she hadn't read; if she gave birth here, she would have plenty of time over the next thirty-two weeks to take a closer look.) Next to the bookcase was a large white fireplace with a painting of a couple sitting together in a birth tub, a ceramic bust of a female torso on the mantel. Light streamed through the windows that faced the main road and shined onto a coffee table stacked with glossy Anne

Geddes photography books. Surrounded by art and plants and books, T'Nika felt at home. Even the air smelled good, like a spa instead of the sterile, antiseptic smell she was used to from her shifts at a long-term-care nursing facility.

Moments later, a woman with her graying hair pulled back in a clip and crafty dangling earrings entered, a client by her side. She guided her to the front desk to make a follow-up appointment with Jillian and then strode with purpose over to T'Nika and Daniel to shake their hands. She looked T'Nika square in the eyes, her voice blending genuine and gentle with seasoned assertiveness as she introduced herself as Marilyn. Immediately, T'Nika felt like she was in good hands. Before even venturing past the lobby for a tour, she was pretty sure this was where she wanted to have her baby.

The Andaluz building had four birthing suites, Marilyn explained as she guided them out of the waiting area, each color-coordinated and named: Tierra, Brisa, and Solana—all on the ground floor—and Clara upstairs. (The Florencia suite, also upstairs, was set up for prenatals but not births.) Tierra was the first room, closest to reception and decorated in a plant motif. The walls were sage green with a queen-size bed covered in a sage comforter and throw pillows, an upholstered armchair, and a capacious tub in the corner covered in green mosaic tiles. Brisa, Marilyn said, pointing it out as they walked by, was the smallest.

In the hallway, a tray of essential oils sat on a white dresser next to a diffuser and a hand lotion pump. Above it was a framed bulletin board filled with baby announcements and photos. Across the hall was the storage closet, filled floor to ceiling with labeled plastic bins containing medical supplies like instruments, suturing equipment, gloves, lidocaine, pulse oximeters, heel lancets, wipes, and oxygen tanks. Each room, T'Nika and Daniel learned, had its own rolling cart with supplies and dressers for storing items like diapers.

Adjacent to the supply closest was the Sonora suite, the biggest and most popular because of its size and corner windows, which looked out onto the back parking lot. The room was decorated in desert earth tones, and like the others, it had a spacious, tiled tub in the corner and a large bathroom with a handicap-accessible toilet and shower. When someone was in labor, Marilyn explained, the midwives hung up a pink laminated sign that read, "Birth in Progress—Do Not Disturb," on the door of whatever suite they were in. The doors were thick, but groans, moans, yells, and yowls could occasionally be heard in the kitchen across the hall. Clients and their families were welcome to spend time in the kitchen, which was painted a henna hue. A ragged and overwhelmed-looking father-to-be might wander into the kitchen on occasion, looking lost, but it was primarily where the midwives and students hung out, chatting around the table, making coffee between appointments, and snacking on the trail mix and dried fruit stored in large glass canisters. From the hallway, T'Nika could see a kitchen counter with a blender (midwives used it to make smoothies, their go-to sustenance for people in labor) and an area where midwives brewed tea and herbal baths meant to promote the healing of delicate areas.

After each birth, Marilyn continued, Andaluz ordered food delivery from the restaurant of the new parents' choosing and would transfer the hot meals to plates and place them on TV trays to bring into the suites, filling the kitchen with the aromas of curried lentils, bowls of chili, and grilled chicken salads. The back door to the birth center was next to the kitchen, perpetually opening and closing as the midwives arrived at work, students returned from errands, and clients' family members bustled in for visits.

In the middle of the hallway, T'Nika could see a wide staircase that led upstairs and down. The basement wasn't included on the tour, but it was where the birth center stored supply reserves, along with an autoclave, backup oxygen and nitrous tanks, laundry machines, and a narrow bed where midwives could crash after staying awake all night at a birth. There was also a fridge with a sign on the freezer that read, "Not

For Food." That was where placentas were stored, the sign thanks in part to an urban legend about a midwife's son (or husband or wife or friend or neighbor or nephew) who had defrosted a placenta thinking it was a frozen pizza.

On the second floor, they were brought into Clara. The birthing suite was on the smaller side, but it offered the added privacy of being upstairs and connected to a large common room. The common room, carpeted and lined with brown couches, was where Andaluz held its monthly midwife meetings and childbirth classes. It was also a space where big families could hang out while someone labored. T'Nika could see her and Daniel's families gathering up there while they waited for her baby to be born.

After the tour, Marilyn, T'Nika, and Daniel settled back downstairs into the Tierra suite, Marilyn's favorite room, so she could explain how the birth center worked. Andaluz had five or six midwives on staff who worked on schedules of three months on and one month off, she began. In addition to the birth center in Portland, there was a small birthing cottage in Dundee, about a one-hour drive south. Depending on where T'Nika planned to give birth and her due date, she would see at least three different midwives throughout her prenatal care. It was important to Andaluz that each client was attended in birth by a person they knew, but birth was unpredictable, which meant midwife schedules were too. To account for that, T'Nika would get to know a few midwives and rank her first, second, and third choice. When in labor, she'd call her first choice, and if that midwife was unavailable (usually due to being at another birth), she'd move down the list. No matter what, the midwife would have two apprentices assisting her at the birth. She'd rank her preferences for birthing suites as well.

That system made sense to T'Nika. She appreciated the opportunity to get to know multiple midwives and that the rotating schedule gave them a break; she knew from her own experience how burned-out healthcare providers could get. T'Nika also got a good vibe from Marilyn. She seemed like the sort of wise, hippie grandma she wanted to guide her through this experience.

After finishing her spiel, Marilyn asked if T'Nika had any questions. T'Nika took a deep breath. She did. Before committing to Andaluz, she needed to know how much it would cost. She really wanted to give birth there, but she was nervous that it would be out of her price range.

Midwifery services, at home or at a birth center, generally cost between $3,000 to $9,000, including prenatal and postpartum care and labor and delivery services. That's a fraction of the cost of a hospital birth, though it often ends up costing more money for clients due to inadequate insurance coverage. While all insurance carriers, both public and private, cover hospital births, few cover community births.* As a result of gaps in insurance coverage, two-thirds of planned home births and one-third of birth center births are self-paid, compared to only 3.4 percent of hospital births. Oregon was more friendly to midwives than most states—T'Nika had heard that multiple private insurance carriers in the state covered birth centers, and the public insurance program, Oregon Health Plan (OHP), extended coverage to qualifying out-of-hospital births as well—but she wasn't sure if her insurer covered Andaluz. She figured a boutique environment like Andaluz would cost a premium.

She and Daniel were prepared for the fact that having a baby in America was expensive, regardless of the environment. They earned comfortable incomes and had private health insurance, but they didn't want to put themselves in a financial situation that would sap their savings. They hoped to buy a house someday. Marilyn said that she understood their concern, and if their insurance covered Andaluz (which, it turned out, it did), the out-of-pocket cost for prenatal, labor and delivery, and postpartum care would likely be around $3,000. Three thousand dollars was a hefty amount of money, but T'Nika knew it wasn't necessarily more than she'd pay if she went to a hospital. People with employer-sponsored health insurance paid an average of $4,500 out-of-pocket for labor and delivery, and between her own history with medical bills and her nursing ed-

---

* Private insurance companies cover 49.6 percent of births in the US, and Medicaid finances 42.3 percent, making it the dominant payer of births.

ucation, she knew how costs could sneak up and accumulate in hospitals. She had recently read an article about a woman who went into a hospital to give birth and received in her bill a fee for "skin-to-skin contact"—charged to hold her own baby.

T'Nika and Daniel discussed it and decided they were willing to pay for Andaluz. If they had to pay thousands of dollars one way or the other, they might as well pay for an environment they liked. On their way out, they scheduled T'Nika's next appointment for four weeks later. Her due date, like Jillian's, was March 20.

CHAPTER 3
Jillian

Jillian had not always known she wanted to be a midwife. Growing up, she hadn't even known what a midwife was. Born outside of Houston, Texas, she moved to the St. Louis area when she was a child with her family. As a teenager, she started working as soon as she was old enough to do so, hostessing at Outback Steakhouse and babysitting for families in her neighborhood. When she graduated from high school, Jillian wasn't sure what she wanted to do with her life but was drawn to the idea of working with moms and babies. She signed up for nursing prerequisite classes at Maryville, a community college near her home, and worked part-time as a hospital technician in an emergency room.

Right away, she realized that nursing, or at least ER nursing, was not for her. It wasn't the medical stuff—she was fine with the sight of blood and sticking people with needles—so much as the hierarchy and atmosphere. She saw doctors and nurses talking over patients, ignoring them, and charging ahead with medical tasks or procedures without explanation or consent—what she thought of as the "power-over" dynamic. She wanted an environment that felt more nurturing and collaborative and began casting around for another path to take.

Around the same time, she met a boy named Chris and followed him to Florida. She transferred her job at Outback Steakhouse to a location near Leesburg, a town in the middle of the state, and the couple adopted a sweet gray pit bull named Diesel. When they broke up a little over a year later, Jillian was not interested in returning to Missouri, so she and Diesel moved in with an aunt in St. Augustine. Even though the ER technician job hadn't clicked, she signed up for more nursing prerequisite classes, thinking she might enjoy working on a labor and delivery ward or in an OB/GYN office someday.

With its history, charm, and old Spanish fort, St. Augustine teemed with tourists, which paid off handsomely in waitressing tips. The city was also filled with young people who loved the beach and loved to party. Jillian, twenty-one years old and newly single, decided to take a break from school. She wanted to have fun and not think about human anatomy or chemistry. She waitressed at a family-owned southern food restaurant and moved into an apartment with roommates who hit the bars every night.

It was great, until one day at work, about a year later, when she found herself reeling from a swell of nausea. She puked in the bathroom, which prompted one of her coworkers to joke that she might be pregnant. Jillian laughed it off; she had been hooking up with a musician friend on and off, but it was casual, and she had a NuvaRing, so the prospect that she was pregnant, though not impossible, seemed unlikely. Despite her doubts, she drove to a drugstore after her shift to buy a pregnancy test and took it at her apartment.

When the result came back positive, Jillian stared at the test stick, stunned. She didn't know how to feel or what to do. There were so many things she wanted before having a baby. She was young, un-partnered, and had yet to finish school. She was living paycheck to paycheck. She was still forming who she was, who she would be, as an adult. When she thought about having to tell her parents she was pregnant, her stomach twisted. And then twisted again when she thought about telling the father. Jillian had no idea how he would react. There was a solid chance she would have to navigate this journey without him.

For a brief, fleeting moment, she considered whether she would end the pregnancy. She supported access to abortion and didn't believe anyone had a right to make that decision but the pregnant person themselves. But for her, in that moment, she wasn't sure that was the choice she wanted to make. She decided to continue the pregnancy, whether or not she was ready, and turned her attention to the relentless, dizzying barrage of practical considerations and logistics. Where would she live? How would she do this without nearby family support? Should she leave Florida? Should she stay? If she stayed, she'd have to move into a place better suited for a baby. How was she going to work? She was on a hiatus from college—would she ever be able to go back to school? How would she afford it? Would she and the father try to coparent or be together as a couple? What would that look like?

It was overwhelming and not a little terrifying, but in quiet moments, when she stopped panicking about the practicals, she could envision herself as a happy and dedicated mom. Jillian had always known she wanted to be a parent someday. If, at twenty-two years old, it was earlier than she anticipated, maybe that was okay. She was a determined and gritty person and trusted herself to make the best of the situation. When she told the father, he wasn't exactly thrilled, but he said he wanted to be involved and make it work.

Because Jillian didn't have health insurance, she went to a clinic run by the local health department to confirm her pregnancy with a blood test and an ultrasound. She was about nine weeks along. That was further than she'd thought, but it also made sense—her menstrual cycle hadn't been regular since she went on contraceptives, and a couple of months without a period hadn't caught her notice. The only symptom she had experienced was the one time she threw up at work.

The clinic recommended she seek prenatal care right away, and Jillian began looking into public healthcare options. Around the same time, she was offered an office job with better pay, stable hours, and health insurance coverage. To Jillian, it felt like a sign that everything would work out. She still hadn't broken the news to her parents, but she was glad that when she did, she could at least share a coherent plan to show she was prepared for the responsibility. Just as she was mustering the courage to call her mom, miscarriage symptoms began.

It started with cramping. Then, when she went to the bathroom, she saw spotting in her underwear—not a lot, but enough to give her pause. Throughout the rest of the day, the cramping and spotting continued, getting heavier. She drove to an urgent care center after her shift, but it was closed, so she kept driving to the ER.

The waiting room was not crowded when she arrived. Jillian checked in and told the intake staff what was going on—that she was pregnant, in her first trimester, and she'd been cramping and bleeding all day. They told her to take a seat. Assuming she wouldn't have to wait long, she called her friend Hallie to wait with her. They sat in uncomfortable chairs under fluorescent lights, watching people with broken bones and mysterious rashes come and go for hours, as Jillian continued to bleed. Periodically, she walked up to the reception desk, but they kept telling her she had to keep waiting. After seven hours stuck in the purgatory of the emergency room lobby, with little to no communication, Hallie stormed up to the desk.

"EXCUSE ME. SHE IS BLEEDING ALL OVER HER CLOTHES. SHE NEEDS A PAIR OF SCRUBS. GET US BACK THERE!" she yelled.

Fifteen minutes later, a nurse gave Jillian a pair of scrub pants and brought her back to an exam room. When the door opened again, a male doctor walked in. Jillian balked at first. She had always had—and preferred—female physicians, but after seven hours of waiting, there didn't seem to be much of a choice.

"Can I do a pelvic exam?" the doctor asked.

"Is that necessary?" Jillian said.

"It is," he said. "I have to see if your cervix is dilating at all."

Jillian agreed and laid back on the exam table. The doctor said her cervix was closed and there were large blood clots in her vagina, which he removed. It was a "threatened miscarriage," he explained, meaning that she was still pregnant but possibly faced a higher risk of miscarriage. He advised her to rest, stay home from work, and avoid physical activity. The next week, she should return to the hospital to see an OB/GYN and get an ultrasound.

Jillian trudged back through the hospital doors, feeling confused, relieved, annoyed, freaked out, and exhausted. Following the doctor's instructions, she called work and asked for time off. She felt okay for the next few days, but bleeding and cramping started again over the weekend. She went back to the ER, and this time she waited only twenty minutes before a doctor—a woman this time—sent her for a transvaginal ultrasound. The ultrasound technician stuck the large probe into her vagina and maintained a tense and awkward silence.

"What's going on?" Jillian asked nervously. "What are we seeing? What are we not seeing?"

The technician responded that he could not interpret the images because he was not a doctor. When he finished the scan, Jillian was sent back downstairs to an exam room to wait. A nurse drew blood and gave her an IV, and two hours later, the doctor came in.

"The pregnancy is no longer viable," she said matter-of-factly, her face impassive. "I recommend that you follow up with an OB/GYN, but you don't need a D&C. The miscarriage has completed on its own."*

The news was a whiplash. Not only was the pregnancy not viable, but it had *already* passed? Jillian said nothing, staring at the woman in front of her.

"Make sure to do that follow-up appointment and have a good day," the doctor said as she walked out of the room.

Moments passed, but Jillian stayed still. She was taken aback. *That's*

---

* A D&C, which stands for "dilation and curettage," is a common procedure for removing tissue from the uterus. It's used in both miscarriage management and abortion care.

it? That's how they deliver this news? She was young and alone. The doctor had just dropped this bomb and left. After all she'd been through over the past few weeks, the existential project of reimagining her entire life was suddenly no longer necessary. What was she supposed to do now? Return to her normal, prepregnancy life like nothing had happened? As she began to gather her things, she called the father, who spouted a few awkward platitudes and said he had to get back to work. (She later heard that he celebrated that weekend like a man freed from prison, buying rounds of drinks at the bar and taking a series of women home with him.)

All she could do next was go home. She took a shower, crawled into bed, and slept for a long time.

For months, Jillian distracted herself to avoid processing what had happened. She felt moments of grief but reminded herself that she was young and resilient, and some part of her felt a sense of reprieve. *Fuck it,* she thought. *I'm just going to party.*

She drank, she dated, and she didn't take care of herself, emotionally or physically. She contracted pyelonephritis, an infection that occurs after a urinary tract infection, which, when left untreated, can spread to the kidneys. The pain was intense, like getting stabbed in the back with a sharp knife. She visited the public health clinic (the same place she had gone for the pregnancy test), had the problem treated with antibiotics and fluids, and continued her partying streak.

Three months later, she met an older man, a divorced father of two. When he got into a bad motorcycle accident, she threw herself into being his caregiver, supporting them financially and taking care of his health needs. Yet again, her life was veering in a direction she hadn't anticipated. As she sunk deeper into what she thought of as her Florence Nightingale role, she worried that if she didn't carve out a path of her own, she would continue to be batted about by the whims of fate. She moved back to Missouri at the end of 2011, right around Christmas. She planned to live with her mother, stepdad, and younger siblings at first, and took a job at the front desk of the medical office where her mother worked as a healthcare biller. Far away from all that had happened in Florida, Jillian had space to decompress, to process, and to mull over what she wanted to do next. To find a sense of purpose.

Six months later, she got the news that one of her best friends from Florida, Bethany, was pregnant. The two spoke regularly, and during their long phone calls, Jillian learned that Bethany wasn't thrilled with her OB, who was prone to brushing off her concerns and treating her questions with impatience during their short, fifteen-minute appointments. She had stuck with him thus far because he was her doctor and she wasn't sure where else to go. That changed, however, during her third trimester, when the doctor announced he would start performing weekly vaginal checks. When Bethany said she was uncomfortable with that approach, the doctor said that in that case, he couldn't continue as her provider. Indignant and unwilling to concede, Bethany booked a consultation with a midwifery practice in town. She loved everything about it, she told Jillian on one of their calls—how much time the midwives spent with her, how they wanted to get to know her, and how they encouraged her to ask questions and make her own decisions.

"I think you would be really good at that," Bethany said.

"I've never even heard of midwifery," Jillian replied. "How could I be good at it?"

Bethany told Jillian to watch *The Business of Being Born*, a 2008 documentary produced by talk show host Ricki Lake that covered the history of obstetrics, modern-day midwifery practice, and hospital versus home birth, with a heavy slant toward the latter. After work one night at her apartment (the new job paid enough that she was able to leave her parents' place), Jillian curled up on the couch under a blanket and played the documentary. By the credits, she had bawled her eyes out. The film addressed some of the darker aspects of the US maternal healthcare system, like the overuse of cesarean surgeries and rising maternal mortality rates, and shared the stories of women who were unsatisfied, or even traumatized, by their hospital birth experiences. Midwives, it explained, provide an alternative type of care. Ina May Gaskin, a legendary midwife in the US, was featured in the documentary, as were visceral scenes of home birth that involved plenty of mess and full-frontal nudity.

Suddenly, it hit Jillian like a ton of bricks. Something about hospital birth had always felt off to her, and the documentary had finally brought into focus the reason why: birth was not an injury or a disease or a medical crisis. To Jillian, it was a rite of passage, but the system, as it stood, seemed to treat women like they were broken and needed to be fixed. What if they didn't have to be treated that way? What if Jillian could become a midwife? How did a person even become a midwife? And why hadn't she known about them before?

This is what I want to do, she thought.

The origins of the modern midwifery system in the US can be traced back to the 1600s, when ships sailing from West Africa and from Europe arrived in the "New World." The former carried enslaved African women who had midwifery experience from the lives they were taken from or who became midwives by necessity, and who continued to practice midwifery throughout their lives in bondage and beyond. The latter sailed with white colonists, one of whom was a doctor's wife named Bridget Lee Fuller. During the crossing of the *Mayflower* in 1620, she assisted with three births and continued to practice midwifery in Plymouth for the next fifty years, as more women populated the colonies.

During this era, and for white women in particular, childbirth was a social event. Women gave birth at home, attended by a midwife—usually an esteemed and trusted older woman who had already given birth to her own children—and surrounded by female family members, friends, and neighbors. It was an occasion for women to come together and care for one another, providing support, solidarity, comfort, and practical aid.

Still, birth was extremely dangerous. Anatomical knowledge was limited, there were no antibiotics or basic standards of hygiene, and the overall health of the population was poor. Women went into pregnancy acutely aware that they or their child might not survive. The conditions and perils of childbirth were even more dire for enslaved women, who had a limited ability to control the circumstances under which they got pregnant and gave birth, and for whom their children would be born into slavery. It's estimated that 50 percent of their infants were stillborn or died within the first year of life. "The essence of Black women's experience during slavery was the brutal denial of autonomy over reproduction," wrote the scholar Dorothy Roberts in her seminal book *Killing the Black Body*. "Female slaves were commercially valuable to their masters not only for their labor, but also for their ability to produce more slaves."

Midwives did what they could under the circumstances, guiding their charges through the ordeal with skilled and steady hands. Healing traditions and practices could also serve as forms of solidarity and resistance. Attending births was one of the only ways that enslaved women were allowed to travel, and as midwives circulated between plantations and communities, some transmitted messages between separated families and loved ones. They helped to spread culture and knowledge, known as "motherwit," and shared methods for contraception, spacing out pregnancies, and abortion, such as the use of cotton root to induce menstruation.

After the Civil War and Emancipation, through Reconstruction and Jim Crow, many African American midwives continued to practice, delivering babies across the South for the next one hundred years. Aside from the fact that doctors were expensive and scarce, use of midwifery remained strong in southern Black communities due to a profound suspicion of white healthcare providers, who had a long history of racism, coercion, and abuse. During the twentieth century, more than sixty thousand people—overwhelmingly people of color—were forcibly sterilized. The practice was so common that civil rights activist Fannie Lou Hamer coined the term "Mississippi appendectomy" after she went into a hospital for a tumor removal and was sterilized without her consent.

Outside of the South, there were white elder midwives practicing in Appalachia and the Ozarks, as well as Cajun midwives in Louisiana, Tejano midwives (known as *parteras*) in Texas, and Indigenous and Native American midwives in pockets across the country. They represented the practice of "lay" or "traditional" midwifery—women without formal education who learned and trained through observation, apprenticeship, and practice. They were sometimes referred to as "baby catchers," since much of midwifery involved patiently waiting until the baby made its appearance and then catching it out of the birth canal.

During the nineteenth and early twentieth centuries, immigrant women became a significant part of the American midwife population. Most trained and practiced in their countries of origin and continued to serve women from similar ethnic and class backgrounds in their new homes. Irish midwives, for instance, abounded in Boston, Jewish midwives from Eastern Europe set up shop in New York, and German midwives had thriving practices in Midwestern cities like Milwaukee. In 1908, 86 percent of laboring Italian-immigrant women in Chicago used midwives. In the Pacific Northwest, California, and Hawaii, hundreds of trained Japanese midwives called *sanba* assisted local Japanese residents. Midwifery schools opened in St. Louis, New York, and Chicago, offering courses in multiple languages, but they were relatively short-lived, and a robust educational system dedicated to midwifery—like those in the UK, Denmark, Germany, and Japan—never developed in the US.

Around 1900, white women were turning away from midwifery and toward physicians, who still attended them at home. Doctors, however, were largely unwilling to take on patients who were not white (or considered white at the time), who lived in remote areas, and who could not afford their higher fees. As a result, the practice further divided along ethnic and racial lines, and the midwives who remained were primarily immigrant women and Black women who served members of their own communities.

The more midwifery came to be associated with immigrant women, poor women, and Black women, the easier it became for the powers that be to demonize and criminalize it. In 1905, a Finnish midwife named Hanna Porn who practiced in Gardner, Massachusetts, was charged with the crime of practicing medicine without a license. Porn had attended the Chicago Midwife Institute and was well-known within her neighborhood. She served a clientele that was 99 percent working-class immigrant women—69 percent Finnish, 12 percent Russian, 11 percent Swedish—married to husbands who worked as chair makers and laborers in furniture factories. Her neonatal mortality rates were less than half the rates of local physicians, who charged three times as much for their services. But in Massachusetts at the time, there was no designated midwifery license, and so Porn was treated like a rogue, unlicensed obstetrician. She was put on trial, fined, and sent to jail, again and again, until her death. The Massachusetts Supreme Court used her case to make midwifery illegal in the state. In 1913, 40 percent of births in the area were attended by midwives, but as authorities began making arrests, the numbers declined precipitously. Other states, primarily in the North and Midwest, followed suit.

For decades, doctors had publicly played on prejudice, wielding xenophobia, racism, and sexism in a bid to eradicate midwifery altogether and claim dominion over childbirth. However, their unwillingness to serve poor Black women in rural areas meant midwives remained a tolerated necessity in some parts of the country. In 1921, the US passed the Sheppard-Towner Maternity and Infancy Act, which was meant to benefit poor women and children with prenatal and child health clinics and improve funding for nutrition and hygiene education, as well as regulate midwifery training in rural areas. At this point, most northern women were giving birth in hospitals. Of the sixty thousand midwives who still practiced in the US, most lived in the South. The practice of lay midwifery rested almost entirely in the hands of African American "grand" midwives like Onnie Lee Logan and Margaret Charles Smith, who delivered thousands of babies over the course of their careers.

Midwives like Logan and Smith were highly skilled, trusted, and respected figures who served any mother, regardless of where she lived or if she was able to pay. Logan was born around 1910 near Sweet

Water, Alabama, the fourteenth of sixteen children. Logan's mother and grandmother were midwives, and she went to births with her mother from a young age. At twenty-one, she began practicing on her own, but because she mostly attended poor families who could not pay much for her services, she earned income through domestic work for white families, as many grand midwives did. Then, in 1949, Logan received a midwifery license from the Alabama Board of Health and served as the primary maternal healthcare provider for Prichard and Crichton, predominately Black areas around Mobile. She lost only one baby in forty years of practice.

Smith got her start in midwifery when she was just five years old, after catching a neighbor's baby before the midwife arrived in her town of Eutaw, Alabama, about 165 miles north of Mobile. Smith also received a midwifery permit in 1949 and went on to practice for thirty-five years, attending nearly three thousand births. She became known as the midwife "who never lost a mother and rarely lost a baby."

The outstanding records of both of these grand midwives were even more impressive given the conditions under which they worked. They were sometimes called to deliver babies in isolated homes without running water or electricity and had to be resourceful and adaptable. (One clever technique to gauge whether a cloth had been adequately sterilized was to put a potato in the oven along with it—when the potato was cooked through, the cloth was safe to use.) And they had limited options for what to do if there were serious complications. Because local hospitals would not accept Black patients, Smith had to transport women to the Tuskegee hospital—170 miles away—in the event of an emergency.

There were strict state guidelines they had to follow as well, which limited the scope of their practice. They could not use instruments or administer drugs. They were subject to strict uniform and bag inspections and discouraged from maintaining traditional or folk practices, such as using herbal teas to augment labor. The rules helped legitimize the profession, and many midwives embraced them because protocols around hygiene and asepsis helped to reduce infection rates and save lives, but the intense supervision and hierarchy was also patronizing, and contributed to the idea that midwifery was inferior to obstetrics.

By 1938, there were thirty-five thousand midwives left in thirty-four states; they attended 9 percent of all births: 3 percent white, 9 percent "other" races, 50 percent Black. Midwives continued to practice in the South in mid-century America, but their numbers—and those of their clientele—steadily dwindled. By the 1960s, it was almost unheard of for women to deliver with a lay midwife at home outside of isolated rural areas and specific religious communities, like the Mennonite and Amish. Fewer than 1 percent of births each year happened outside the hospital, which had become the norm for women across geographies, races and ethnicities, income levels, and social classes.

Then the hippie, feminist, civil rights, and anti-war movements of the late 1960s and '70s arrived. The counterculture sowed a widespread distrust of authority and a willingness to challenge the establishment, leading to a surge in consumer activism and an interest in the ideal of more natural, authentic living through getting back to the land, which led to a renewed interest in midwifery.

Around 1970, a group of hippies formed a community around a spiritual leader named Stephen Gaskin. Three hundred of his followers left San Francisco in a caravan of fifty remodeled school buses and vans to follow him on a lecture tour around the country. Several of the women in the caravan, including Stephen's wife, Ina May, were pregnant when they set off. When the caravan arrived at Northwestern University, Stephen was preparing to give a lecture when a soon-to-be father asked for his assistance for his laboring wife, since Stephen had first-aid skills from his military experience. Stephen had the lecture to get to, so Ina May stepped in to help. The birth went quickly and smoothly. In her book, *Spiritual Midwifery,* Ina May recalled staying in a "state of amazement" for several days and feeling called to become a midwife.

Eleven babies were born as the caravan continued on the road. When the settlers arrived in Summertown, Tennessee, in 1971, they set to work creating a commune on over one thousand acres of land, known as the Farm. Fifty babies were born the first year. The Farm midwives did not have any kind of official certification or licensing, but the local hospitals and health departments, accustomed to the home birth traditions of the nearby Amish community, were willing to help when needed. By 1974, when the commune was at its peak, with close to 1,200 members, 25 to 30 babies were born there a month—a higher volume than at the county hospital. The midwives provided minimal medical intervention and their outcomes were good. (The first hospital transfer was birth 56, because the baby was coming bottom first. The first cesarean birth was baby 188.)

In 1976, Ina May published the first edition of *Spiritual Midwifery*, which went on to become a canonical text for lay midwives and the women who sought their services. The book offered a vision of childbirth that was profoundly different from the hospital norm, which relied extensively on instruments, tools, and technology. Unmedicated birth, Gaskin argued, was and should be a spiritual experience, akin to a psychedelic trip or an energetic journey along an astral plane (and, for the lucky, orgasmic). Laboring women "smooched" with their husbands to make labor go faster and "swapped bodies" with each other so a friend could telepathically take over for a few contractions. Instead of viewing birth as painful, Ina May and the Farm midwives urged women to let go of the "pleasure-pain sensation continuum" and experience "surges" and "rushes" instead of contractions. Giving birth was the ultimate high, and doing it without anesthesia, outside of the hospital, was portrayed as transgressive and groovy.

Before long, pregnant women of all backgrounds and beliefs started showing up at the Farm to give birth. In other parts of the country, hippie midwives operated underground or in legal gray areas. This was partly because they claimed to offer freedom from the "paid paranoia" of mainstream maternal healthcare, but also because many states no longer had systems in place for legal, out-of-hospital midwifery. In 1974, the midwife Raven Lang had her birth center in Santa Cruz raided by police in an undercover sting operation, in which plainclothes police arrested two midwives for practicing medicine without a license. Their court case ultimately led to California passing a law that allowed midwives to practice, as long as they were certified by the state.

When lay midwifery reemerged onto the national stage in the 1970s, it reemerged as a primarily white, middle-class phenomenon. There were midwives, activists, and advocates, like the midwife Shafia Monroe, who promoted Black midwifery and home birth as part of a larger effort to promote health activism and self-reliance within African American communities, but for the most part, preferences were moving in the opposite direction. The passage of the Civil Rights Act and Medicare and Medicaid in the mid-'60s made hospitals more accessible, which, according to the anthropology professor Dr. Gertrude Fraser, "signaled a symbolic if not fully realized inclusion in the field of vision of a health-care bureaucracy that had until then largely ignored the health needs of African Americans." The opportunity to give birth in a hospital was seen as a sign of progress. Midwives were no longer needed to fill in gaps in care, which created an opportunity for states to pass laws outlawing the practice for good. In 1976, Alabama—where Logan and Smith served their communities for decades—stopped issuing licenses to new midwives, stopped renewing the licenses of current midwives, and revoked licenses outright. Over 150 senior midwives—all Black women—were forced to retire. "Nothing in my life has ever made me feel so little," Logan said about the retirement letter she received.

Facing steep opposition from regulatory health boards and medical institutions, a cadre of lay midwives (mostly white) began to organize, forming the Midwives Alliance of North America (MANA) in 1982. Five years later, MANA created the North American Registry of Midwives (NARM), which established standards for education and training and administered certification for a new midwifery credential—certified professional midwife, or CPM—which was first offered in 1994. Since then, NARM has issued approximately 4,000 CPM certifications. As of 2020, 2,572 CPMs have active certifications from NARM—a tiny number relative to the population.

As Jillian read everything she could about midwifery, a whole new world opened up, one she hadn't been aware of, but one that existed alongside the birth system as she knew it. Seeing the profession as part of a long and rich tradition, one that was valuable and yet minimized—oppressed, even—solidified her interest in the field.

Before long, the question in Jillian's mind had evolved from "Do I want to be a midwife?" to "What kind of midwife do I want to be?" There were two main options that she considered: a certified nurse-midwife (CNM) or a certified professional midwife (CPM). CNMs were nurses who earned a midwifery credential and primarily practiced in hospitals. CPMs were direct-entry midwives, also known as lay or traditional midwives, and they were the primary attendants for births that took place outside of hospitals, in homes and birth centers.

CPMs, Jillian learned, were not required to be nurses. Instead, they developed their skills by attending dedicated midwifery schools and/or apprenticing with senior midwives. Then, they took a lengthy exam and earned credentials from NARM, and, depending on where they lived, applied for a state license as well. Thirty-seven states had some kind of legal recognition for CPMs, while thirteen states, as well as Puerto Rico, Guam, and the US Virgin Islands, still had laws on the books that criminalized the practice of direct-entry midwifery. In those states, some families chose to travel across state lines to access midwifery care, going to great lengths to avoid the hospital. (While there are direct-entry midwives who practice without the CPM credential, it is the primary, official form of national certification for the category.)

Direct-entry seemed like the more obvious route for Jillian, but she was drawn to nurse-midwifery because it offered a broader scope of practice and more flexibility. Direct-entry midwives were less understood and less accepted by mainstream medicine, not to mention mainstream society, and she didn't want to go to all the effort of becoming a midwife only to find it prohibitively difficult to practice. She didn't know anyone who was a midwife, but she knew plenty of nurses; they were well-respected and a known entity. She was nervous about committing to a profession where people could reasonably say, "Wait, those still exist?"

For the next two years, Jillian worked at the medical office in Missouri and took community college classes as she considered her next steps. She went back and forth, again and again, before finally arriving at a decision: direct-entry. That way, she could root her training in holistic care and be independent from hospitals, enacting the "heart- and hand-centered way" those midwives approached their work. Pursuing the CPM credential felt like more of a gamble, but it was a risk she was willing to take.

She focused her research and found there were fewer than a dozen accredited direct-entry midwifery schools in the country, and none in Missouri. There was one in Florida, but Jillian didn't want to go back there; another was in Maine, but she worried about the cold. A school in Texas served the border communities of El Paso and Juárez, but Jillian didn't speak Spanish. There were a few distance-learning programs, but she wanted a more hands-on, in-person environment.

Finally, she settled on the Birthingway College of Midwifery in Portland, Oregon, as her top choice.* In the prospective-student materials, the school recommended that people complete a doula workshop before applying. Jillian didn't know what a doula was but looked up the word and learned that they provided emotional and physical support to people in labor, helping them to get more comfortable, navigate the environment they were in, and express their wishes and needs. She found a two-day workshop in the St. Louis area that was held in the home of a doula trainer named Kim. There were ten participants representing a blend of ages and backgrounds. There were people with kids and people without; people who had experience attending births and people who had never seen a birth before. The workshop covered the physiological aspects of

* In 2018, Birthingway announced that it would no longer admit new classes of students—the rising cost of higher education and dropping enrollment numbers had become financially unsustainable.

birth, like the three stages of labor and how babies rotated like a screw as they descended the birth canal, and went over simple measures, like hip squeezes and immersion in water, that could help relieve pain during contractions. Jillian relished every second, and in the six months following the workshop, she attended six births as a doula, finding clients through word of mouth.

It was a powerful learning experience.

The first time she arrived at the hospital with a client, the staff immediately started the expectant mother on Pitocin, a synthetic hormone used to stimulate contractions, without asking her if doing so was okay. That pattern continued throughout the birth, the classic "cascade of interventions" that Jillian had learned about during her doula training (and in documentaries and books). She noticed that the care providers seemed to use a lot of scare tactics and didn't talk to her client about what they were doing. There was no offering of options or giving her a moment to think things through. It was the same "power-over" dynamic Jillian had observed years before at her job in the ER.

Another one of Jillian's clients went into her birth with one main goal: to avoid an episiotomy, a surgical cutting of the perineum. Episiotomies were routine for a long time in obstetrics until research showed that they should be used only in emergent situations. This client had had one during her first birth, followed by an arduous recovery, and was terrified about going through it again. Just as the baby was crowning, Jillian spotted the doctor pulling out a pair of scissors. She was not a medical expert, but nothing and no one, at any point, had indicated that the baby was in distress. Jillian knew the doctor had an ethical obligation to get her client's informed consent before performing a procedure, which included explaining the risks and benefits. It was not okay to whip out the scissors without saying a word.

"I believe she explicitly said she didn't want an episiotomy unless it was absolutely necessary," Jillian said.

The doctor gave Jillian a look and then turned to the mom.

"Do you consent to an episiotomy?" he asked.

The client, in the throes of the end of labor, desperate to be done, said yes. Later, after the baby was born, she told Jillian she had appreciated the effort she'd made to speak up, but Jillian still felt like she had failed. After the training course, she had wondered if doula work might be a better fit for her than midwifery, especially since the barriers to entry were lower. She would be able to start building a doula practice right away, whereas becoming a licensed midwife required years of education and a lot of money. But standing by those hospital beds, feeling powerless, reinforced that midwifery was the career she wanted to pursue. Doulas provided a valuable and impactful service, but it seemed to Jillian that doctors went ahead and did what they wanted anyway. She couldn't stop a steamroller, but maybe she could provide a different kind of care in a different environment.

CHAPTER 4
Alison

Alison woke up one day in June 2020 and went through her morning routine. She got out of bed, brushed her teeth, and took a pregnancy test from a box of twenty-five she'd bought on Amazon. After struggling to get pregnant and a miscarriage earlier that year, Alison wasn't expecting to get good news. She and her husband had only just started trying to conceive again, and she figured it would take months. She walked to the kitchen to make coffee and then returned to the bathroom, where the test was waiting on the counter. It was positive.

Alison and her husband, Steve, had first started trying to get pregnant in June 2019, a little less than a year after their wedding. The timing seemed right: Steve had a new job, they liked where they lived, and their dog, Barry, was no longer a puppy. Excited to start the process, Alison had made an appointment to have her IUD taken out and get preconception counseling. (The concept amused her, because what were they going to tell her other than *have sex, good luck*?) Since she was young and healthy, she expected she would get pregnant easily. Her birthday was in May, and she loved the idea of a baby with a birthday close to hers.

So, when they didn't get pregnant right away, it almost felt like a bird crashing into a glass window it didn't know was there.

Determined, Alison began using a period-tracking app to monitor her menstrual cycle, wanting to leave as little as possible to chance. At first, the tracking was fun, almost like a game, but then a month passed, and her period came. And then another month. And then another month. The tracking became edgier, a little more compulsive. Every morning, the first thing she did when she woke up was enter her stats into the app. She treated it like an oracle. On the days when the app said she was ovulating, she and Steve had sex, which meant that instead of treating sex as a fun, romantic activity and doing it when they wanted to (or not), it sometimes felt like a chore.

Alison strove to follow what the app advised with scientific rigor, as if the fate of their family depended on it. She spent hours on fertility websites and message boards, wondering if she should be drinking certain teas or eating certain foods. Every time she got her period, it felt like a failure, and as time went on, the dynamic put a strain on their relationship. Steve felt like Alison was being too aggressive and anxious, trying to force the situation. As she looked at her apps and mused about what she saw, he started to tune her out. He didn't understand why she was freaking out so much when, in the grand scheme of things, they hadn't been trying to conceive that long. To Alison, it felt like Steve was withholding, like he wasn't as invested in having a baby as she was. She wanted him to feel that the stakes were as high as she did.

For all the worries that one missed birth control pill can result in pregnancy, a lot has to go right for conception to happen: a viable egg has to meet viable sperm at just the right time. Infertility is defined as not being able to conceive after one year or longer of unprotected sex. It is extremely common, affecting one in eight couples in the US, or 7.3 million people. 12 percent of reproductive-aged women have trouble having a baby. (In one-third of heterosexual couples struggling with infertility, the issue is with the female partner; in one-third, the issue is with the male partner; and in another one-third, the issue is unidentified or with both partners.) Sometimes, nothing is amiss and the journey to conceive just takes a while. Sometimes, couples need a boost in the form of medication or assisted reproductive technology (ART). Fertility medicine exists in an odd space where sophisticated science meets crapshoot. Sometimes, infertility is unexplained, and no amount of testing or treatment yields an answer. To grapple with it is to live in a state of uncertainty, and there's more than just an emotional cost. Fertility treatments are exorbitantly expensive, with the average IVF cycle costing $12,000 to $17,000, not including medication. With prescriptions, the cost can reach $25,000, and many people require multiple rounds. More often than not, infertility treatments are not covered by insurance and must be paid for out-of-pocket, which has made them "a luxury for a privileged class."

Queer families, too, can face a number of barriers and stigma if they want to have biological children, including high costs, discrimination, and restrictive laws around measures like surrogacy, not to mention a fertility system that is generally oriented around cisgender, heterosexual couples. It wasn't all that long ago that sperm banks and other fertility service purveyors turned away people who weren't in conventional, straight marriages.

For just about everyone, navigating fertility medicine, assuming they're able to do so, is a stressful, draining process. It can also be an isolating and stigmatizing one. People don't want to share what they're going through because they feel like something is wrong with them. For those who want to conceive and can't, the experience can be one of powerlessness, like being in an earthquake. Parenthood is not a guarantee, and trying hard does not mean it will work out. When it doesn't, Dr. Janet Jaffe, a clinical psychologist and co-founder of the Center for Reproductive Psychology, said that can lead some people to feel defective and inadequate in a way that poor vision or bad knees do not. They may end up facing existential and identity crises that make them question who they are, what they want, and their place in the world.

For Alison, in the limbo phase of trying-to-get-pregnant-but-not-being-pregnant, she felt like she had to be constantly vigilant. Soon, her fears started to cast a shadow over the rest of her life. During a bachelorette party weekend in Nashville, she was so stressed about drinking—because what if she was pregnant?—that it was hard to enjoy herself. Even though they had only been trying to get pregnant for six months, Alison began to wonder what their options would be if a year or eighteen months passed. What would that mean for her? And for her and Steve as a couple? Would they go see a fertility doctor? Would they find any problems if she went through testing? Would she have to take hormones or medication? Would she do intrauterine insemination, or IUI (the so-called "turkey baster" method)? Would they or could they spend tens of thousands of dollars on IVF? Would they try to adopt? Would she join the ranks of groups like #IVFWarriors, tight-knit social media communities where every missed period or trigger shot is documented in meticulous detail? The path she'd had so much faith in no longer felt assured, and she felt adrift.

That morning in June 2020 had started out just like a morning six months before—the last time Alison had seen a positive pregnancy test. In late December 2019, Alison woke up, showered, and took a pregnancy test from a big box she'd purchased online, before going to make coffee. On this particular morning, Steve had already left the house. He had gone to work and then was headed to meet up with Alison's dad and brother, so they could drive together to the Rose Bowl.

Alison was going about her usual day, until she went back to the bathroom. She bent over the counter and stopped in her tracks. The test was positive. She couldn't believe her eyes. After months of negative tests, it seemed like a mirage. *Positive?* She looked again. *Positive!* Her heart pounded as she kept staring at the test, filled with glee. She jittered around the bathroom, not sure how to channel her excitement. What should she *do*?

The first thing was to text Steve.

Steve texted back and said, *"Oh my God, that's so exciting!"* They agreed to wait to share the news with their families together, when Alison was further along. In the meantime, they'd try to keep it a secret. That wouldn't be difficult for Steve, who was quiet and shy to begin with, but Alison was prone to exuberance. Her mother was planning to drive up to Portland for the weekend, to spend time with Alison while the men were at the game, and Alison resolved to keep her lips sealed.

That evening, she and her mother painted the guest bedroom and then went out to dinner. As they chatted over bowls of pasta, Alison found herself unable to stay focused. How could she think—or talk—about anything else when such a monumental thing was happening? Suddenly, she blurted out her news. Her mother, of course, was thrilled. This would be her first grandchild. Once the cat was out of the bag, Alison texted Steve that he could tell her dad and brother if he wanted. He replied that he might need time to work up to it—the idea of telling her father that he and Alison had made a baby just felt so awkward—but he mustered his nerve and broached the subject on the long car ride home. Alison's brother, who was snoozing in the back seat, sat straight up and said, "What?!"

The whole family was elated, as was Steve's when they shared the news with them too.

When the eight-week mark rolled around, Alison and Steve met with a nurse at a local OB clinic that Alison found via an internet search. (She had been about four weeks along when she called for information but was told that was too early for a prenatal appointment.) The nurse asked a lineup of routine health and medical history questions and handed her a packet outlining what foods she should and should not eat, as well as the risks of pregnancy. She told Steve and Alison that the physicians in the practice delivered at a hospital in Vancouver, the Portland suburb where they lived, and shared details about hospital policies, like prohibiting video recordings during births. To Alison, the appointment felt anticlimactic. It was supposed to be an exciting, warm moment—her first-ever prenatal appointment—and the focus was on whether she was a smoker (no) and hospital rules.

She scheduled her next appointment for twelve weeks. In the meantime, she continued to read and research online, surprised by how many options and perspectives and opinions were out there. Alison had always assumed that pregnancy was fairly clear-cut, with black-and-white guidelines. Some things were good, and others were bad: Don't drink alcohol. Take vitamins. Get an epidural. But through her research, and in particular through a book called *Expecting Better*, by an economics professor at Brown University named Emily Oster, Alison realized that most choices were infinitely more complicated. Certain accepted tenets of pregnancy dogma were not actually rooted in evidence, and different people with different priorities and circumstances might make different (but fine) decisions. The process of weighing upsides and downsides was more subjective than Alison had ever realized. Part of that lesson felt liberating, and part of it felt like an overwhelming responsibility. It meant there were a lot more things to consider.

In anticipation of her twelve-week ultrasound, Alison prepared a long list of questions to ask the OB, including about unmedicated birth. Everyone she knew who had given birth had received an epidural in a hospital, but she was intrigued by the prospect of doing it without anesthesia. Less technology and fewer medical interventions appealed to her: she usually tried to avoid sedatives when she could because she didn't like to feel out of control. She also thought a "natural" birth fit with her values—she ate vegetarian, composted, owned chickens, and was committed to minimizing waste. But during the appointment, when she asked the OB about whether foregoing an epidural in the hospital was an option, the doctor had a startling response.

"Not to be crass, but you're going to be pushing a watermelon out of your vagina. That is going to hurt a lot."

Alison was taken aback. The answer seemed patronizing and even combative, especially for a first-time mother. She forged ahead with her other questions, but she could tell the OB wasn't listening closely, her eyes trained on the ultrasound screen as she mechanically rolled the Doppler over Alison's stomach. And then she stopped.

After a moment, she told Alison and Steve she was having a hard time finding a heartbeat. Within seconds, Alison went from feeling peeved to battling a sinking, thudding dread. Without the repetitive, recognizable thumping she'd expected to hear, the room seemed to fill with static. The doctor moved the wand around again and paused in various spots, but still nothing. She said she was going to try a different ultrasound machine. Alison held back tears as they waited, mentally trying to dam her panic until there was definitive news. Steve reassured her that it could be nothing, and that she shouldn't be too worried yet. The doctor returned with a new machine. Still no heartbeat. Next, she sent Alison and Steve to a dedicated ultrasound room where a technician would do a transvaginal ultrasound. The room, with its low lighting, felt ominous, as did the silence as the technician began to work.

After a few moments, he confirmed that there was no cardiac activity. Alison yelped and started to cry, and Steve tried to console her.

And then, he fainted.

The ultrasound tech ran out to get help, and other medical personnel rushed into the room. All the attention went from Alison—who still had the ultrasound probe in her body—to Steve. He came around quickly, and when he did, the first thing he saw was the doctor looking at him, horrified. The staff put an oxygen meter on his finger, and he seemed fine (he hadn't eaten much that day, he explained), but the doctor insisted he go to the emergency room. The appointment was over. As Alison and Steve gathered their things, the doctor said to call the next day to schedule bloodwork. A nurse put Steve in a wheelchair and dropped him off at the entrance to the ER, which was on the same campus as the OB clinic. As Alison and Steve walked up to the admittance desk, Steve looked at Alison.

"Let's just go," he said.

So they did.

The emotional experience around miscarriage can be complicated and confusing, a reminder of just how precarious life is and the ever-present specter of mortality. It's also a reminder that bodies behave in ways that are outside of people's control. It's estimated that 10 to 15 percent of known pregnancies end in miscarriage. For some, a miscarriage means the body is doing what it is supposed to do, that the pregnancy wasn't meant to be, a part of the reproductive journey as normal and natural as a period. For others, it's a catastrophe, devastating and traumatic in its impact, with responses that run the gamut from anger to disappointment, relief, anguish, ambivalence, frustration, confusion, despair, and peace. Like any grief experience, it is ever-evolving. People may feel one way on one day and another way on another or have different reactions to different pregnancies.

Once at home, safe inside with the door closed behind them, this tsunami of loss hit Alison and Steve. They cried, then stopped, and then the grief swept in again and they kept crying. Alison felt like her insides were hollowing out. She returned to the clinic later in the week, feeling like a nervous wreck, and had her blood drawn. Later that day, the doctor called to report that Alison's hCG (human chorionic gonadotropin, also known as the pregnancy hormone) levels were not going down, which likely meant that, though the fetus had stopped growing and the pregnancy was no longer viable, the miscarriage hadn't started to pass. She advised Alison that the best course of action was to perform a D&C. They scheduled the procedure for that Saturday, March 7, at 9:00 a.m.*

Alison was devastated. To her, the loss of the pregnancy felt like the loss of a specific future, the loss of a world with that specific child in it. She never expected to go through this. It was all happening so fast, and no one in the clinic seemed to view the tragedy as anything more than routine. She was undergoing an emotional crisis, and the doctor was focused on scheduling and logistics, as if this were a simple medical problem with a simple medical solution, and not the dissolution of Alison's hopes and dreams for her family.

---

* In states that ban abortion, women who miscarry may find themselves criminalized for their pregnancies and find routine care for miscarriage management—which is essentially the same as abortion care—unavailable to them, putting their lives at serious risk.

To prepare for their next steps, Alison and Steve researched D&Cs and informed their immediate circle of friends and family. In an effort to be reassuring, people kept saying that miscarriage was normal, that the surgery was minor, and that it was nothing to worry about, but Alison didn't find those words comforting. Miscarriage might happen every day, but it didn't happen to *her* every day. To be told that it was not a big deal felt trivializing. It also didn't help with her nerves, which increased as the procedure approached.

She arrived at the hospital early on Saturday morning. It didn't quite hit her that she was about to have surgery until the nurses inserted an IV and gave her socks for the cold OR. Then she found out the doctor's plan was to administer general anesthesia. Alison was alarmed. She had always been adamant about not wanting it, out of fear that if she was put under, she might not wake up. Immediately, she broke down. She didn't want to do this. She didn't want to be here. And she did not, she told her OB in no uncertain terms, want to go under general anesthesia. She repeated her preference to the anesthesiologist, and both agreed to honor it, but they also told her that she should sign a consent form in case she changed her mind.

"You seem kind of high maintenance," the anesthesiologist told her. "For people who are type A, it's best to do more anesthesia. I would really recommend that for you." He also commented on her job—an elementary school teacher—calling it "rough."

Alison was insulted. She wanted to push back and stand her ground, but everything seemed to be moving full steam ahead, regardless of what she said or wanted. There was nothing she felt she could do. No one was listening to her. In the end, she was given general anesthesia, which she only fully realized once she'd woken up from the procedure.

Meanwhile, Steve was out in the waiting room. No one else was there, and most of the lights were off. A little screen flashed code names with the state of the various procedures that were ongoing, but he didn't know which code name was Alison's. She had gone into the OR around 11:30 a.m., and it was supposed to be a ten-minute procedure, so when fifteen minutes, twenty minutes, and then thirty minutes came and went, he started to pace around in panic. After forty-five minutes, the OB walked into the waiting area wearing her winter coat, like she was on her way out. Steve called out to her, and she paused. She told him the procedure went fine and then kept walking. After some searching, Steve found Alison in a recovery room.

The couple made their way home with a prescription for oxycodone and the odd sensation of being tricked. Of having something taken from them. In the days following, Alison was a wreck. She felt pulverized, the blow of the pregnancy loss only the first of many over the course of her experience. She and Steve spent the rest of the weekend watching movies on the couch, but her mind kept wandering back to how she had felt mistreated by the medical professionals involved in her care. Alison had never had reason to distrust the healthcare system before, but now, it was as if the wool had been pulled off her eyes.

She returned to school on Tuesday morning, struggling to keep it together. A colleague asked Alison if she was okay, and the simple query sent her reeling. Alison replied that she was having an emergency and needed to leave immediately, but then she quickly started to panic that her unceremonious exit would cost her her job. She called the OB's office, asking for a letter expressing that she needed to take a medical leave of absence—she was hysterical, not functioning, and crying herself to sleep. They scheduled her an appointment for the next day, during which the doctor agreed to write a Xanax prescription for ten pills. When Alison asked if there were any counselors or support groups she could talk to (schools offered an array of wraparound services, so she assumed a medical practice would too), the doctor said she wasn't aware of any but found Alison a referral for a counselor and for a support group that met at a church. Then she touched Alison's shoulder and said words that were meant to be reassuring but didn't quite land as intended: "I just want you to know that this is very hard. It will be okay. We will do everything we can so you can be pregnant again."

As with infertility, pregnancy loss is not widely discussed. That has started to shift with more people, including celebrities like Meghan Markle and Chrissy Teigen, sharing their experiences publicly, but feelings of shame, guilt, and self-blame are still very common. A 2015 study found that most women believed that miscarriage was a rare or preventable occurrence (which it isn't), and when asked how they felt about their experiences of miscarriage, 47 percent of people polled reported feeling guilty, 41 percent reported feeling that they had done something wrong, 41 percent felt alone, and 28 percent felt ashamed.

As the psychologist Jessica Zucker wrote in her memoir, *I Had a Miscarriage*, the length of gestation does not necessarily or automatically create a hierarchy or progression of grief. For people like Alison who experience intense grief around their miscarriage, there can be a sense that they are not entitled to their feelings, especially if they miscarried early. They feel crushed, which is only made worse if people around them shrug or minimize what they're going through. "We cannot assume the stage of gestation will automatically determine the potential impact of a pregnancy loss—it does not," Zucker wrote. "We also have the right to feel relieved, or even indifferent, about a loss without feeling judged."

Zucker referred to a "strident trifecta" of silence, stigma, and shame that perpetuates the taboo-ness of pregnancy loss. In the US, it's regular practice for people not to share that they are pregnant until after twelve weeks, when the chance of miscarriage is lower. From one perspective, this makes sense. It might be traumatic for someone who has shared that they are pregnant to then share that they miscarried, or later to field questions about how their pregnancy is going from people who don't know about the loss. But that also means miscarriages are kept quiet, which can lead to and reinforce feelings of isolation and loneliness, as well as uncertainty on behalf of friends and family about how to react. This, combined with other factors, has led one in six women who experience pregnancy loss to develop long-term post-traumatic stress.

It took Alison months to start feeling better. She saw a counselor and leaned on friends and family for support, but self-care was a daily struggle. She couldn't stop thinking about how it didn't have to be this way—not the miscarriage; she eventually came to accept that she hadn't had control over that—but rather what happened afterward. She and Steve had felt blindsided by the lack of communication and compassion at the hospital and during their doctors' visits. They hadn't been given the chance to ask questions, to understand what was happening. When things had started to go wrong, they had been brushed aside and decisions had been made *for* them. Alison felt like her agency, her dignity, had been snatched away. It made her think of something she hadn't thought about for a long time, another experience with pregnancy that she'd had in college.

During her senior year, she had woken up on New Year's Day feeling horribly, inordinately hungover, and couldn't stop vomiting. A friend asked if she might be pregnant, which hadn't occurred to Alison, but she took a test and it was positive. Right away, she knew she did not want to be pregnant or to have a baby. She was an ambitious college student who loved to travel, and she didn't know the father all that well. It was definitely not the right time or situation. Her friend found the contact information for a local abortion clinic in Eugene, gave Alison the phone number, and Alison scheduled the appointment for the following week.

The clinic was very Eugene, with a "crunchy, granola, earthy vibe." The doctor seemed like a nerdy hippie dad—professional, empathetic, gentle, and kind. Alison received a mild anesthetic, and the tissue was extracted using manual vacuum aspiration (MVA), a procedure that uses suction to empty the uterus. The whole process was quick, straightforward, and relatively painless. At no point along the way had she felt judged or pressured by any of the healthcare providers—in fact, the prevailing emotions she felt were relief and gratitude. She hadn't struggled with the decision to get an abortion at the time or since, but with a pregnancy she yearned for, the emotions around its ending were completely different. Everything changed with the wanting. As the grief ebbed, it was replaced by indignation and even anger. At that abortion clinic, she had felt respected, safe, and cared for. Why had the treatment she received around the miscarriage felt so different? If she got pregnant again, she would be more deliberate about who she involved in her care.

Now, two months after the D&C, as she looked at a new positive pregnancy test on her bathroom counter, every emotion came back to the surface. She'd never thought of having a baby as an act of bravery, but as she and Steve had started trying to conceive again after the loss, she realized that there was a good amount of courage required to foray into the unknown, to willingly submit to the mysteries and vagaries of a situation with no assured outcomes. In some ways, to try to conceive again was to invite heartbreak.

Despite those worries, Alison had been more relaxed about the conception process the second time around. She had emerged from her post-miscarriage "woe is me" phase in April, and she and Steve had started trying again for a baby. They accepted that the process would not conform to what they wanted, and for whatever reason, she got pregnant much faster. Alison was euphoric and relieved, but the anxiety about not getting pregnant again was almost immediately supplanted by anxiety that it wouldn't stick. She didn't want to get her hopes up or get too invested before knowing whether the pregnancy was viable.

This time around, Alison pledged to fiercely advocate for herself and her preferences. She was not about to Google where to go for care or prioritize proximity. Nor was she going to wait to be seen for prenatal care. She wouldn't just sit around, waiting and wondering, until then. If the pregnancy wasn't progressing, she wanted to know sooner rather than later. Alison had never considered giving birth anywhere other than in a hospital before. But now that she'd been exposed to a glimpse of what that might look like, she didn't want to go that route again. Not after what she'd been through.

At that moment, she decided: She was going to try something new. She was going to consider a birth center.

CHAPTER 5
Jillian

In the summer of 2014, Jillian sent an application in to the Birthingway College of Midwifery in Portland. She was invited to an interview and meet-and-greet for prospective students in November. Jillian had never been to Oregon—she'd never been west of the Kansas-Colorado border—and was excited for the adventure. The event was held at the Birthingway "campus," a converted home far on the east side of town. The quaint white building had dark green shutters and a columned porch. It was easy to miss, tucked under leafy trees and set back from the road by a stone-walled garden. The house seemed out of place on a busy street lined with automotive repair shops and industrial warehouses.

The interview and the meet-and-greet were a blur, but an exhilarating one. As she had in the doula workshop, Jillian felt herself come alive around people who shared her interests and way of looking at the world. She and another applicant named Alysa gravitated toward each other and became fast friends. Like Jillian, Alysa had entertained becoming a nurse and wasn't aware of midwives until she took a class on human sexuality at Western Oregon University. During the unit on labor and birth, the teacher covered birth centers and home birth, in addition to hospital birth, and assigned students *The Business of Being Born*. Alysa was twenty weeks pregnant at the time, and the documentary moved her. She had been seeing a nurse practitioner for her prenatal care, but upon watching the movie, she switched to a midwifery practice near her home. After Alysa's daughter was born, she asked the student who assisted at her birth how to become a midwife, and the student told Alysa about Birthingway.

At the end of the meet-and-greet day, Alysa and Jillian exchanged phone numbers; not long after, they both received word that they'd gotten in. They were going to become midwives. Jillian was ecstatic and prepared to move across the country before the semester started in April. She didn't have much money in savings and had racked up debt while living in Florida, which she was still working to pay off, so her budget would be tight. Her parents offered to help with tuition, but with the condition that Jillian cover her own living expenses. To help, Alysa connected Jillian with a friend who had an affordable room for rent.

With eighteen people, Jillian's class was one of the largest Birthingway had ever had. The full "core" days of classes started at 9:00 a.m. and ended at 5:00 p.m. Students attended three and a half hours of theory in the mornings, which covered antepartum care and pregnancy-related conditions like preeclampsia. Jillian soon learned an encyclopedia of definitions, signs and symptoms, risk factors and rule-outs, and what to do if a client showed signs of having them. After lunch, skills lessons covered how to perform physical exams, how to fill out lab slips, hematology, and IV insertion. The students practiced their skills, including vaginal exams, on one another. It was intimate and nerve-wracking, but studying midwifery had a way of scraping away inhibitions about the human body.

Oddly, receiving a vaginal exam from a classmate was not the most challenging aspect of midwifery school. That turned out to be the lunch break. Each week, a rotating group was tasked with bringing food and preparing a meal for everyone to eat together. Jillian's class found it impossible to identify meals that everyone could eat, thanks to different dietary restrictions, beliefs, and personalities. Even a dish as simple as rice and beans could be controversial. Instead of engaging with that particular brand of chaos, Jillian and Alysa started going for midday walks, just the two of them. Powell Butte Nature Park was less than a ten-minute drive away and offered a well-maintained trail system, with panoramic views and wildflowers blooming in the spring. On those walks, they dreamed out loud about their post-school plans.

Alysa, who identified as Indigenous and Latina, wanted to build a practice that would make midwifery more accessible to her community and to other women of color who thought of midwifery as a "white lady" thing. 80 to 85 percent of midwives are white, and most midwifery schools are run and staffed by white midwives, which can be a barrier to people of color interested in the field. Alysa hoped that by becoming a midwife herself, she could inspire others to pursue midwifery, both as a career and as clients.

A major obstacle, however, was the steep expense of formal midwifery education. Full-time programs are expensive, and the apprenticeship process, while critical to midwifery training, requires hundreds, if not thousands, of hours of unpaid labor. The cost and time commitment mean that people without a fair amount of financial privilege can struggle to earn their credentials. It was a problem with which Jillian and Alysa were intimately familiar. Both had a tough time supporting themselves while in school. Alysa and her husband and kids lived with both sets of parents, and spent a brief stint in a "janky" trailer that her in-laws fixed up, because money was tight. Jillian, even with her parents paying her tuition, was also barely getting by. She had applied for waitressing jobs and to coffee shops (a serious business in Portland) and medical offices, but her school schedule made working regular office hours difficult.

Finally, through a posting on a bulletin board at Birthingway, Jillian found a nannying job with flexible hours. She lived as frugally as she could, eating rice and beans for dinner almost every night. On rare flush weeks, she bought ground turkey. She felt exhausted and run-down, constantly unsure whether she'd be able to pay her rent, afford gas, and buy food. One unexpected bill could derail everything.

Life as a midwifery student was stressful, but the end goal was worth it. The more Jillian and Alysa talked, shared, and planned, the clearer their vision became: once they graduated and became CPMs, they would open a home birth midwifery practice called Blooming Dahlia Midwifery. Their understanding of the barriers to midwifery care, combined with the skills they were developing in school, would inform how they would approach their work—and, they hoped, the way people viewed the profession more broadly.

Jillian and Chad got married in June 2020, not long after she graduated from midwifery school. Their plan was to wait to start a family because Jillian wanted to get her midwifery license first. She had been off hormonal birth control for years, and the couple typically relied on condoms and the natural family planning methods she'd learned in school. But, on the night of their wedding, they had unprotected sex. Jillian later realized she had been ovulating, but between moving and the wedding, tracking her cycle hadn't been front of mind. She took an initial pregnancy test, but it came out negative.

A few weeks later, during a "mini moon" camping trip to Crater Lake, Jillian felt cramping, which she assumed to be her period. But days later, it still hadn't arrived. She figured it was stress but decided to take another pregnancy test just in case.

This time when she peed on the stick, the word "Pregnant" appeared immediately. Jillian stared at it. *Ah shit,* she thought. She smiled. This was good news. Unexpected, but good.

CHAPTER 6
T'Nika

T'Nika had always looked forward to having children of her own. Growing up as one of five kids in an overwhelmingly white place like Eugene, Oregon, family was everything to her, and her family was tight-knit. T'Nika's mother and father had met at a high school track meet, as members of different teams. They started dating later while attending Lane Community College and got married in their early twenties.

Throughout T'Nika's childhood, her mother had worked as a certified nursing assistant (CNA). Her father was a jazz musician and an artist who made glassworks, and later became the executive director of the Eugene/Springfield NAACP chapter. Her parents were deeply interested in their African and African American heritage, and her dad held discussion groups at the house, making it a priority to teach his kids about politics, music, history, and religion. Their home brimmed with books, and T'Nika grew up loving to read, especially sci-fi and fantasy books like *The Hobbit*. All the children participated in multiple extracurriculars like sports and music. T'Nika ran track and played the viola, and she later sang gospel in college.

When T'Nika was in seventh grade, her family moved to Hawaii for a year. After staying with her uncle for a while, the family moved into a house on the west side of the island of Oahu, in Waianae, which was more affordable than Honolulu. There was only one road in and out of the neighborhood, and it was constantly congested with traffic. The family had one car, so every morning, everyone had to be up and out of the house by 5:30 a.m. so her dad could drop off T'Nika's mom for her shift at the hospital, and then drop all the kids off at school, before driving to his shift at a 7-Eleven.

T'Nika loved Hawaii—the warmth, the ocean, the diversity—but as much as the family wanted to make it work, the circumstances weren't sustainable. After a year, they moved back to Oregon and T'Nika returned to the same middle school she'd left. It was hard at first because middle schoolers could be tribal, and everyone seemed to have cliqued up while T'Nika was gone. She was teased for wearing the same pair of jeans every day (flared, with hot pink stitching) and did not have a solid group of friends to which she belonged, but that didn't last for long. A charming, chatty kid, she soon rebuilt friendships and got involved with school activities, which allowed her to bounce between social communities.

And then there was Daniel. When she had moved to Hawaii, T'Nika had brought her sixth-grade yearbook with her, mainly so she could look at the photos of the dozen or so boys she had crushes on. Daniel was one of them. In his yearbook photo, he wore a Hawaiian shirt, which she'd taken as a sign that they were meant to be and drew hearts around his picture. Though they'd met in sixth grade, it wasn't until high school that they started to spend real time together. They were both on the track team and involved in the Black Student Union, co-hosting the Martin Luther King Jr. Day assembly. T'Nika wasn't shy about her feelings—she gave him Snickers bars and sent her girlfriends as emissaries to ask him out—but he always said no. Still, they remained friends and partnered up for cross-country runs, during which Daniel would run ahead on the bark trails and unwittingly spray dirt all over T'Nika's face.

During their senior year, a friend of Daniel's snuck T'Nika out of her house to a party. After everyone else had fallen asleep, T'Nika and Daniel stayed up watching *The Fresh Prince of Bel-Air* and talking late into the night. A week later, T'Nika sent a friend, once again, across the track to ask Daniel out. This time, he said yes.

For their first date, T'Nika brought her favorite Star Wars podracing game over to Daniel's house to play on his Nintendo 64. They played for hours, until Daniel's mother poked her head downstairs to invite T'Nika to stay for dinner and watch the Grammy Awards, which were airing later that night. T'Nika was in heaven. She had had a crush on Daniel for so long, and finally he was interested in her too. The next time she went over, they cuddled for hours. With their lives ahead of them, the idea of already finding their soul mate seemed crazy, but she knew he was the One.

As extroverted as T'Nika was, Daniel was introverted and enjoyed solitude. The two balanced each other out but had lots of things in common. Both were self-professed and proud nerds who loved video games and board games. He lent her books like Harry Potter, *The Da Vinci Code, The Golden Compass,* and *The Lord of the Rings.* They read the Game of Thrones series together and were big fans of anime. They continued dating after high school even though Daniel was headed to Claremont McKenna in Southern California and T'Nika was going to the University of Oregon, the first person in her immediate family to attend a four-year college. After freshman year, Daniel transferred to Lewis & Clark College in Portland, and after graduating in 2013, the couple moved to Boston. They wanted to try living someplace that wasn't Oregon and took jobs working for an organization that ran play-based recess and after-school programs for elementary school kids in low-income, urban areas.

T'Nika quickly came to feel ambivalent about the work. She could do it, and do it well, but it didn't feel challenging or fulfilling in a way she craved. It wasn't what she wanted to spend her life doing. She had always dreamed of becoming a nurse.

During her first semester of college, she had signed up for Human Physiology 101, a nursing prerequisite, and it was tough—an intense load of memorizing muscle systems and tiny bones. She'd earned a C–, which stung, but she knew plenty of students failed the class outright, so she didn't make too much of the grade. When she found out that the University of Oregon offered a transfer program to Oregon Health and Science University (OHSU) for nursing, T'Nika asked her school counselor about it, but he quickly squashed her plans, advising her against applying to the program and against pursuing nursing in general. T'Nika wanted to give him the benefit of the doubt. *Maybe he knows something I don't know,* she thought. *He's worked with lots of other low-income students, so maybe he doesn't want me to waste my time and money on a course of study that I wouldn't succeed in.* At the same time, she didn't think he knew her well enough to make that judgment call. His response was dismissive at best, and it was demoralizing and dejecting to be put off by someone who was meant to encourage her. That interaction led T'Nika to question whether she had what it took to become a nurse. Ultimately, she decided to keep to her original plan of studying education and spent all four years of college working at the day-care center with infants and toddlers.

As she worked at the schools in Boston, the idea of becoming a nurse hovered stubbornly in her mind. She befriended a school nurse and asked her a volley of questions about her career path and day-to-day life. Talking with the nurse, and with Daniel, T'Nika realized that she'd given up on her dream because someone who barely knew her thought she couldn't hack it. She couldn't let one conversation with a person who didn't know what she was capable of dictate the course of her career. She decided to give nursing another go, and she'd see for herself whether she could make it work. In her early twenties, she signed up for nursing prerequisite classes at a community college in the Boston area: human physiology again, along with microbiology and statistics. The anatomy and physiology classes continued to be a struggle—there was so much to memorize—but Daniel pushed her to keep going. He reminded her that it was okay if the material didn't come easily, and that just because the course was hard did not mean she couldn't do it.

One spring day, the couple took a ferry to a nearby island to stroll around. Daniel said he wanted to set up his camera to take a picture.

T'Nika sat, looking around and people watching, wondering what was taking him so long. Then, with a view of the city in the background, and with the camera secretly running video, Daniel pulled a sock out of his pocket. T'Nika was confused, until he reached into the sock and pulled out a ring.

That summer, T'Nika and Daniel moved back to Oregon, where she enrolled in a twelve-month licensed practical nurse (LPN) program, with plans to go on to a registered nurse (RN) program. The following year, in July 2016, they got married in a big wedding at the Mount Pisgah Arboretum in Eugene on a hot and windy day, surrounded by their families and friends. T'Nika walked up the aisle to the song "Someday My Prince Will Come," and they danced back down it together to the Jamie Foxx rendition of "I Don't Need Anything But You" from the Black version of *Annie*.

In 2018, T'Nika received her LPN license and took a job at a long-term-care nursing facility. She also started a sixteen-month RN course at Concordia University in Portland. After years of taking prerequisite classes and going to LPN school, the anatomy and human physiology courses no longer felt so arduous, and she discovered that the clinical aspect of the education and training—the skills and lessons around actually caring for the patients—came naturally to her. Where some students felt awkward and tongue-tied at a bedside, T'Nika intuitively knew the right things to say to people in pain and could make them smile. She loved to help people.

In nursing school, T'Nika's favorite units had been those dedicated to maternal health. As her education progressed, her specific career ambitions came into focus: she wanted to be a labor and delivery nurse, and maybe someday a nurse-midwife herself. She had always been obsessed with anything birth related—consuming every episode of *A Baby Story* on TLC, reading books like Ina May Gaskin's *Spiritual Midwifery* for fun, watching *The Business of Being Born*, and listening to podcasts about birth—and she aspired to make a difference. As a Black woman working in maternal healthcare, she could support her community and ensure that other Black women, along with anyone who was more likely to face discrimination in hospitals, received equitable treatment, with "all the bells and whistles."

Even before she pursued nursing in earnest, this mission had always been important to her. In college, T'Nika had worked on a group project that involved creating support groups and holding informational sessions for pregnant teens. The girls she worked with said they often felt like people in hospitals looked at them sternly, discrediting and blaming them for their situation and treating their pregnancies as negative and shameful. This was something T'Nika immediately understood—she had three cousins who gave birth as teenagers. One cousin had talked frequently about her experiences, feeling like her pain was underacknowledged by the hospital staff and like there was an acute focus on her being young and unmarried.

T'Nika thought about how different those birth experiences could have been if there were more Black women working on the L&D units. She imagined that as a nurse, and later as a nurse-midwife, she could be the person in the room who would take the time to understand where people were coming from, listening and guiding patients through the often confusing and overwhelming world of hospitals. She could help women in labor feel respected and achieve their goals in situations where other healthcare providers might say, "This is how it's done, even if you don't want it."

When it came time for students to apply for clinical rotations, T'Nika set her sights on an assignment on an L&D floor. Despite all the content she'd consumed about birth, she'd never actually been present at one, and she was eager for the opportunity. It was what she'd been working toward. Clinical rotations were competitive because there were more nursing students in Portland than rotation slots, so to make assignments, program administrators talked with the students' clinical instructors about their grades, their skills, and their interests. T'Nika had made her intentions clear to her teachers and peers from the beginning, and between her affinity for the specialty and her school records, she had a good shot.

Then the assignments were released. She was placed at a day-care center, a typical overflow assignment. She couldn't believe it. She'd gotten her last-choice placement, one that wasn't even on a hospital unit. That might have been fine for some students, but it was not fine with T'Nika, who had pursued nursing specifically to move past working in day care. After all the hard work and time and money, it was like she was being sent back to where she started.

She resolved not to accept the assignment without resistance. She emailed the administrators, asking why she had been placed at a day care and outlining the case for why it wasn't a good use of her time, reemphasizing her interest in L&D. The administrators responded, telling her that if a space opened up, they would let her know. It didn't sound like a sure thing, but T'Nika held out hope and continued to check and recheck the rotation assignments, until one day when her name appeared in group six of a hospital's L&D rotations. T'Nika was elated but curious about what happened. She messaged the other members in the group, who said a student had failed the semester. T'Nika, whose grades were good, wondered why someone at risk of failing had been assigned to a coveted L&D rotation in the first place but shrugged it off. At least she'd gotten the placement she wanted.

She had completed just one full shift before the coronavirus pandemic broke out. Clinical rotations were canceled, and hospitals became dangerous transmission points. No extraneous people were being allowed in, including the partners of women who entered the hospital to give birth (and nursing students). T'Nika was disappointed, but as she neared the end of her nursing program, her mind turned to starting a family of her own. Even though it was in the middle of a pandemic, when so much was uncertain, she felt like it was time. She was ready, or as ready as she'd ever be. Every time she saw her nieces and nephews, she felt a surge of "baby fever."

In spring 2020, T'Nika told Daniel that she wanted to get pregnant before she turned thirty. The transition from not trying to have a baby to trying to have a baby was a subtle one, more mental than anything, a willingness to take a leap. (She had gone off birth control two years earlier, sick of the way it made her feel.) Now, she started tracking her cycle in a low-key way and figured she would be more rigorous about it if they had a hard time conceiving. Then, after a couple of months, her period didn't come. She was pregnant.

T'Nika had always thought that she'd like to have her baby at a birth center. T'Nika and her siblings had been born at a birth center, and she was drawn to the idea of carrying on that tradition. Some of her earliest memories were of lolling in the hammock at the birth center while her mother was in labor down the hall, and she remembered bumping into the midwife who delivered her when she and her mom were out running errands. She appreciated that the birth center and midwife were a part of her family's story and wanted that for herself as well. Once she confirmed she was pregnant, those preferences crystallized. She had no real interest in finding an OB or looking into hospitals, and she started browsing around online for birth centers.

Beyond her family history, birth centers appealed to T'Nika because they seemed to have more options for *how* to give birth. One of her top priorities was to labor in a birth tub. She had grown up swimming, playing water polo, and taking trips to the river, and as soon as she heard the term "water birth," it appealed to her. T'Nika felt at home in the water—weightless, relaxed, and protected.

She also wanted the option of nitrous oxide, or laughing gas, for pain relief. She did not want an epidural, or at least did not want it to be the default expectation. She knew that might be naive, given that she'd never experienced childbirth before, but she hated the idea of her legs not working; thinking about being numbed from the waist down and unable to move made her feel anxious and panicky. She had a fear, she joked, about getting an epidural right before a zombie apocalypse hit, making it impossible for her to run with her brand-new baby. Nitrous oxide was temporary, self-administered, and allowed people to maintain a full range of motion.

More than anything, though, T'Nika hoped that giving birth outside of a hospital would minimize the chance of a cesarean section. C-sections were major abdominal surgery, and she knew they could lead to difficult recoveries and lasting complications. At the long-term-care nursing facility where she worked as an LPN, she had cared for patients recuperating from surgery, dressing wounds and administering antibiotics, drawing up pain medications and helping people get back and forth to the bathroom, and knew firsthand how taxing it could be. She wanted to avoid that if she could, along with the hospital environment in general, even though it was the norm.

In the US, the transition of childbirth out of the home and into the hospital began when male medical practitioners decided to get involved. Birth, up to that point, had been considered private, messy, women's work to be handled by female midwives. The men who were interested, so-called man-midwives, tended to be of dubious repute and questionable skill. The respected midwife Elizabeth Nihell referred to them as "broken barbers, tailors, or even pork butchers" who spent half their lives stuffing sausages before they turned their attentions to midwifery. There were no medical schools in early America, so men with serious medical ambitions traveled to Europe to study.

In 1762, a physician named William Shippen returned to Philadelphia after years of studying medicine in London and Edinburgh and launched a midwifery practice for Philadelphia's elite families, as well as the first organized series of lectures on midwifery in America. Medicine was an increasingly competitive field, and physicians striving to grow their fledgling practices realized that in pregnant women, there were golden business opportunities. They attempted to recruit patients away from midwives, but with key differences in how they practiced: male doctors and man-midwives tended to be less patient and more willing to use tools and technologies to intervene. They deployed a range of seemingly advanced techniques, from bloodletting and manually breaking waters to using ergot to stimulate contractions and tobacco infusions to encourage the cervix to dilate.

Before the twentieth century, birth was a largely housebound, non-surgical practice: hands, cloths, and baskets and bowls were the primary tools used, and obstetrical instruments came into play only in cases where barber-surgeons had to extract a fetus by any means necessary to save the life of the mother. Forceps changed that process forever in the 1700s by providing a way to free a fetus from its mother without killing it. As awareness of forceps spread throughout England and France and beyond, male midwives embraced them more ardently than their female counterparts, wielding them as a "talisman of ability and a panacea for every difficulty in birth." Educated midwives like Nihell, however, were skeptical of what they saw as injudicious use. Laboring women, too, were wary of the invention, which led some male doctors to extremes to have them available at births. One forceps proponent, William Smellie, was known to don a woman's nightcap and capacious gown in order to smuggle the tool into deliveries. Nihell, with a flair for insult and not a Smellie fan, referred to him as a "great horse God-mother of a he-midwife."

By most measures, the ministrations of male midwives were inferior to those of female midwives. The exceptions were with patients whose births required more aggressive, surgical rescue efforts. In those cases, forceps could be a life-saving tool—if used appropriately. To promote their safe use, Smellie published the three-volume *Treatise on the Theory and Practice of Midwifery* between 1752 and 1764. The idea of intervening with tools changed how birth was thought of, nudging it further into the domain of men.

In 1817, Princess Charlotte Augusta, the only child of the Prince of Wales, died after a prolonged labor attended by a man-midwife. The case was highly publicized and the man-midwife was denounced for failing to use forceps, which might have saved the princess's life. This tragedy convinced leading physicians that their reputations could suffer if they were seen as not doing enough during labor. A new era of unusual birthing gadgets began, and while the popularity of some contraptions like the *tractions soutenues* (which enabled doctors to maneuver forceps using a pulley system from three feet away) were short-lived, they helped doctors establish their superior status over other types of practitioners.

The prospect of death or permanent injury was something every woman faced as she prepared to give birth, which most would do again and again over the course of their childbearing years. Families who could afford it wanted the safety that the educated, professional male physician with his book learning and bag of tools seemed to offer. As their approach to childbirth became more aligned with surgery than with midwifery, physicians wanted a label that reflected that divergence. Practitioners of the type of medicine now thought of as "Western," "modern," or "allopathic" campaigned for licensing laws that would regulate medical practice and stamp out the competition. In 1828, an English doctor suggested the term "obstetrician," which came from the Latin root of the verb "to stand opposite."

Despite its growing influence, the emerging specialty of obstetrics and gynecology was still disparaged by the broader medical community in the early days, viewed as an unscientific field in which men with formal educations were doing the same job as uneducated, illiterate women. Physicians pursuing obstetrics and gynecology strove to enhance the prestige of their specialty by advancing medical research and pioneering new techniques. To achieve that goal, they sought out people from vulnerable populations to experiment on.

Thanks to increasing industrialization, cities had become filled with squalid living and working conditions that bred injury and disease. The first maternity clinics in the US were opened to serve the growing numbers of poor, unmarried women who had no other place to go. Delivery in these wards was free, but in exchange the women might be used as "obstetrical guinea pigs" and treated as subhuman. Wards were hotbeds of infection where puerperal, or "childbed," fever spread like wildfire, and conditions were dangerous. One particularly horrifying tale involved a thirty-one-year-old unmarried Irish housekeeper named Mary Connor, who checked into Bellevue, New York's first "lying-in" hospital. Connor was barely conscious when she gave birth, and nearby patients called out to the staff for help. When the doctor finally arrived, his examination revealed that the newborn had been mutilated by rats in the interim. Some lying-in hospitals saw as many as 75 percent of new mothers die from infections. In the North, doctors practiced on poor immigrants, often Irish-born women. In the South, they practiced on enslaved women. Though Black midwives were the primary birth attendants, slave owners sometimes called on white doctors for particular types of assistance, such as to investigate infertility or to fix a problem that interfered with someone's ability to work.

J. Marion Sims, historically referred to as the "father of modern gynecology," was one such physician. Between 1844 and 1849, he performed gruesome, painful surgeries on enslaved women—notably three named Anarcha, Betsy, and Lucy—without anesthesia, dozens of times, to find a method of repairing fistulas, a debilitating complication of prolonged labor. (The experiments were underlined by the racist belief that his subjects could not feel pain as acutely as white women.) In 1849, after thirty surgeries, he successfully repaired Anarcha's fistula and went on to replicate the technique with other patients. "Slavery's existence allowed for the rapid development of this branch of medicine," wrote Dr. Deirdre Cooper Owens in her book, *Medical Bondage*. "Black women were used . . . for the benefit of white women's reproductive health." In 1852, Sims published a paper with his findings in the *American Journal of Medical Sciences* and then moved to New York, where he climbed his way to renown as a top gynecological surgeon, serving as president of the American Medical Association and founding the American Gynecological Society. He is also credited with inventing the speculum by using a pewter spoon.

Sims's experiments occurred around the same time that chloroform and ether emerged as pain-relief options for women who could afford doctors, namely white women. The prospect of meaningful pain relief during childbirth felt like a holy grail, but there were no standards for how to administer it, and the side effects could be dangerous, which led to reluctance among some physicians. There was also religious and moral pushback from the church, which saw pain and sorrow during childbirth as a burden women should bear. The use of the drug remained the subject of hot debate until 1853, when Queen Victoria used it during one of her births and it became fashionably known as "chloroform *a la Reine*." Women were asking for chloroform, and physicians realized they would lose business if they did not oblige. It became another service they could offer to middle- and upper-class women that midwives could not.

As the practice of medicine advanced, so did efforts to formalize and legitimize the field. In 1848, the American Medical Association was founded, and medical journals proliferated as forums for sharing knowledge, reinforcing the prestige of university-educated doctors over their lay (and female and non-white) peers. Physicians collaborated and organized against alternative, sectarian practitioners, including midwives, whom they impugned at every opportunity. In articles and lectures and speeches about the "midwife problem," physicians claimed that midwives were dirty, ignorant, clumsy, amateur, foreign, feeble-minded, superstitious, and outdated, among other aspersions. They also called them "abortionists." As male doctors grappled to gain greater oversight and control over women's bodies, campaigns to outlaw abortion and to outlaw midwives worked hand in hand to achieve that goal. Doctors presented themselves as paternalistic protectors and guardians, encouraging their patients to be submissive, yield to their wisdom, and not ask too many questions.

Over time, physicians became more adept at addressing certain obstetrical issues, which helped advance their cause. Most notably, advancements in germ theory led to the introduction of sanitizing protocols into hospitals in 1885. Physicians were starting to realize that hospital birth could be beneficial for all women, not just the indigent, as well as for physicians themselves, and thus hoped to expand their appeal. Hospitals offered convenience because physicians could see their patients in one place instead of schlepping to homes all over town. It also meant birth happened on their turf, in an environment governed by their own ideas, preferences, and rules. And clinical environments made it easier to maintain strict sterilization and sanitization protocols. Attempts at "scrupulous cleanliness" emboldened physicians to intervene more actively in birth because of the protection they thought that cleanliness provided.

For many women at the time, the prospect of childbirth that was less susceptible to the whims of cruel and impartial fate, and instead managed by capable men of science, was deeply appealing. "The lure of medicine and the progress it symbolized captured large numbers of birthing women as the nineteenth century progressed and the twentieth began," said the historian Judith Leavitt. "Women's increasing use of physicians and their increasing acceptance of medical solutions to their childbed problems combined to create the milieu in which the twentieth-century move to the hospital occurred."

Despite numerous medical and scientific advances, and the generalized improvements to hygiene and disease prevention in the United States, death during childbirth remained prevalent in the early twentieth century. In 1906, at the height of the Progressive Era, the government initiated a study into infant mortality and found that the US lagged behind peer countries in Europe. Something had to be done. In an effort to restructure and improve the medical field, the American Medical Association commissioned a report into the state of medical education, led by a teacher named Abraham Flexner. The Flexner Report, an in-depth evaluation of 155 medical schools in the US and Canada, was published in 1910 and served as a final, harsh blow for sectarian medicine. It described some medical schools as "indescribably foul . . . the plague spot of the nation" and proposed sweeping medical reforms such as prerequisites for medical training and a standardized curriculum grounded in physiology and biochemistry. Though the document would ultimately improve the quality of medical care in the US, it also had the effect of excluding just about everyone who was not a white man from entering the field.

By 1910, the US had more than four thousand hospitals in operation, and the numbers of women giving birth in them became a "flood," jumping from less than 5 percent in 1900 to over half of all women by 1939. After World War I, an almost military posture of routine and control was applied to birth—one of "manipulation, intervention, and active combat," stated the historians Dorothy and Richard Wertz. In the first volume of the *American Journal of Obstetrics & Gynecology*, the highly influential physician Dr. Joseph DeLee argued that nature did not intend for human birth to be "analogous to that of the salmon, which dies after spawning"—a "normal" delivery, one that did not require intervention, was considered exceedingly rare. DeLee came up with systems for standardizing delivery that involved giving every woman an episiotomy and extracting babies with forceps. As the journalist Jennifer Block wrote in her book *Pushed*, he precipitated the "transformation of childbirth from a sequence the woman's body executes into a procedure the physician performs."

In 1914, word of a new, miraculous method for pain relief made its way stateside. Pioneered in Freiburg, Germany, in a clinic at the edge of the Black Forest, *Dämmerschlaf*, or twilight sleep, was the combination of a drug called scopolamine, an alkaloid of belladonna, and morphine and could knock women out without compromising their muscle function. When used in the process of childbirth, patients would still feel pain, but they wouldn't remember it. Belladonna wasn't new—the ancient Greeks used it for medical purposes—but German doctors had figured out how to calibrate lesser doses. Upper-class women from the US and around Europe descended on Freiburg in droves and evangelized about their experiences back home.

Before long, the suffragist movement, which had gained steam in the US, was connecting women's liberation from the pain of childbirth to their argument for political liberation and the right to vote. They accused doctors of being callous and narrow-minded for being hesitant to administer twilight sleep widely and waged a nationwide consumer campaign to promote it, holding meetings in department stores and even opening their own clinics. Physicians chafed at the argument, stating that the concerns were medical and related to the newness of the method and questions about administration and dosage. It required careful monitoring and supervision, and some clinics actually built dedicated facilities with padded walls and doors, restraints, and "crib-beds" to contain patients' thrashing. The doctors who opposed twilight sleep were loath to be "dragooned" or "stampeded" by "misguided ladies" with their silly demands, but once again, an advantage presented itself: because of the need for facilities, equipment, and expert care in the administration of scopolamine, twilight sleep had to happen in a clinical environment.* Doctors would no longer have to negotiate their decision-making with pregnant patients because they would have complete control from the start. The drug went mainstream, trickling down from the province of the wealthy and elite to become the standard for hospital birth.

By the early 1930s, a concentrated campaign to get women in hospitals resulted in 60 to 75 percent of city births taking place there. (In rural areas, hospitals were still too few and far between to be a viable option for everyone.) Popular literature of the 1920s and '30s was filled with heart-wrenching stories of women whose lives could have been saved by hospitals. They had tipped over from the place only the most destitute went to palaces of obstetric achievement that elevated birth out of darkness.

And yet, mortality rates still had not improved.

In 1933, the White House published a report about maternal and infant death that found that rates of fatalities due to birth injuries had not declined between 1915 and 1930, despite the increase in hospitalization and adoption of aseptic techniques. In fact, they had increased significantly. The report cited two main reasons: first, inadequate prenatal care and overlooked complications; and second, excessive and often improperly performed interventions. The report embarrassed doctors, who

---

* Scopolamine has the effect of lowering inhibitions and has also been used as a truth serum and a date-rape drug.

quickly moved to increase regulation and cut down on the overuse and misuse of the tools at their disposal. That shift, while improving safety, created a hospital birth environment that was even more rigid and said to resemble a factory assembly line.

By 1945, the percentage of hospital births jumped to 80 percent when the federal government began to pay for the healthcare of women married to service members during and after World War II, and the private insurance market expanded, helping more families afford hospital care. The Hill-Burton Act of 1946 ushered in the next wave by providing federal funds for the construction of hospitals in rural areas around the country, particularly in the South, which gained five hundred thousand hospital beds. Between 1936 and 1955, the rates of maternal mortality dropped precipitously, in large part thanks to the arrival of blood banks, oxytocic drugs (which can stimulate contractions), and new screening tools and anesthetics.

More hospital beds, however, could not counteract hundreds of years of systematic oppression and the poorer health conditions that racism wrought. Though hospital birth had become more accessible to Black women, the enduring presence of segregation and Jim Crow meant that Black hospitals remained generally underfunded and under-resourced, as did the segregated wards in general hospitals. Moreover, Black doctors were systematically excluded from access to medical education, internships, and residency programs, as well as from membership in medical societies like the AMA. Black mothers and infants continued to face rates of maternal and infant mortality that were nearly double those of white mothers and infants.

Finally, in the mid-1960s, Congress passed the Medicare and Medicaid Act, which enabled lower-income communities to access the private medical care system, and the Civil Rights Act, which meant Black patients were no longer relegated to segregated hospitals or wards. After desegregation, Black women embraced the opportunity to give birth in modern institutions with up-to-date facilities and medical technologies, and they were encouraged to do so by organizations like the NAACP.

All these policies and changes, along with concerted campaigns to eliminate midwives, completed the transition from home to hospital. Hospital birth was the norm, but the norms within the hospital continued to evolve. Epidurals, inductions, and fetal monitoring, for instance, became commonplace in the 1980s, as did childbirth classes and birth plans. Today, the desire for preparedness has only continued to grow more pronounced, due in part to the rise of the internet and social media, wider access to information about childbirth, and increased awareness about inequities and risks. Those factors are also driving a spike into out-of-hospital births.

T'Nika knew much of this history from all the reading she'd done, and it informed how she thought about birth. She saw that the evolution of birth out of the home and into the hospital, away from midwives and toward doctors, didn't necessarily follow some clear ladder of progress, where things just got better and better. Especially not for Black women. She just didn't see a hospital as an obvious or inevitable place to give birth. She was committed to giving birth with a provider and in an environment that made more sense to her—one where clinical interventions weren't the default and where she and her care provider could build a meaningful relationship.

CHAPTER 7
Alison

Almost immediately after her positive pregnancy test, Alison made an appointment for an ultrasound at a birth center near her house. Sitting with a nurse-midwife, she explained her history with miscarriage and shared how nervous she was. Her last ultrasound had been traumatic, and she was bracing herself for bad news. As the midwife prepared to perform the scan, Alison trembled, trying to hold back tears and keep herself calm.

After what felt like hours, the midwife spoke up. She confirmed that Alison was pregnant and about six weeks along.

"I see a heartbeat—" she said.

Oh, thank God, Alison thought, exhaling all the breath she'd been holding.

"But you can never be sure."

Alison looked up in dismay at the woman in front of her. *What?* Why would she say such a thing and taint the happy news?

"Until twelve weeks, you never know," the midwife continued. "Anything can happen."

Alison stayed quiet for a moment. Intellectually, logically, rationally, she knew what the midwife was saying was true, but the disclaimer felt callous and unnecessary, especially given the history she'd just disclosed. She did not need someone to remind her that there were no guarantees, as if she wasn't aware of that every second of every day.

That exchange was just one of the things that felt off to her. When Alison asked about whether it was okay to maintain her vegetarian diet during pregnancy, the nurse-midwife acted like it was unusual that Alison was a vegetarian (never mind that the Portland area was something of a vegan and vegetarian utopia) and offered to Google it since she wasn't sure. Then there was the décor. The wallpaper and curtains were fusty, and one suite had an inexplicable nautical motif. Alison knew aesthetics were not a good reason to decide against a place, but it was hard to imagine wanting to spend time there. It reminded her of an escape room, but with drapes everywhere and potpourri in the bathroom. This couldn't be the place where she had her baby.

Disappointed and stressed, Alison wasn't sure where to turn next. Then she remembered that a friend from college named AlexAnn had trained as a nurse-midwife at OHSU. They hadn't talked in a few years, but Alison felt comfortable enough sending her a message to say hello, explaining she was pregnant and interested in midwifery. She asked if AlexAnn would talk to her on the phone, and AlexAnn agreed.

During the call, Alison walked AlexAnn through everything she'd experienced with the miscarriage and the doctors who were involved. AlexAnn murmured in agreement and said she wasn't surprised—those kinds of dissonant interactions happened all the time. She told Alison that she deserved to see a provider she trusted, who listened to her and made her feel comfortable, and who would give her the support and information she needed. The desire to provide that kind of care was part of why AlexAnn had become a midwife herself.

Alison told AlexAnn that she was reluctant to go back to a hospital or use any kind of anesthesia, but she was not interested in a home birth either—because of all her anxiety that something would go wrong, she wanted to know that medical support was close by. AlexAnn pointed out that, given Alison's interest in unmedicated birth, her ambivalence toward hospitals, and her worries about coercion, her instinct to explore going to a birth center with a midwife seemed spot-on. Just because Alison didn't like the birth center near her house didn't mean she wouldn't like any of them. There were plenty of other options, including practices staffed entirely by nurse-midwives.

Nurse-midwifery emerged in the US as debates about the future of midwifery in the country heated up. In the 1920s, a nurse named Mary Breckinridge founded the Frontier Nursing Service (FNS) in Appalachian Kentucky, with the goal of carving out a new category in the US that existed somewhere between obstetrician and lay midwife—following the professional medical model while also emphasizing midwifery's focus on physiological birth and client-centered holistic care.

Breckinridge was born to a powerful Southern political dynasty with male family members who fought in the Confederate Army and served high up in the US government. In 1904, at the age of twenty-three, she married a lawyer from Arkansas who died two years later from complications of appendicitis. Women had always taken on the duty of caring for the sick, but professional nursing training didn't become widespread until the turn of the century. As the numbers of hospitals grew in the US, so did the need for trained healthcare workers, and by 1910, one out of every four hospitals offered a nurse training program. Breckinridge, a young widow with no children, attended St. Luke's Hospital School of Nursing in New York City.

She remarried in 1912 and had two children, a daughter who died as a newborn and a son nicknamed Breckie who died at the age of four. Ravaged by those losses, Breckinridge dedicated her life to infant welfare, working for the newly formed Children's Bureau, which aimed to curb infant and maternal mortality. (During that period, she also left and divorced her second husband.)

In the aftermath of the First World War, Breckinridge applied to work with the Comité Américain pour les Régions Dévastées de la France, a small group of American women who volunteered to help the French Third Republic recover from the war. She arrived in France in 1919 and served as director of child hygiene and district nursing, working closely with British nurse-midwives. She was impressed by their skills and by the British midwifery system at large, in which nurse-midwives handled normal deliveries and called in doctors to handle complications. As Breckinridge built "a well-oiled visiting nursing service" in France, she realized the potential for a similar rural health service in the US. America's comparatively high rates of maternal and infant mortality, in her view, were a national disgrace, and once she returned to the US, she wanted to focus her efforts on aiding rural, poor American women. She enrolled as a student at London's British Hospital for Mothers and Babies to become a nurse-midwife herself. In 1925, she launched the Frontier Nursing Service.

According to her biographer Melanie Beals Goan, Breckinridge's Confederate roots, along with the popularity of the eugenics movement at the time, meant that supporting the health and growth of "pure" American families—as in white—was core to her mission. She emphasized this as part of her fundraising efforts, soliciting wealthy donors who shared those beliefs, and recruited her staff accordingly. She wanted to build a cadre of educated white midwives who would be viewed as legitimate practitioners by educated white doctors, and keep white patients and their babies alive as the nation's population changed. "Her plan to make maternity safer for the women of Appalachia succeeded in large part because she capitalized on the nation's paranoia that the white race was in danger," wrote Goan.

From the start, Breckinridge was drawn to Kentucky as a testing ground for her service because her family was well-known and well-connected in the state. Leslie County, where the FNS first put down roots, had no licensed medical doctors and was extremely remote. In the early days, Breckinridge's midwives traveled by horseback through the mountains to see patients, often through darkness and rain, and the conditions were perilous. Over rushing rivers, rickety bridges, and icy mountain passes, the "angels on horseback" carried forty-eight-pound midwifery bags, which included a rubber apron, an operating gown, soap, a scrub brush, gloves, a thermometer, scissors, basins, and pharmaceuticals—everything they might need to attend births in rustic backwoods homes.

Local families did not immediately embrace the Fronter Nursing Service midwives—their practices differed from those of the local lay midwives, and they were seen as outsiders. Over time, however, the FNS gained the trust of the community, once their dedication and skill became apparent. Outposts were opened in neighboring counties and grew until more than one thousand families over a seven-hundred-square-mile area relied on the service for healthcare. In 1937, the FNS registered its three-thousandth maternity case, with only two maternal deaths at a time when the national average was closer to six deaths per thousand. Of the three thousand cases, FNS nurses performed six emergency cesarean surgeries and used forceps, which were routinely used in hospitals, only fourteen times. The FNS delivered more than 14,500 babies, with only eleven maternal deaths, over the course of four decades.

As the organization grew, so did its need for trained nurse-midwives, of which the US had few. In 1939, eighteen of the service's twenty-two nurse-midwives were British, and Breckinridge soon realized this was not sustainable. She needed a pipeline of nurse-midwives that didn't require them to come from or be trained abroad, so she opened the Frontier Graduate School of Midwifery (a program that still exists today as Frontier Nursing University), which matriculated thirty-six American nurse-midwives by 1945.

Back then, the only other nurse-midwifery program in the US was part of the Maternity Center Association in New York City, which had begun serving patients as a maternity hospital in 1918, modeled after the Chicago Maternity Center opened by Dr. DeLee in 1895. When the MCA announced its plans to open a nurse-midwifery school, nursing leaders immediately voiced opposition, worried that associating public health nursing with midwifery would taint nursing's reputation. Still, the

MCA forged ahead and opened its nurse-midwifery training program in 1931, graduating its first class two years later.

In 1935, as the federal government started funding nurse-midwifery education through the Social Security Act, nurses from all over the country traveled to New York to participate in the MCA's program and then returned to serve their home communities. Nurse-midwifery training programs could be costly and time-consuming, and they often required applicants to pass a literacy test and meet certain educational requirements, which prevented aspirants from underserved and under-resourced communities from applying. Regulations varied from state to state, but for the most part, the primary role of nurse-midwives, who were mostly white, was to ensure that lay midwives, who were mostly women of color, followed the state's midwifery regulations and guidelines. That tiered model was intended to promote safety, accountability, and professionalism, but it also reinforced a midwifery caste system that was divided by race and class.

To address those divisions, a fourth nurse-midwifery training program in the country opened at the Tuskegee College School of Nursing in 1941. It was the first nurse-midwifery school at a historically Black college and trained thirty-one nurse-midwives between 1941 and 1946. In 1951, *Life* magazine ran a feature and photo spread titled "Nurse Midwife: Maude Callen Eases Pain of Birth, Life, and Death" featuring Callen, a missionary nurse and Tuskegee graduate who served as a skilled and beloved nurse-midwife to the rural community of Berkeley, South Carolina. The article portrayed nurse-midwives as the antithesis of the lay midwife, emphasizing that Callen was a highly trained professional who practiced in a modern, scientific way.

A few years later, in 1955, the Maternity Center Association published its twenty-year report, which showed that its nurse-midwifery program had led to dramatic reductions in mortality and morbidity statistics. That same year, Columbia-Presbyterian-Sloan Hospital in New York City became the first major medical institution to open its doors to nurse-midwives, and the founding meeting of the American College of Nurse-Midwives (ACNM) was held. (The organization had folded in Breckinridge's American Association of Nurse Midwives, which, when it was founded in 1941, had excluded Black midwives from membership.) ACNM did not bar members based on race, but one midwife of color referred to it as "a sea of whiteness that could be quite intimidating" and minority nurse-midwives working in hospitals faced sustained discrimination.

In 1971, there were 1,200 certified nurse-midwives (CNMs) in the US, and the American College of Obstetricians and Gynecologists (ACOG) approved nurse-midwifery for uncomplicated cases.* With legal lay midwifery effectively eradicated and nurse-midwives practicing primarily in hospitals and public health clinics, women who wanted a home birth were left with few options—namely, find a midwife operating under the radar or give birth without medical assistance. It was around this same time that midwifery was coming back into vogue. In 1975, the writer and advocate Suzanne Arms published her groundbreaking bestseller *Immaculate Deception*, which reported how women in childbirth were still routinely separated from their partners, physically restrained at the wrists and ankles, shaved and scrubbed, lowered into the stirruped lithotomy position (on their backs), administered drugs without their consent, given episiotomies without their consent, discouraged from breastfeeding, and denied their babies following delivery. The book, released in the wake of the women's liberation movement and second-wave feminism, and two years after *Roe v. Wade*, struck a chord. Combined with the hippie renewal of midwifery, the calls for childbirth experiences that balanced medical management with humane treatment were getting louder. This manifested in a number of ways, including in the growth of the so-called natural childbirth movement and in the establishment of freestanding birth centers.

---

* ACOG, founded in 1951, is the leading professional membership organization for obstetricians and gynecologists, and publishes practice guidelines and recommendations for clinicians working in women's health.

In 1933, a British doctor named Grantly Dick-Read wrote a book called *Natural Childbirth,* in which he argued that "excessive" pain in labor was the result of fear of the birthing process. He also postulated that medical interventions interfered with labor and made women feel anxious, which tensed their muscles, which increased pain and slowed down labor, ideas that were roundly mocked and led to his being kicked out of his London practice. Undeterred, he wrote a second book, titled *Childbirth Without Fear*. The book was a hit, and in 1947, Dick-Read embarked on a book tour across the US. He espoused the view that birth was a physiologic, rather than a pathogenic, process, akin to defecation, inspiring a vocal vanguard of privileged women who demanded to be awake and alert during birth.

Despite his focus on improving birth experiences, Dick-Read was not what one might call a feminist icon. By all accounts, he was an arrogant male chauvinist who believed that women were "made primarily in order that children might be born . . . yet somehow we don't always feel that women are quite as proud of that magnificent gift as they should be." In the era of Freudian psychology, he perpetuated the idea that intense labor pain was a female delusion caused by selfishness or resistance to motherhood. He also endeavored to capitalize on his popularity by attaching his name to a line of maternity lingerie consisting of, as described by Randi Hutter Epstein in her book *Get Me Out,* "a bra attached to humongous underpants with a complicated series of suspenders." He and other advocates of physiological childbirth like Dr. Fernand Lamaze did not encourage women to give birth outside of hospitals or to work with midwives. Instead, their schools of thought focused more on how women in hospitals could manage labor pain without anesthesia, and these ideas took hold in American society.

The Lamaze movement originated in the postwar Soviet Union, where women did not have access to pharmaceutical pain relief during childbirth. Building off Pavlovian theory about behavioral conditioning,

Russian doctors developed a method they called "psychoprophylaxis," drawing on midwifery folk practices, which aimed to override pain signals to the brain through techniques like deep breathing. In 1951, two French doctors, including Lamaze, studied the techniques in Russia and created a simplified version back in Paris that involved rapid "small dog" panting breaths.

An American woman named Marjorie Karmel, who had used the Lamaze technique while living in Paris, published a book in 1959 called *Thank You, Dr. Lamaze* about her experience. Like *Childbirth Without Fear*, the book was a hit, and word spread like wildfire. One reader, named Elisabeth Bing, was so moved by what she read that she contacted Karmel, who happened to live just on the other side of Central Park. The two became friends and teamed up in 1960 to launch the American Society for Psychoprophylaxis in Obstetrics (ASPO), which promoted the Lamaze method in the US. The duo procured a copy of a film from France called *Naissance* and arranged a small, private viewing at Karmel's apartment. The film showed a woman giving birth without drugs or anesthesia with the French flair for "anatomical candor." In the US, it was considered obscene, borderline pornographic, but word got out. Karmel and Bing held film screenings for interested couples, kicking off the ascendence of childbirth classes.

This marked a paradigm shift. Instead of perceiving birth as an event that befell someone and that hospital staff would manage for them, it became an event people could prepare for. It was an exam, a performance, and a team sport. Women led campaigns to overturn long-standing hospital practices they found objectionable, like restraints and bans on partners in delivery rooms. As they grew more motivated and equipped to assert their needs in labor, healthcare providers had to adapt accordingly. In some cases, this meant hospitals reorganized labor and delivery wards to allow for rooming-in, the practice of letting babies stay with their mothers after birth. Others opened their own birth centers where unmedicated, lower-intervention childbirth was the default.

Soon, birth centers were cropping up outside of hospitals. One of the first modern birth centers opened in 1975 in an Upper East Side town house in New York. Called the Childbearing Center, it was run by the Maternity Center Association and staffed by nurse-midwives and OBs. The building had a garden, an oriental carpet, and sculptures of fetal development placed around the lobby. The women who went there could labor in any position they wanted. They were not subjected to routine enemas, shaving, episiotomies, or sedatives, and they could stay with their babies after birth. The facility was equipped to handle medical emergencies and transfer patients to the nearby Lenox Hill Hospital if needed. Desperate to keep up, hospitals like San Francisco General also jumped to open their own birth centers, housed within the same building. In her memoir *Baby Catcher: Chronicles of a Modern Midwife*, the nurse-midwife Peggy Vincent described how the medical establishment "swayed and then buckled to the wishes of the pregnant population," afraid they'd lose business if they didn't. "In Berkeley, in 1977, it seemed common sense to suppose that any hospital boasting a birth center with liberal policies would pull in the money," she wrote.

In 1983, the National Association of Childbearing Centers, now the American Association of Birth Centers (AABC), formed to standardize, regulate, and accredit birth centers. Best-practice guidelines included that birth centers serve only low-risk women, that they promote reimbursement for services, and that they secure liability insurance. When Mutual Fire, Marine and Inland Insurance Company, the only carrier to provide group liability insurance for nurse-midwives, withdrew from the market in 1985, birth centers were dealt "an almost fatal blow," blocking the openings of new birth centers, threatening the survival of established ones, and causing at least a dozen existing birth centers to close. Throughout the 1990s, the number of birth centers dwindled, due to the skyrocketing costs of malpractice insurance and decreasing reimbursement rates. "It was as if the gains we'd made in that magical decade of the eighties had been erased," Vincent recalled. "Not even a trace of chalk dust remained on the blackboard."

Today, there are around 385 freestanding birth centers in the US (meaning they are not attached to or housed within a hospital) in forty different states. They may employ only CPMs, only CNMs, or a combination of both, but of the twelve thousand CNMs practicing in the US today, 94 percent work in hospitals. The number of birth centers has doubled since 2010, and although representing just 0.5 percent overall, the number of people giving birth at a birth center each year has grown by 60 percent in the same time period—a time period in which the annual number of births overall decreased by 12 percent. Around twenty thousand people give birth at a birth center each year, and according to Kate Bauer, the executive director of the AABC, that number is positioned to rise as more families seek alternatives to the hospital. "For a long time, it was very slow growth," said Bauer, whose mother was a midwife who trained with the Frontier Nursing Service. "Maybe about ten to fifteen years ago, we really started to see the numbers begin to climb more dramatically, and now there's steady growth at a much higher rate."

By the time Alison was looking for a birth center, there were about half a dozen options in the Portland area, not including nurse-midwifery practices within hospitals. To narrow down her selection, AlexAnn encouraged Alison to outline her practical requirements and then do some research to find birth centers that met those needs. At a minimum, Alison's priorities were a place that accepted her insurance and was reasonably close to her house, as she had no desire to battle traffic to and from appointments. Once she'd narrowed down the list, AlexAnn recommended that Alison book appointments for tours and interview midwives before making her final choice, and suggested a few key questions to ask: Where did you do your midwifery education and training? How long have you been a midwife? How many births have you attended? What is your transfer rate?

Alison eagerly took AlexAnn's advice. She searched the internet for birth centers in the vicinity and called a handful, including one called Andaluz, to schedule tours.

CHAPTER 8
Alison

From Alison's home in Vancouver, Washington, it was a straight shot down I-5 to get to Andaluz. Once she arrived in the hilly, residential neighborhood and found the building, Alison walked up to the front steps. There was a sticky note on the buzzer that read, "Please Knock." When she did, a receptionist named Jillian, a tall woman about her age with blue eyes and light brown hair, opened the door and welcomed her into the lobby.

The interior, she noted, reminded her of a quaint bed-and-breakfast. There were big couches, books, and a fireplace with a painting hanging above it, and the front desk had all the accoutrements of a medical office, with file cabinets, a computer, a printer, and stacks of neatly organized folders and papers. Jillian said a midwife named Marilyn would be right out to take her for a tour, but until then, Alison could sit on one of the couches.

A few minutes later, a woman—Marilyn, she assumed—entered, walking right toward her. She shook Alison's hand, introduced herself, and invited her to follow her into the back. As they walked down a long hallway lined with suites, each room color-coordinated and named, Alison noticed with appreciation the big tubs and queen-size beds inside—there were no exam tables or hospital beds, and all the medical supplies were tucked away.

During the tour, Marilyn asked Alison what drew her to birth center care. Alison explained that she wanted a care provider who respected her preferences. She was worried about being pressured into things she didn't want. Marilyn listened carefully and nodded her head in agreement as they continued on, patiently answering all of Alison's questions. Nothing was dismissed as trivial, though the looseness of some of Marilyn's answers—many variations of "It's up to you," including when it came to wearing a mask—felt surprising. To Alison, who was concerned and cautious about Covid (especially while pregnant) and always wore her mask indoors, that kind of flexibility seemed ill-advised. When she asked if the birth center had a relationship with a specific hospital in the event of a transfer, Marilyn replied that all clients created a transfer plan and could choose which backup hospital they wanted to go to. OHSU was just up the hill, but Providence or Legacy Emmanuel were also options. Again, it would be her choice. *That seems odd,* Alison thought. *Shouldn't there be a protocol set in place based on the relationship the center has to a hospital?*

Alison wanted a practice where clients were equal, active participants in their care. She wanted to feel in control and not have other people making decisions for her, but at the same time, she liked structure, policies, and guidelines. She knew that without a codified plan in place, honed by professionals and experts, she would be anxious.

As she said goodbye to Marilyn and left Andaluz, Alison felt like it was probably not the right place for her. She understood its appeal: the inside was lovely, the midwives had decades of experience, and it was clear they cared. But things felt a little *too* comfortable. Marilyn had called her "honey" and "sweetie" as they chatted, which was a nice change from the brusque, distant tone she'd experienced with her last OB, but pet names felt so informal to her. Ultimately, the whole thing had felt too "woo-woo," she told Steve. Later that week, she had an appointment for another tour, this time at a birth center in East Portland run by a local network of OB/GYN clinics called Women's Healthcare Associates. AlexAnn had mentioned the practice on the phone because she thought its distinct emphasis on close collaboration between doctors and midwives might strike the right balance for Alison.

WHA's Midwifery Birth Center was housed in a yellow building, situated off a busy road lined with strip malls and big-box stores (in a previous life, it had been the Acapulco Mexican Restaurant Y Cantina). Through the front entrance was an airy check-in desk and lobby with doors on either side; to the left was the Midwifery Birth Center, and to the right was a regular OB/GYN clinic run by WHA, allowing both patients and staff to move between as needed.

Alison liked the birth center's vibe from the moment she walked in. The first room through the door into the birth center was a waiting room, bright with mid-century modern furniture—with a couch, small dining table, and galley kitchen, it resembled a tasteful Airbnb. The rest of the facility extended off that room along a long, wide hallway with white walls, wood floors, and artwork from a local artist. The four birthing suites were on the left, with frosted windows that ran parallel to the road outside. Each room had white walls with colorful abstract prints, a prominent white tub, a queen-size bed, and bureaus where birthing equipment and supplies were tucked away. Like Andaluz, each suite had a name—Iris, Azalea, Lotus, and Cypress—and was cozy yet spare, with nothing extra or out of place. The en suite bathrooms were spacious, with sliding doors and clean white towels folded neatly on the shelves. On the other side of the hallway was another small lounge area, generally used by family members taking a breather, and a nursing station with large computer monitors, files, and cabinets filled with labeled plastic tubs. Everything was streamlined and simple, without feeling austere. There was nothing "woo-woo" about it, but nothing intimidatingly clinical either.

The Women's Healthcare Associates network, Alison learned, included fifteen OB/GYN specialty clinics and a team of more than 120 clinicians around the Portland metro area. Though it was a birth center, the idea to open it came from one of WHA's obstetricians, Dr. Greg Eilers, who had been searching for innovative ways to lower the costs of maternal healthcare.

Born and raised in the Portland area, Eilers had done his OB/GYN residency at OHSU. Like many physicians, he had been initially biased against out-of-hospital birth after seeing patients who transferred to the hospital during labor when something went wrong, for what he often thought were preventable reasons. Then, one day, a patient was transferred from home, accompanied by her midwife, who explained the situation to Eilers outside the hospital room. The midwife clearly knew exactly what was going on with the patient and exactly what the patient needed. Eilers was impressed. They walked back in together, started the patient on Pitocin to get labor going again, and the baby was born safe and healthy. That night as he drove home, he marveled to himself, *Wow, that went really well.*

The experience stuck in his mind, and he was reminded of it again a few weeks later while reviewing cases for the hospital in order to identify areas for improvement. There were two births that had gone badly—one had taken place in a hospital, and the other had been a community birth transfer. In looking over the files, it seemed to Eilers that the issue was a mismatch of care: if the hospital birth patient had been at home (or at a birth center) and the home birth patient had started at the hospital, maybe, just maybe, both labors would have gone more smoothly. He dug into the literature and was surprised to find compelling evidence showing that out-of-hospital birth could be managed safely and efficiently. Perhaps, Eilers considered, the hospital wasn't always the best option.

Inevitably, the first question asked about out-of-hospital birth is: Is it safe? The answer: It depends.

Hospitals, with their squads of doctors, arsenal of technologies, and proximity to operating rooms, are widely seen as the safest places to give birth. In the event a complication emerges during labor or delivery, there is an entire infrastructure dedicated to acting fast and responding to the crisis. But that crisis-waiting-to-happen mindset can cause problems of its own. Obstetricians are surgeons trained to manage high-risk cases, but that can also enhance the perception that all births are high-risk and should be managed accordingly. "It's like an auto mechanic who sees only the Fords that have broken down and have been brought to his shop, so he ends up thinking that all Fords are in imminent danger of breaking down," said Dr. Marsden Wagner in his book *Born in the USA*. "He forgets that he never sees all the Fords on the road that are running just fine."

The counterpart to this view is that giving birth outside of a hospital, away from those resources, is reckless and naive. Even though community and unmedicated birth have become trendier, a stigma against out-of-hospital birth persists. "When the women in our study decided to pursue an out-of-hospital birth, they frequently met with judgment, rejection or panic from family members," said the authors of a report on Black women's birth experiences in California. "Media images misrepresent labor as fast-moving and urgent, with women being rushed to the hospital in speeding cars as soon as their water breaks. As a result, many of us assume that giving birth in a home or facility without immediate access to a surgeon and operating theater in case of an emergency is unsafe and irresponsible."

That may be true in some cases, but certainly not in all.

For low-risk people having uncomplicated pregnancies, who work with trained and licensed midwives who have relationships with nearby hospitals, out-of-hospital birth can be about as safe as hospital birth. In 1989, *The New England Journal of Medicine* published the results of the National Birth Center Study, a landmark survey of 11,814 low-risk women across eighty-four birth centers. "Few innovations in health service promise lower cost, greater availability, and a high degree of satisfaction with a comparable degree of safety," the report concluded. In a study of 16,924 women that the Midwives Alliance of North America (MANA) collected of planned, midwife-led home birth in the US, it found a 93.6 percent rate of vaginal birth and low rates of intervention with no increase in adverse outcomes or maternal or infant mortality.

Many other studies, too, show that planned home births and birth center births are associated with fewer procedures, easier recoveries, fewer vaginal tears, and lower infection rates. "Increasingly better observational studies suggest that planned hospital birth is not any safer than planned home birth assisted by an experienced midwife with collaborative medical back up, but may lead to more interventions and more complications," concluded a Cochrane meta-review.

However, for every study showing that community birth has comparable outcomes, there are others that find that the neonatal or infant mortality rate for home births is double or triple or quadruple that of hospital births in the US. In part, these discrepancies could be due to the state of the country's maternal data, which has been described as "in shambles." For example, in some states, all home births are lumped into the same statistical category, meaning the outcomes of someone with a "planned" home birth—where a trained and licensed midwife came equipped with oxygen and iodine and suturing kits and Pitocin in the event of a hemorrhage—are grouped with someone who gave birth unassisted at home or didn't make it to the hospital in time and gave birth in a car, and those are very different scenarios.

Even Emily Oster found existing data to be inconclusive, a plenitude of poorly designed studies with different methodologies and inconsistencies: "To be frank, it seems very unlikely that there isn't some added risk to home birth. . . . How much is not something we can address with logic alone, and thus far it's really not something answered in the medical literature." The National Academies of Sciences, Engineering, and Medicine reached a similar conclusion, finding that "adequate data is not available to make comparisons across birth settings regarding perinatal death."

The American maternal health landscape is so fragmented and the data collection so motley that it's impossible to make sweeping, comparative statements; there are simply too many variables. How far away someone lives from a hospital, for instance, impacts how quickly they can access emergency care. So can the variation within the field of midwifery. Not all midwives are trained or certified in the same way or operate using the same scope-of-practice guidelines, and midwifery regulations vary from state to state. In one state, a direct-entry midwife may be able to serve clients with a previous cesarean, while being barred from doing so in the state next door. In other states, direct-entry midwives (even if they are NARM certified) cannot legally practice at all. A midwife practicing underground is operating in a different context than a midwife with a state license because, among other reasons, licensure enables smoother transfers to the hospital. For an underground midwife, transferring a client to the hospital means exposure to legal jeopardy, and the fear of being caught can lead to delays and limits open communication between providers, which is key to safety. "Right now, we have a hodgepodge of what defines midwifery," said Dr. Mimi Niles, a nurse-midwife and professor of midwifery at NYU. "And that's problematic because it's asynchronous with the global community. I believe we need licensing and education that meets the international standard of what a midwife is."

Malpractice insurance is another issue. In some states, no professional liability carrier offers policies to independent midwives or the coverage that is available is too expensive to maintain. That means that a midwife's options are either to not practice at all or to "ride bare," meaning to practice without coverage, which leaves no safety net if they get sued. "This is such a profound barrier for out-of-hospital providers," said Dr. Niles. "So many regulatory and structural gatekeeping mechanisms are designed to keep us out of the system." It's also not great for families in the event they want to bring a malpractice suit against a midwife.

All this fragmentation and variation has led to claims that direct-entry midwifery is a "Wild West landscape where anything goes," where there aren't standards for training or practice, or mechanisms for accountability. In 2018, GateHouse Media published a nine-month investigation, which found that state regulatory boards "rarely take serious action against midwives, even in cases that result in death or permanent injury," and that midwives who have been censured or barred from practicing in one state can cross state lines and practice elsewhere.

A key part of ensuring that out-of-hospital birth is safe is screening clients for eligibility, to make sure they are low-risk. Most pregnancies are uncomplicated, but approximately 8 percent involve complications that, if left untreated, may harm the mother or the baby, according to Johns Hopkins. Even among eligible clients, approximately 11 percent of planned home births and 16 percent of birth center births result in transfers to a higher level of care, with first-time mothers transferring more often. Part of a midwife's job is to identify complications and refer clients to a higher level of care as needed at all stages of the process. During pregnancy, a complication could be a condition like dangerously high blood pressure, known as preeclampsia, or placenta previa, a condition in which the placenta covers the cervix. During labor, a complication could be a cord prolapse, in which the umbilical cord gets compressed between the fetus and the cervix, or fetal heart rate decelerations. Not all transfers are due to complications or emergencies—sometimes, people in labor simply hit a point where they need more potent pain relief.

Life-or-death situations are not always predictable, and hospitals tend to be better equipped to handle them. But even in states where certified midwives can legally practice, the transfers can be rocky. Acrimony between hospital staff and midwives leads to delays and breakdowns in communication. It's not uncommon for midwives to face hostility, harassment, and persecution when they go into a hospital, making them understandably wary to do so. Hospital staff members may report a midwife for negligence, even if she followed protocol and best practices exactly. Factions on both sides remain prone to mudslinging, and parents can get caught in the middle, unsure of who or what to trust. This dynamic is harmful, as research shows that the more deeply embedded midwives are into the system, the better the outcomes are. "In the United States, integration of midwifery into the maternity care delivery system is fragmented, coverage is not available for all women or for all birth providers, and care is poorly coordinated, contributing to adverse perinatal outcomes," said the 2020 *Birth Settings* report. "Poor communication, disagreement, and lack of clarity around provider roles are identified as primary determinant of these adverse outcomes."

The debate over midwives and out-of-hospital birth remains fierce. The patchwork of state legislation, the confusing "alphabet soup" of midwifery credentialing, and the vagaries of insurance coverage have created a byzantine system that is illegible and inaccessible to many. For clients like Alison, it can be confusing and overwhelming to figure out. It's hard to know the right questions to ask and what opinions to trust.

What Eilers came to believe, as he did his research, was that the divisions between hospitals and community settings, between doctors and midwives, didn't have to be as pronounced as they were. In 2013, he had a radical idea—what if WHA opened a birth center where doctors and midwives worked closely together? Eilers was a member of a group within WHA focused on achieving the "triple aim" of obstetrics—how to improve outcomes and patient experiences while lowering costs—and one day he floated the birth center idea with someone else in the group. The response was along the lines of "That's crazy. Keep it to yourself." Eilers was undeterred. He saw that a birth center could be the answer to many of the problems plaguing his field, starting with cost.

Most of the money paid in maternal and newborn care goes to hospital facility fees, as the cumulative expenses of the staff and equipment and medicine and tools and procedures and administration and insurance add up. Eilers thought of the problem in terms of "Patient A" and "Patient B." Typically, in a hospital, a low-risk patient in spontaneous labor at full-term, Patient A, might be in labor next door to a woman with preeclampsia and preterm labor, Patient B. Both patients had access to the same resources, and someone—the hospital, the insurance company, the patient, or, most likely, a combination of all three—was paying a premium for ready access to them. But there was an exceedingly low chance that Patient A would require the same resources as Patient B, and so wasn't deploying those resources for every single patient, regardless of need, inefficient and wasteful? And wouldn't it make more sense for Patient A to give birth in a lower-cost environment where all those resources weren't unilaterally marshaled? Where their go-to care provider wasn't a surgeon? A birth center, Eilers realized, was a powerful vehicle for cost reduction.

If just an additional 10 percent of births in the US took place in private homes or freestanding birth centers, the country would save almost $11 billion per year without compromising safety.

Eilers started talking to a nurse-midwife who also worked for WHA and was also interested in the prospect of opening a birth center. It took a few years and intense lobbying, but in 2017, the Midwifery Birth Center opened its doors, with the goal of building a practice where each patient could get the appropriate amount of intervention they needed, where midwives were the experts in physiologic birth, and doctors were experts in higher-risk situations, forming links in a chain that people were moved up or down as required.

In 2021, the Midwifery Birth Center surpassed Andaluz with the highest number of births per year in the state. On average, the birth center has about twenty patients with due dates each month: 70 percent give birth at the birth center, 10 percent transfer to the hospital in labor, and the other 20 percent transfer during pregnancy for another reason, such as gestational hypertension or their water breaking early. And because WHA was part of a larger healthcare network that had existing relationships with insurers—and because their protocols are strict (people with a previous cesarean, for instance, could not give birth there, because of an increased risk of uterine rupture)—the Midwifery Birth Center accepted public insurance and most of the private insurers in the state.*

For Alison, all the WHA midwife's talk of evidence-based practice and protocols and guidelines, in an environment that felt like a cool new condo, was a good fit. Her insurance covered the birth center, and the overall cost, both out-of-pocket and in total, would be cheaper than the hospital.

She scheduled her initial prenatal visit for July 30. Her due date was March 3.

---

* In 2022, WHA announced that it was closing the Midwifery Birth Center, as part of a larger plan to consolidate its services in the region.

GESTATION

But pregnancy is above all a drama playing itself out
inside the woman between her and herself.
She experiences it both as an enrichment and a mutilation.
—Simone de Beauvoir, *The Second Sex*

CHAPTER 9
Jillian

Even though Jillian had apprenticed at Andaluz and continued to work at the birth center, she had known from the start that she wanted to have her baby at home if she could. She was a creature of comfort and loved being in her own familiar, unrestricted space.

She also knew that she wanted Alysa to be her midwife. Though the Andaluz midwives did attend home births, Jillian wasn't sure how it would feel for her coworkers to be her care providers. She had close personal relationships with them, but that was different from being naked around them. She liked the idea that her best friend and future midwifery partner, who already knew her and Chad so well, would help her deliver her baby.

There was also the not-insignificant issue of cost. Even as an employee, Jillian wasn't sure she could afford Andaluz. She was on Oregon Health Plan, the state's public insurance, and even though OHP ostensibly covered community birth, Andaluz (along with other local practices) had stopped accepting it after finding that coverage requests were routinely denied or inadequately reimbursed. Jillian and Chad, who didn't have thousands of dollars just set aside, were willing to pay out-of-pocket if they had to, but only with a midwife who was open to a long payment plan.

One afternoon in August, Alysa drove to Jillian's house for their first prenatal appointment. Sitting in Jillian's living room, with the sun streaming through the windows and the dogs snoozing nearby, they reviewed her vital signs, as well as personal health and family history. They talked about what Jillian could expect over the coming months, and Alysa asked about her personal preferences, like if she wanted an early ultrasound and to labor in water. For both, it was a notable shift in their dynamic: Alysa already knew some of the answers from their years of friendship, but it was different to pose them as a midwife asking a client, rather than as a friend asking a friend.

Then, they relocated to the bedroom, where Alysa felt Jillian's belly and listened to the fetal heart tones with her handheld Doppler. It was a milestone, a marker of how far they had come since they first met at Birthingway as midwifery applicants. As Alysa located her baby's heartbeat, Jillian found it touching that her friend was a licensed midwife who was taking care of someone, and that someone was her. The past five years of her life, and maybe longer, seemed to have been leading to this moment.

Around the same time, the nausea—relentless and unsparing—hit hard. She felt sick from the start of every day to its finish. Her appetite was gone, and she was perpetually poised on the precipice of vomiting. Keeping food down was a struggle. She tried to keep her spirits up by reminding herself that she was growing a human, but that was not easy to do while hunched over a toilet bowl. As another wave rolled through, Jillian thought back to every time she'd listened to clients talk about how miserable they were and told them it would all be worth it. Her intention had been to be encouraging and provide a sense of perspective, but now she wondered if those words had been dismissive. Jillian had felt compassion for those clients, of course, but she hadn't really understood the visceral reality of their misery until now. How could they have listened to her giving advice, without having experienced the process herself, and not rolled their eyes? This was *awful.*

In addition to the nausea, she was tired all the time. The smallest, simplest tasks drained her of energy, and getting out of bed felt like a momentous feat, especially in the summertime heat. She was irritable and self-conscious, worried that her colleagues would think she was slacking off because she wasn't running at her usual lively pace. At the end of every workday, Jillian collapsed onto her couch at home and stayed there until it was time for bed, sinking deeper and deeper into its cushions like a stone sinking in the sea.

During her second prenatal appointment with Alysa in September, they talked about ways Jillian could keep nausea at bay, like eating every two hours, integrating more protein into her diet, and keeping snacks by the bed. She tried them all, and none of them worked. All the tips and tricks Jillian had learned in midwifery school failed her—ginger didn't help, and neither did Sea-Bands or acupressure massage. Meals became a chore and a gamble. Chicken, which she used to eat regularly, became repulsive. The world was riddled with olfactory land mines that turned her stomach in an instant. Sometimes eating made her feel better, and sometimes it made her feel worse, and though she knew she had to, sometimes she didn't want to eat at all. Sure, at the end of her pregnancy she'd have her baby, but that felt so far away. Right now, she was focused on when she'd see a sliver of relief.

One day at work, feeling like she was reaching the end of her rope, Jillian asked Marilyn for advice. She was still the only person at the birth center who knew what Jillian was going through, and she had decades of experience working with nauseated, grumpy pregnant women who had to forge through their everyday lives as if nothing had changed. Marilyn suggested she try a combination of Unisom and B_6. The supplements didn't get rid of Jillian's nausea entirely, but they made a palpable difference. Through trial and error, she eventually managed to find a limited array of foods she could stomach, including peanut butter and crackers on the nightstand and, randomly, hamburgers from McDonald's. Jillian hadn't eaten much fast food before her pregnancy, but now it was all she craved.

As the exhaustion and nausea continued, another reality made itself apparent, one Jillian had been reluctant to face. The more she thought about it, the more she understood that the grand plans she and Alysa had for Blooming Dahlia Midwifery would have to be put on hold.

When Jillian arrived as an apprentice in September 2018, Andaluz midwives were handling around 120 births a year. By October 2019, after a year of intense and grueling work, Jillian had logged all the clinical training she needed, clocking 55 births and around one thousand hours, which also included prenatal and postpartum care. Her plan had been to apply for her midwifery credential with NARM, apply for her Oregon license, and work on opening Blooming Dahlia with Alysa straightaway, but then Jennifer, Andaluz's founder, had mentioned that the birth center needed someone to replace their current office manager and staff the front desk. Jennifer knew Jillian had medical office experience from Missouri and thought she would be great at the role, if she was interested.

At first, Jillian wasn't sure. She loved going to births, and after so many years striving to become a midwife, she was eager to get started with her own practice. But she was also burned out from the intensity of midwifery school and wanted to make space in her life for other things. The prospect of staying involved with midwifery and birth work, without having to be on call (which meant no wine with dinner or out-of-town trips), was tempting. Jillian took the job and started as Andaluz's office manager in December 2019. She reasoned that it was a chance to learn the behind-the-scenes mechanics of running a midwifery practice—the administrative and business stuff that kept it afloat—which would come in handy for Blooming Dahlia. Part of her yearned to be more hands-on with clients, but she was organized, efficient, proactive, and adept at multitasking, which made her a phenomenal office manager. She also appreciated the stability. For so long, she had counted every penny and budgeted in survival mode, where one surprise bill could be a disaster. Now, she had steady hours, a steady paycheck, and could treat herself to everyday things she would never have allowed herself before, like her favorite brand of nitrate-free, thick-cut bacon. She had been proud of herself for persevering and putting that more precarious phase of her life behind her, and for giving herself a moment to breathe before making the next big move.

She had never intended for the office manager work to be a long-term thing. Now that she was pregnant, though, her priorities had changed. The prospect of giving up the consistency of an office manager job in order to start a business with significant financial investment and risk, as well as a high demand on time (being on call to attend births 24/7, scheduling and coordinating prenatals, managing apprentices), on top of caring for a new baby, seemed unworkable. On some level, she had known from the moment she saw the positive pregnancy test that Blooming Dahlia would have to wait. Although the reasons for delaying made sense on just about every practical level, it was a hard reality to face. Jillian trusted that Alysa would understand, but it still didn't feel fair that she had worked hard to enter her prime professional years, only for them to overlap with her prime reproductive ones. To have come so far, only to have to stop, or at least to delay, her career before it really got started—that was a profound disappointment. Instead of becoming a midwife, she was becoming a client.

Once she'd made her decision, Jillian asked Alysa to meet for lunch at a café in Salem. They sat across from each other at the table, and Jillian apologetically explained that she didn't think she could be a new midwife, a new business owner, and a new mom at the same time. That would all be too much. Alysa was gracious and kind and told Jillian she thought she was making the right choice. And, she added, just because the timing wasn't right now did not mean it never would be. Until then, Alysa would keep working with a birth center in Salem and start taking on home birth clients of her own. And she would still be Jillian's midwife.

When she hit twelve weeks, with no complications arising, Jillian finally told Carrie, the Andaluz midwife she'd apprenticed with during midwifery school (her "preceptor"), that she was pregnant.

"Well, I got knocked up on my wedding night," she said.

Carrie laughed at how unceremonious she was about it—Jillian hadn't done some big reveal; she'd just dropped the news into casual conversation in a self-deprecating and lighthearted way. Carrie said she was excited for her and knew Jillian would be a great mom. The next person she wanted to tell was Jennifer, but she was in Haiti, working at the midwifery clinic she'd founded there in the aftermath of the 2010 earthquake. When Jennifer returned, Jillian shared the news while they were working together in Jennifer's home office. They didn't talk in depth during that conversation because there were other people around, but they picked up the thread again a week later. One night, Jillian swung by the birth cottage on Jennifer's property to drop off supplies after a birth, and Jennifer asked her to stick around.

"How are you?" she asked. "Tell me about things."

Jillian told her about the nausea, which hadn't abated even though she was beginning her second trimester. She also mentioned that her best friend, Alysa, was going to be her midwife, but that she hoped to charge full price, which Jillian wasn't sure she could afford. Jennifer pushed back and asked why Jillian wasn't getting care from Andaluz.

"I can provide you the care," she said, as if it were the most obvious thing in the world. "You work for me. It's the least I can do!"

Jennifer offered right there to provide the midwifery services at a discount and on a payment plan, if that was what Jillian needed. It wasn't an unusual offer, as Andaluz provided dozens of births a year at a discount or for free to clients who couldn't afford to pay out-of-pocket. After Jennifer's own experience struggling to afford midwifery care, she didn't want cost to be a barrier for anyone.

Jennifer had been a midwife for over thirty years. She was born in Puerto Rico and spent most of her childhood in Central America with her family, who were members of the Church of Jesus Christ of Latter-day Saints. Jennifer went to college in the US, where she majored in piano performance, but also considered nursing school. When she was pregnant with her first child, she and her husband, Fernando, were living in Utah, barely scraping by, which made it difficult to find an OB practice to take her on as a patient. Finally, at seven months pregnant, she walked into an ER to see a doctor, unsure of how else to find prenatal care she could afford. She didn't appreciate how she was treated throughout the final weeks of her pregnancy and labor, feeling that she received inferior treatment because she was young and poor.

By the time she became pregnant with her second baby, she and Fernando were living in California, and the idea of going back to a hospital was unappealing. Her sister suggested a midwife, but her Medicaid insurance didn't cover that kind of care. Jennifer contacted a midwife anyway and explained her financial situation. The midwife said she would take Jennifer as a client and take payment in installments of $150 a month. The attention and nurturing she received were life-changing. Jennifer got an hour of "loving care" (as she called it) at every appointment, and the midwife answered all her questions. She decided she wanted to become a midwife herself.

Not long after, Jennifer, Fernando, and their two kids moved to Guatemala City to be closer to her family. She attended midwifery school and worked at a public clinic that handled around five hundred births a month, a number that paled in comparison to the local hospital, where the births numbered in the thousands. Many patients who attended the clinic said they were afraid to go to the hospital because the cesarean rate was so high. Jennifer had heard horror stories, so when she got pregnant again, she decided to give birth unassisted. It was risky—and later, she herself would call it reckless—but both she and the baby came through healthy. In 1994, Jennifer began to practice independently as a midwife, strapping her infant to her back and venturing out to people's homes, often at night and often in neighborhoods with high rates of violent crime.

The more she practiced, the more worried Fernando grew about her safety, so they decided to convert their house into a birth center—the original Andaluz—and move the family into a room in the back of the house next to the kitchen, originally built as a maid's quarters. All five of them slept in one king-size bed while Jennifer used the three front rooms to see clients and deliver babies. It was a tight squeeze. Within six months, everyone had grown tired of being confined to one room, and the kids didn't have an area to play, so they moved into a bigger house two doors down. There were still three rooms for the birth center, but now the family had two spacious rooms as their living space instead of one. Jennifer attended about fifteen births a month there, helped by local midwives and midwifery students who flew down from the US to train.

In the late 1990s, with violence escalating in the country, Jennifer, Fernando, and their growing brood left Guatemala with $20,000 in savings to start over with in the US. Once they arrived, they used seven thousand of those precious dollars to buy a car and hit the road for Oregon. The car turned out to be a lemon, breaking down almost as soon as they arrived in the state, but it was enough to get them to their destination of Tualatin, a suburb south of Portland. They checked into a Motel 6 on a Wednesday afternoon, ready to start their new life. The hotel room had no kitchen, and without a car they couldn't get groceries, so Jennifer ordered pizza delivery every night. Within a few days, even the kids were sick of it. On Sunday morning, the Gallardo family attended a church service, and when members of the congregation asked what brought them to Oregon, Jennifer (who had earned her NARM credential in 1997) told them she was going to open a birth center. It was a long shot and she had no idea how she would pull it off, but she believed saying plans out loud would help them come to fruition.

With $1,400 left of their fast-dwindling savings, the Gallardos moved into an apartment. They had a broken car, hungry kids, and no furniture, and after a few nights of sleeping on blankets on the floor, Jennifer took $200 and went to PJ Sleep Shop to buy the cheapest mattress she could find. The family signed up for government assistance to help pay for food, and Jennifer set off to build her birth center. The sooner she could get a practice off the ground, the sooner the family could find its footing. After some searching, she found a medical office suite she liked in the Whitney Professional Building in Tualatin and contacted the rental property manager. He wouldn't let Jennifer come in for a meeting because of her finances—no credit score, no savings, no existing business track record—

but she managed to circumvent him and appeal directly to the building's owner, telling him that all she needed was one birth a month to cover the rent. Impressed by the spunky, small blonde in front of him clutching a portfolio, he agreed to give her a lease.

They needed the birth center to succeed, and fast. To get the operation off the ground, Jennifer and Fernando opened lines of credit at multiple furniture stores, accruing $17,000 in furniture debt. Jennifer attended midwifery meetings to recruit employees and chased pregnant women down in the grocery store to ask when they were due and hand them a business card. When Andaluz opened in June 1999, she had, against all odds, managed to get twenty-five clients on board.

Given mainstream medicine's long history of antagonism toward midwifery, it was rather audacious to open a birth center in a building filled with doctors. Andaluz's neighbors were a kidney dialysis center and an orthodontist. The Andaluz office suite didn't have a stove, so the midwives cooked breakfast for their postpartum clients using a hot plate, leading the other tenants to complain that the smell of French toast and bacon permeated the building. Andaluz started as a scrappy operation, but the early momentum that Jennifer generated never flagged. When the Gallardos found an old firehouse in Portland for sale, right off the highway and down the hill from OHSU, they decided to open a Portland location, which would connect them to a bigger market and enable the birth center to take on more clients.

The Portland Andaluz location opened in 2008, and like Tualatin, it was consistently busy. Certainly, there were bumps in the road—battles with local hospitals; a malpractice suit filed by a family whose baby died two days after labor, alleging the midwives were at fault; disagreements with the state about Oregon Health Plan and reimbursement—but overall the journey had been rewarding, and Jennifer knew she'd built something special.* Jillian thought so too.

---

* In 2017, Jennifer closed the Tualatin location. In 2022, she sold Andaluz Portland to new owners.

After her conversation with Jennifer, Jillian went home and discussed her offer with Chad. It was certainly appealing from a financial perspective, and though Chad knew and trusted Alysa, he felt more comfortable using midwives who had decades of experiences over someone who had recently gotten her license. Jillian told Alysa that she loved her and wanted her to be involved in her pregnancy and birth, but the Andaluz opportunity was too good to pass up. Alysa replied that, if she were in Jillian's position, she'd be making the same decision. She did want to have a conversation, though, about what it would be like for Jillian to have her boss and preceptor as her care providers, as that was a consideration Jillian had raised before. It would change the dynamics of those relationships, and Alysa worried that Jillian wouldn't feel as open to sharing intimate, sensitive details of her personal life or her body with people she knew on a professional level. She wanted Jillian to feel comfortable blurting out whatever she was thinking or feeling, and Jillian assured her that she would.

When she was around fifteen weeks pregnant, Jillian transferred her care to Andaluz.

CHAPTER 10
T'Nika

One day at work in August, T'Nika was following her nursing preceptor around the floor and took a step that caused a jolt of pain to her stomach. It was like she'd stepped down *too* hard and was now hunched over, feeling like she'd been kicked in the gut. All she could do was waddle behind her preceptor and try to keep up, but the fact that she was dragging herself around like Quasimodo attracted attention. One nurse said to T'Nika's preceptor, "Is your student okay?" and all T'Nika could do was grimace, nod, and try to keep going, stepping as lightly as she could.

T'Nika was about five weeks pregnant at the time, and during those five weeks, she'd been experiencing the worst constipation of her life. It felt like her bowels had gone on strike. She could physically feel the blockage, like a boulder that couldn't be moved. She tried taking MiraLAX, but that didn't help, and one night, in an attempt to relieve the pressure, she lay in the shower and let the hot water hit her abdomen, but that didn't do much either. Even though she was so early in her pregnancy, T'Nika told her preceptor what was going on to explain her bizarre behavior.

As time went on, the pain became so acute that T'Nika feared she was having an ectopic pregnancy.* She called Andaluz, where she'd already had her tour and initial appointment, to share her concerns. The midwife suggested she get an ultrasound at a nearby clinic as soon as possible, so T'Nika scheduled an appointment for later that week and left work early, nervous for what the results might show. Almost immediately, the ultrasound technician told her that the problem wasn't an ectopic pregnancy—the fetus looked fine. The problem was, in fact, poop. The technician said she could see that T'Nika's bowels were "undulating with turds" on the screen. The surges in progesterone, an active hormone in pregnancy, had slowed down her gut and caused severe constipation. *You've got to be kidding me,* T'Nika thought. She was relieved that the problem wasn't more serious, but it felt like an absurd problem to have. At least it was a solvable one. T'Nika called Andaluz to report the ultrasound's findings, and Marilyn suggested additional supplements to get things moving. She started adding senna, magnesium powder, flaxseed, and a dandelion root tincture to her use of MiraLAX, which helped.

But then, just when she started feeling better, at around nine weeks, the headaches arrived. Bad ones. She first told Marilyn about them at an August appointment. The good news, Marilyn said after a quick physical examination, was that her blood pressure was normal. She wondered if T'Nika's headaches could be related to tension, as she'd experienced tension headaches in the past and was currently finishing nursing school while also working at a healthcare facility that was understaffed and weathering a global pandemic. There was plenty to be tense about. By the end of August, nothing had changed. In fact, the headaches had gotten even worse. Portland was blanketed in thick smoke due to raging wildfires in the Pacific Northwest, and the air quality index in the city was the worst in the world for about a week, and it was so bad that it was deemed dangerous to go outside because the smoke was so unhealthy.

---

* Ectopic pregnancies, in which the embryo implants outside the uterus (usually in a Fallopian tube), can be life-threatening if not caught and addressed early due to the threat of rupture.

Even after the smoke was gone and T'Nika had finished school, though, the headaches lingered, as did other symptoms. It felt like if it wasn't one thing, it was another. Between the constipation, the morning sickness, and the migraines, she was losing weight. She weighed less at the end of her first trimester than she had when she started care at Andaluz in July.

Despite these setbacks, T'Nika appreciated that her team of midwives listened to her complaints, communicated with one another about her case, and worked with her to come up with solutions. That treatment stood in stark contrast to the treatment she'd received a few years before for gastrointestinal ailments. T'Nika had always had a fickle stomach, something her family teased her about since childhood as she waddled around Dollar Tree looking for a bathroom or squirmed in the back seat of the family car on the way home from Izzy's Pizza. They had never been incapacitating until she and Daniel were living in Boston. Suddenly, it was difficult for her to eat without being in pain. She was nauseated all the time and grew weaker and malnourished. At one point, the symptoms were so bad—a jabbing pain in her abdomen—that T'Nika went to the emergency room, worried something might be wrong with her kidneys or appendix. The doctors ran a slew of tests ($5,000 worth of them), but other than ruling out any problems with those organs, they couldn't identify a source, so they referred her to a gastrointestinal (GI) specialist, who ran T'Nika through colonoscopies, endoscopies, and a barium swallow study.

No answers emerged. None of the doctors seemed to know what was going on, floating Crohn's disease or maybe ulcerative colitis as possible causes. Finally, Daniel's uncle, a GI doctor in California, referred T'Nika to a well-known specialist outside of Boston. She was hopeful the specialist would be the game-changer, but that doctor didn't seem to have any more insight than the others. She prescribed T'Nika additional medications, including a drug that she had to stop taking because it gave her heart palpitations. With every doctor she saw, T'Nika left the appointment questioning whether she had been taken seriously. The providers she saw often made her feel like she was complaining, overreacting, or annoying. They seemed to distrust her accounting of her symptoms, as if she wasn't a reliable reporter of what was going on in her body. One doctor had even asked her, "Are you sure you are actually feeling these symptoms?"

The question had shocked her. She was a recent college graduate—why in the world would she rack up thousands of dollars in medical debt unless she really was in pain? As the medical bills piled up, T'Nika began to worry that she'd never get better. Her job required her to be active, which she was increasingly unable to do. She was taking so many medications that sometimes just walking down the school's hallways lined with fluorescent lights made her feel woozy. The experience was affecting her not only physically, but also mentally, and altered the way she approached her health. The next time she experienced crippling, alarming pain, she did not want to go back to the ER. If the doctors couldn't help the first time, she doubted the second time would be any different, and she didn't want to be billed hundreds or even thousands of dollars for another dead end. She tried an urgent care clinic first, but they didn't have an appointment available for three weeks and said they weren't equipped to handle her issue. When the pain didn't abate after four days, T'Nika reluctantly returned to the ER, where they advised her to see a specialist. She felt like she was being pawned off.

Finally, after months of struggling, T'Nika's mother made her an appointment to see a gastroenterologist with whom she worked as an endoscopy technician in Eugene. He ran a slew of tests, and to T'Nika's immense relief, he found something: a Helicobacter pylori (H. pylori) bacterial infection, which, when left untreated, could cause peptic ulcers. T'Nika had tested negative for H. pylori in Boston, but this doctor had used a different type of test—a stool sample instead of a blood test that identified antibodies. She was also diagnosed with IBS and gastroparesis, a motility disorder in which food digests slowly, and given a strict nutritional regimen to follow.

Finally, after over a year, she had answers and a path forward toward feeling better. But one takeaway from the whole saga lingered in the back of her mind. It seemed that the only reason she'd finally found answers and a personalized, effective treatment plan was because her family had a connection to the doctor, and so he went above and beyond to help her. T'Nika never forgot the way the doctors in Boston had made her feel, and she believed that was in no small part due to her race.

Racial bias in healthcare—also known as medical racism—is a well-documented phenomenon. In 2002, the Institute of Medicine published *Unequal Treatment: Confronting Racial and Ethnic Disparities in Health Care,* a lengthy study that concluded that racial and ethnic minorities experienced a lower quality of health services in the United States and were less likely to receive routine medical procedures than white Americans. The researchers also found that people of color were less likely to be given appropriate medications for heart disease, to undergo coronary bypass surgery, to receive kidney dialysis, and to get a transplant, resulting in higher death rates. Black people were 3.6 times more likely than white people to have their legs and feet amputated as a result of diabetes, even when all other factors were equal. Pain is also undertreated in Black patients for conditions from appendicitis to cancer, and patients who ask for pain relief routinely report being denied it due to racist beliefs about higher pain tolerances and suspicions about "drug-seeking behavior."

In pregnancy care specifically, Black women are subject to care that provides a dangerous combination of too-much-too-soon and too-little-too-late: receiving aggressive interventions they may not need sooner than they might need them, which can lead to complications, or facing complications that they are unable to get taken seriously, resulting in missed opportunities to protect their health and safety. For example, cesarean sections are approximately 35 percent more likely among Black women compared with white women, but Black women are less likely to receive surgical intervention for pregnancy-related hemorrhage. Both too-much-too-soon and too-little-too-late cause harm, and the combination of both can be deadly.

Medical racism also manifests in how patients are treated by healthcare providers. For many Black women and people of color in America, engaging with the healthcare system can involve neglect, indifference, hostility, and contempt. "Like millions of women of color, especially black women, I was churned through a healthcare machine that neglected and ignored me until I was incompetent," the sociologist Tressie McMillan Cottom wrote in her book *Thick*. "When the medical profession systematically denies the existence of black women's pain, underdiagnoses our pain, refuses to alleviate or treat our pain, healthcare marks us as incompetent bureaucratic subjects. Then it serves us accordingly."

As T'Nika sought help for her illness, she'd found herself dismissed and doubted at many points along the way. She saw how healthcare professionals could make a patient feel small and unhinged, how they often seemed to ignore and disregard her pain. What she went through cultivated a sense of skepticism around the idea that modern medicine could solve any problem. History, social dynamics, and culture, she realized, could play as big a role in the medical care someone received as the clinical notes in their hospital chart. She had a lot of respect for the medical profession—she was becoming a nurse, after all—but she had seen that doctors didn't always have the right answers, or the patience, willingness, or capacity to try to find them.

For her maternity care, T'Nika did not want the pregnancy version of her GI journey. Beyond the family tradition and her desire for a water birth, she wanted a midwife because she wanted to be seen and heard. She didn't want to have her guard up, and the fact that she felt listened to during her prenatal appointments was revelatory. She took full advantage by being bracingly honest about her symptoms and ailments. T'Nika had a tendency to turn something small into something big or do the opposite—grin and bear through something serious. Sometimes if she felt a twinge or flash of pain, she told herself to calm down, wait it out, and see if it turned into something bigger. As a nurse, T'Nika knew what it was like to have a large patient load. She also knew what it was like to have patients freak out over nothing. And she knew the midwives were busy, so she tried to reserve her texts for issues that felt genuinely pressing. She joked that her prenatal appointments were forty-five minutes of her complaining and fifteen minutes of clinical checkups, and she loved it that way. She sometimes felt self-conscious that her questions or concerns were silly or minor, but the midwives were reliably receptive, and whenever she did decide to text one of them, she got a response within twenty-four hours and then a follow-up a day or so later. The responsiveness was surprising to her at first, and then came to feel solid and consistent. It was something she could count on.

After twelve weeks, T'Nika and Daniel finally told their families she was pregnant. It had been a hard and lonely secret to keep. She didn't like hiding things from her mother, who could tell something was different. When she noticed that T'Nika wasn't drinking wine at dinner like she normally would, T'Nika had to lie, saying her IBS was acting up and making her stomach hurt. Finally, though, once an ultrasound at Andaluz confirmed that things were progressing well, she and Daniel made a plan to share the news.

On their next visit to Eugene to see their families, the couple ate dinner at Daniel's parents' house. After the meal, they were all standing in the dining room and T'Nika pulled up an image of the ultrasound on her phone.

"Take a look at this art project we've been working on," T'Nika said, handing the phone over to her in-laws.

His parents peered at the phone together. "What is this?"

"It's an ultrasound." T'Nika exclaimed. "We are pregnant!"

Immediately, Daniel's mom started jumping up and down and yelling with glee (so much so that she woke up their sleeping nephews downstairs).

The next day, they went over to T'Nika's parents' house and replayed the scene again—handing over their phone to show an "art project"—but when T'Nika announced the news, her mother was quiet. After a few moments, a smile slowly spread across her face.

"I'll be right back," she said, and walked out of the room in a dreamlike state.

T'Nika's dad spoke up, also grinning. "No way," he said. "Not my baby."

"I'm not your baby anymore. I'm twenty-nine years old," she replied, rolling her eyes with a grin. T'Nika didn't understand why her dad was acting so surprised, as she was almost thirty, and she and Daniel had been married for years. Surely, the news they were having a baby couldn't have been that much of a shock, but in her dad's eyes, she would always be sixteen.

When T'Nika's mom walked back into the room, she handed her a box.

"I've been waiting for this moment," she said quietly.

T'Nika opened the box. Inside was a big stack of Dr. Seuss books—books, her mother explained, that she'd been saving for her first grand-baby. T'Nika was stunned and then immensely moved. How long had her mother been saving these? She clearly hadn't gone out to the garage or dug through a box in the basement to find them. The gift had been easily accessible, as if they'd been stashed under the bed or on a shelf in the closet in anticipation of this exact moment. It was like her mother had sensed something, or maybe T'Nika hadn't kept the secret as well as she thought she had. Either way, it was a relief to not have to hide anymore. T'Nika spent the rest of the weekend on the couch, letting herself be taken care of by her family.

CHAPTER 11
Alison

Alison's first prenatal appointment at the Midwifery Birth Center was on July 20 with a nurse-midwife named Jamie, who explained that the first order of business would be reviewing Alison's medical history and chart in close detail and getting to know Alison and what had brought her to the birth center. Alison shared the relevant health information, talked about her miscarriage experience, and told Jamie that she'd already gotten an ultrasound at six weeks, just to be sure the pregnancy was viable. She was hoping to schedule another one at twelve weeks—she knew her anxiety wouldn't go away entirely after, but there would be relief in making it further with this pregnancy than she had before. She wanted to be able to feel excited, and it was kind of sad to her that she couldn't, at least not yet. The first time, it hadn't really occurred to her that the pregnancy might not work out, and now that awareness hovered over her. It was hard not to fret about the possibility of a loss, as if doing one "wrong" thing might result in a miscarriage.

Alison added that she'd been checking her *What to Expect* app every day and reading various forums. She was paying close attention to every physical sensation and continued to look up information online and in books. She treated the data-driven recommendations from Emily Oster's *Expecting Better* like gospel, meticulously weighing out two hundred milligrams of coffee beans every morning and avoiding soft cheeses. She'd learned her iron levels were low and was vigilant about taking iron supplements. She recognized that, in some ways, control was an illusion, but she liked having guidelines and a road map—it felt preventative in a superstitious or ritualistic way, like if she followed a prescribed set of steps and adhered to certain rules, everything would turn out okay and she would have a healthy baby.

As she spoke, she could tell that Jamie was listening. When she had finished, Jamie replied that she understood how Alison was feeling and that it was normal, especially after what Alison had gone through, to crave reassurance. She proposed that they include the "extra" ultrasound at twelve weeks as part of a broader genetic screening to ensure that insurance would cover it. Alison left the birth center feeling optimistic, like she'd found a practice that accommodated her needs.

After what felt like a period of endless waiting, twelve weeks rolled around. It was time for Alison to get her second ultrasound, and while she hoped for good news, she prepared herself for bad. For weeks she had been dealing with nausea that was escalating in frequency and intensity. Though it hadn't been debilitating, she'd had to work it into her routine. Each morning, she would wake up, throw up, eat some saltines or oyster crackers that she kept by her bedside, and go on with her day. She always felt better after throwing up, but it was frustrating to be unable to participate in the usual activities she enjoyed over the summer because of sickness or exhaustion. She figured once school started again, she would have to budget vomiting time into her schedule. She almost appreciated the morning sickness because it felt like her body's acknowledgment of the pregnancy—surely if the pregnancy wasn't viable, she wouldn't be sick every day—but she was eager for an ultrasound to confirm.

Finally, during the twelve-week ultrasound, she got the news she hoped for. The pregnancy was viable and everything was progressing normally. No red flags popped up on the genetic screen either. Everything looked good, and beyond the sense of relief, what struck her most was the sense of wonder. At one point, she was able to see an arm move on the screen, which felt miraculous.

The scan also confirmed a suspicion she'd had for quite some time: she and Steve were having a boy. They already had a name queued up: Theodore Rob—Theo for short—after Steve's grandfather and Alison's dad. The birth center gave her three pictures to take home, and she and Steve cherished them. A name and an image made the pregnancy feel more real. They could refer to the baby as "Theo" instead of "baby" or "it," and Alison got a thrill every time Steve asked her, "How's Theo doing today?"

Alison and Steve had already told their parents and siblings that they were pregnant following the six-week ultrasound. Alison had realized that if or when she experienced a pregnancy loss, there was no way she wouldn't tell the people she loved, and that if she was going to inform them of a loss anyway, there was no point in waiting to share she was pregnant. With the good news confirmed, the couple shared it with their wider circle, and Alison informed her boss and colleagues at work. Sometimes when people asked Alison which hospital she was going to, she felt shy and apprehensive about saying that she was pursuing an out-of-hospital birth. It felt like revealing an intimate part of herself, and she didn't like the idea that people might judge or pigeonhole her based on that information, especially because she knew it made some people nervous.

Her mother in particular had concerns. Alison and her siblings had all been born via cesarean section, and when Alison's youngest brother was born, a complication had required the baby to be transferred to a hospital in Eugene with a NICU, where he spent ten days. Alison had been nine years old at the time, but she remembered, even as an adult, the moment her grandparents came to stay with her, as well as the fear and trauma that stemmed from the baby being sent forty-five minutes away when time was of the essence. Because of that experience, which felt like a close call, Alison's mother believed it was important to give birth in a hospital with an operating room and a NICU.

Not long after Alison shared that she was pregnant, her mother had said, "Well, I had C-sections with all of you guys; you might want to consider that." Alison responded that she was actually planning to go to a birth center and explained her reasons why. "That's not what I would choose, but it's your life and your decision," her mom said. The conversation was a little tense, and Alison could sense that the birth center plan made her mother uncomfortable. Her mindset seemed to be that Alison should follow whatever the doctors and hospital thought was best and that the more medical involvement, the better, but Alison didn't agree. She knew part of the inspiration behind places like the Midwifery Birth Center and Andaluz was the idea that intense medical management may be appropriate for some patients, but not for all.

The phenomenon where all patients receive a high number of interventions is known as the "over-medicalization" of birth, and its most salient manifestation is the prevalence of cesarean surgeries. Today, one in three people who give birth in America have a C-section, a rate that is roughly twice that of Europe's. In 1965, the national cesarean birth rate was 4.5 percent, and it has increased sevenfold since then, with a dramatic uptick over the past few decades. Entities like the World Health Organization and ACOG estimate that a C-section rate between 10 and 20 percent is the benchmark to strive for—a rate over that range can signal that the surgeries are happening unnecessarily, while a rate below that range can signal that people who need the surgery are not getting it.

C-sections can be life-saving procedures that are critical for people with particular risk factors and under certain circumstances, but there are harmful effects to performing major abdominal surgery on young, healthy people who do not need it. The risk of severe maternal complications is, by some estimates, three times greater than with vaginal birth—particularly for repeat C-sections. The most common complications include hemorrhages, blood clots, and infections. C-sections also increase the risk of uterine rupture in subsequent pregnancies, and multiple surgeries can lead to a dangerous condition called placenta accreta. They result in longer hospital stays and a greater chance of hospital readmission. Babies are impacted as well: systematic reviews have found that babies born via cesarean face an increased risk of breathing problems and chronic diseases such as asthma, Crohn's disease, type 1 diabetes, and allergies.

For too many people giving birth in America—by some estimates, one-third of the people who undergo a C-section—the benefits do not outweigh the risks. They are medically unjustified and the decision to perform operations on people who don't need them is not a neutral act. It can cause what's known as "iatrogenic" problems, meaning harm caused by medical examinations or treatments. As Emily Oster wrote in *Expecting Better*, the data show that "Cesarean sections are a good option in an emergency but shouldn't be your first choice."

So how did a surgery meant for life-threatening situations become a standard of care?

One explanation is a higher incidence of risk factors within the birthing population. Factors like maternal age, weight, and chronic health conditions have changed as time, culture, and technology have progressed. But plenty of other countries have seen similar increases in those risk factors without increasing the cesarean rate. As it turns out, the issue is not so much the patients in the hospital as the hospital itself.

High C-section rates are a direct reflection and result of the way the maternal healthcare system, and the healthcare system in the US writ large, is structured. Instead of prioritizing prevention and physiologic birth, the US follows the "heroic" tradition of relying on medical intervention and surgical rescue. The anthropologist Robbie Davis-Floyd described this as the "technocratic model of childbirth," in which the female body is viewed as an "abnormal," "unpredictable," and "inherently defective machine" that must be closely monitored. "We designed the birth environment to resemble an I.C.U., and 99 percent of American women deliver in environments that look like I.C.U.s, surrounded by surgeons," explained Dr. Neel Shah, assistant professor of obstetrics, gynecology, and reproductive biology at Harvard Medical School.

The hospital environment for anyone, not just people in labor, tends to be stressful. When someone goes in to the hospital to give birth, they may be given vaginal exams, IVs, a catheter, continuous fetal monitoring, Pitocin, and/or have their membranes stripped as a matter of course. There are fluorescent lights and beeping machines and glinting tools and strangers in scrubs and lab coats bustling in and out, all stressors that can slow down labor and increase pain by provoking elevations in epinephrine and norepinephrine—the hormones behind the "fight or flight" response. And if a patient is stressed or in extreme pain and labor is stalled or slowed, that may justify interventions to get things going, and one medical procedure tends to beget another and another, in what is known as the "cascade of interventions." "Women may find that technologies used in labor and birth look a bit like a conveyor belt in a factory," wrote the sociology professor Theresa Morris in her book *Cut It Out*, which examined the C-section "epidemic" in America. "Women may jump or be pushed onto this conveyor belt at a number of points, but once they're on it, they may find it hard to get off until they come to the end of the process."

In one *Listening to Mothers* survey, part of a series of qualitative surveys conducted by the National Partnership for Women & Families, women reported experiencing a median of four interventions during each birth, with 47 percent experiencing five or more and 27 percent experiencing at least six. Take labor induction. About one in three women have their labors induced (a rate that is also thought to be excessively high). Pitocin intensifies contractions, which then typically requires a call to the anesthesiologist for an epidural, assuming there wasn't one in place already, which, then, conversely, can slow down labor for some people, which may prompt even more Pitocin.

Another commonly cited justification for Pitocin and cesareans is "failure to progress," which means that labor is taking too long. This might be because a mother is not dilating fast enough, her contractions don't seem strong enough, and/or the baby is in a less than optimal position. In the 1950s, during the era of twilight sleep, Pitocin protocols were built off the "Friedman curve," a bell graph that tracked the average length of labor to determine whether a patient's progress was outside the norm. For patients in active labor who were not progressing by one centimeter of dilation an hour, doctors could administer Pitocin to push things along. The technique was meant to avoid prolonged labors, which could create complications, but it also meant that labor was expected to progress at a standard speed within a standard duration. It meant there was a ticking clock—and when time ran out, it was time to prep the OR.

Research suggests that labor interventions, such as inducing labor when the cervix is closed, increase the chance of surgical birth for first-time mothers. In fact, women whose labors are induced are twice as likely to have a C-section than those who begin labor spontaneously. Despite this marked increase, 37 percent of respondents in the *Listening to Mothers* survey who had an attempted induction reported that there was either no medical reason given or an unsupported reason.

In 25 percent of C-sections, the cited reason for the surgery is "fetal distress" or "non-reassuring fetal heart tones." Around 84 percent of women have electronic fetal monitoring during their labors, which requires patients to stay in bed and limits their movement. A pattern of dips, or "decelerations," on the monitor's "strip" may lead a maternal care team to call for a C-section, and mothers who have continuous monitoring are 63 percent more likely to have a C-section than those who have hands-on monitoring. However, researchers have not found differences between the two groups in Apgar scores or perinatal death. Continuous monitoring is not known to improve outcomes, but it's impossible to know, with any course of action, what would have happened otherwise—to prove a negative. "Many C-sections done for fetal distress are probably unnecessary, but then a lot of biopsies of breast lumps are also unnecessary in retrospect," wrote the OB-turned-blogger Amy Tuteur in her book *Push Back*. "Unfortunately, it is very difficult to determine which babies are in danger of suffering irreparable damage."

When making medical decisions, a baseline or standard for normalcy is helpful, and standardization is an important component of delivering equitable, evidence-based care. However, measures and tools like continuous monitoring have also meant that the spectrum of what was once considered "normal" in labor—a notoriously individual, varied, and unpredictable process—has narrowed to the point where a high proportion of women fall outside of those boundaries. "You have to almost prove to me that you can have a successful vaginal delivery," one doctor told Morris in *Cut It Out*. "And it used to be the reverse."

Some women go into labor knowing they are going to have a C-section—their baby might be breech, or they are having multiples (twins, triplets, etc.)—in which case surgery is considered the safest option.* A suspected macrosomic baby—one that appears to weigh over eleven pounds (or ten pounds, if the mother is diabetic)—is another reason for planned surgery, although measurements of fetal weight in utero are far from precise. In fact, predictions can be off by as much as 20 percent, or even more. One study found that only one in five US women who were told their babies might be too big ended up delivering babies over the weight threshold.

There are also people for whom the prospect of a schedulable, predictable, and controllable procedure is preferable to the vortex of vaginal birth. A small percentage of women, estimated at around 2.5 percent, ask for elective C-sections, also known as cesarean delivery on maternal request. Some want to make sure their doctor is attending their birth instead of an unfamiliar on-call physician, or they want to schedule their birth for a day when a partner or parent can be present. People with panic or anxiety disorders or who have experienced sexual trauma may request a C-section for mental health reasons.

Once someone has one cesarean, they are more likely to give birth that way again. While research overwhelmingly supports that women with a previous cesarean should be allowed to try for a vaginal birth, only

* There is evidence that challenges some of these protocols. For instance, a major study that found that cesarean surgeries were safer for breech babies—and ushered in a shift in practice norms, away from vaginal breech deliveries—was later called into question for being poorly designed.

13 percent of people who have a cesarean will go on to have a vaginal birth after cesarean, or VBAC. In 1916, Dr. Edwin Cragin coined the axiom "once a cesarean, always a cesarean." Back then, cesarean surgeries were performed with vertical incisions, which had a high likelihood of rupturing in future labors. But after the standard cesarean surgery evolved into a smaller, horizontal surgical cut, which had a much lower risk of rupture, the "once a cesarean, always a cesarean" policy remained the norm, even though women who have a repeat section are much more likely to die from childbirth than are women who attempt a VBAC. While current estimates are hard to pin down, one survey from the International Cesarean Awareness Network (ICAN) found that 30 percent of American hospitals formally banned VBAC attempts, and hundreds more hospitals had de facto bans in place. ACOG supports trying for a VBAC in environments where emergency care is "immediately available," but what constitutes "immediately available" is open to interpretation. Mothers have also reported experiences of a "bait and switch," in which a provider said they supported VBAC and was willing to try, but when the mother showed up in labor, that option was no longer on the table.

The reality is that there is no universal agreement or standards on what necessitates a C-section or when to perform one. C-section rates vary wildly from hospital to hospital, and patient characteristics alone do not account for these swings. A national study on cesarean rates by hospital, which was published in the journal *Health Affairs* in 2015, found that C-section delivery rates at hospitals in the United States varied from 7 percent to 70. As Dr. Shah put it, "Your biggest risk factor for the most common surgery is not your preferences or your medical risks, but which door you walk through."

The decision to operate can be subjective. Different doctors, faced with the same electronic monitoring strip or dilation pattern, make different calls at different times. And there are gaps between what the evidence shows is best and what is practiced. "Because NIH and ACOG have given providers little direction on how to decide whether it is safer for a woman to give birth by a planned c-section or a planned vaginal delivery, maternity providers have been left to assess risk on their own, which, of course, is not an ideal situation," said Morris. "It allows for their own or collective biases, fears, and preferences to affect how risk is assessed and to transfer this perception to women."

Decisions may also be affected by economic and legal considerations, as well as hospital culture and care management. Low-intervention births can be time-intensive and require more hands-on engagement from staff. Continuous electronic monitoring, for instance, enables nurses and care providers to track fetal heart rates at a glance, often from a central station where they can monitor multiple patients at once. In contrast, intermittent monitoring requires a care provider to go into each patient's room and manually check and log the baby's heart rate at regular intervals. Many L&D units don't have the staff resources to do that for every patient. Epidurals can also make it easier to manage people in labor. Patients with epidurals stay in bed, while patients without epidurals tend to be loud and mobile. They may be getting in and out of a birth tub, trying out different positions, squatting on a yoga ball, grabbing on to towel racks, and possibly yelling, moaning, flailing, crying, and tossing out curse words. An unmedicated birth is rarely a quiet or calm process, and hospitals rely on stability and order to function smoothly.

Cost-efficiency is another factor. C-sections take less time than vaginal deliveries, and hospitals can bill more for them. Hospitals, like any organization, have the "rational desire" to maximize resources and maintain profitability, said Professor Elizabeth Kukura, and that rational desire can manifest as efforts to streamline labor and delivery. "Indeed, considerations of financial benefit and convenience may occur subconsciously, shifting behavior without health care providers being aware of the impact of economic concerns on their decision making," Kukura wrote in the *Georgetown Law Journal*. That might sound cynical, but there's evidence to show that differences in cesarean rates hinge on the profit orientation of the hospitals or higher reimbursement rates for cesarean births. In one study out of UCLA, researchers found that "hospitals with higher profits per cesarean procedure were associated with an increased probability of delivering newborns through cesarean birth." Following payment reform in California, the state saw a 20 percent reduction in low-risk cesarean rates.

Hospitals also have legal motivations to perform surgery: obstetricians face some of the highest malpractice insurance rates of any medical specialty, and the specialty is number one in terms of volume of claims, second in terms of rate of indemnity, and third with respect to average expenses paid out (although it has the greatest number of outlier awards). In an ACOG survey on professional liability, 63 percent of respondents reported making one or more practice changes due to the risk or fear of malpractice claims or litigation. From a legal standpoint, it's better to have done something than to have done nothing, and doctors, wanting to avoid being blamed for not doing enough, may practice what's known as defensive medicine. "Because all decisions around birth involve some risk and an opportunity for the maternity providers to make the 'wrong' decision and to be held responsible for it, choices become increasingly narrowed so that fewer and fewer 'bad decisions' can be made," said Morris.

There's no doubt that medical advances and interventions have helped to make childbirth safer, or that doctors want to deliver healthy babies to healthy mothers. But there's also no doubt that the maternal healthcare system in the US is still figuring out how to best deploy these advances and interventions in ways that maximize their benefits. There's a tendency to focus on the dangers of *not* intervening, rather than on the dangers *of* intervening. Or to focus only on the risks to the baby, as if the mother is an incidental conduit who can be patched up later. As a result, many patients find themselves surrendering to an institution, to systems, and to healthcare providers with little room left for their own needs. "Pregnancy becomes an experience in which encountering the medical system means taking your individual particular body, which has always housed your individual particular self, and sometimes, for the first time, having that body be subjected to paperwork and protocols; having it tagged, scanned, and in every way made into a datum," wrote Dr. Karkowsky in *High Risk*. "The modern medical system is like a tank: it is large, it is powerful; it can save lives. But it is also heavy and very difficult to turn around, which means that it can run right over those very same people."

According to a *Listening to Mothers* survey, 59 percent of mothers agreed with the statement "Giving birth is a process that should not be interfered with unless medically necessary," while just 16 percent disagreed. Those numbers represent a marked increase from previous surveys, which "suggests rapid changes in women's views about avoiding unnecessary intervention in a 15-year time span." Interest in so-called "natural birth" has soared, and it has even become a marker of status and privilege in some circles. Whereas in the '90s, the elite had C-sections because, as the cultural narrative would have it, they were "too posh to push" (Elizabeth Hurley, Claudia Schiffer, Victoria Beckham), celebrities now tend to emphasize their commitment to unmedicated birth (Gisele Bündchen, Jessica Alba, Gigi Hadid, Mila Kunis, and Beyoncé). The question of whether to get an epidural or go to a birth center has become more than a decision about healthcare preferences. Increasingly, and especially online, these choices have come to be treated as a referendum on someone's entire worldview, value system, and parenting philosophy. There are strong factions on either side, convinced of their own rightness and ready to judge those who choose differently. And while people who choose out-of-hospital birth have been judged for being reckless and forsaking modernity, so have people who prefer a hospital and the apparatus of modern medicine been judged as rubes who put blind faith into the System and have their birth experiences besmirched. Even the term "natural" is stigmatizing because it implies that the alternative is artificial, inauthentic, and inferior.

To Alison, it all felt so tribal. She did not want to be "run over" by the hospital birth system, but nor did she think that her approach was better than another—it was just better for her. She was confident in the decision to go to a birth center, but it was hard not to question what was, all things considered, an unconventional choice in her world. Like many first-time mothers, her inclination was to try to do the "right" thing, but she was increasingly learning that there often was no "right." The choices were complex, and part of what felt challenging was not only making them in the first place, but also justifying them to herself and to others. If (or when) things went well, anyone's hesitations about the birth center could be forgotten, but if a complication emerged, she might be blamed, or blame herself, in a way that just wouldn't happen if she was in the hospital, doing the expected thing.

During her early appointments, Jamie and the other midwives encouraged Alison to think and talk through this tangle of motivations and feelings. Those types of discussions were a cornerstone of their practice. Patients were always asked why they wanted to use a birth center in the first place and what would help them get through labor without pain medication, so the midwives could gauge where their existing knowledge and expectations about unmedicated birth lay. Jamie didn't sugarcoat, talking to Alison about how labor was relentless, painful, hard work. Once it started, it couldn't be stopped, so if someone's desire to go through it without pain medication was because they were avoiding or afraid of something (like the hospital), that may fly out the window when things got sticky. But, she said, if a patient had a positive foundation, those reasons can be used for motivation and encouragement.

The midwife also asked Alison what she was most nervous about. Alison replied that it was being "risked out" due to a medical reason and ending up in a hospital, where nothing would be familiar and where she felt like she would have to advocate for herself. Jamie assured her that because WHA had such a strong relationship with Providence, any transfers would be seamless because there was a protocol in place. Depending on the reason for the transfer, she'd enter the nurse-midwifery program at the hospital and the staff there would have her birth plan, which eased Alison's mind.

At another appointment, a midwife named Gina asked Alison what characteristics she possessed that could help her make it through an unmedicated birth. She hadn't really thought about it before, she admitted, but her mind immediately went to running. She was a distance runner who ran on the cross-country team in high school, competed in a couple half marathons, and participated in Hood to Coast, an annual long-distance relay race that stretched 199 miles from the top of Mount Hood to the Pacific Coast. She knew she had grit and endurance and the ability to push through pain. She wanted to be awake and alert when she gave birth, to experience it to the fullest.

CHAPTER 12
T'Nika

At twelve weeks, sharing the news of a baby coming and seeing the joy it brought to her whole family felt like the only antidote to the unrelenting medical ailments T'Nika continued to endure. The constipation had gone away, but she was still dealing with some morning sickness. From her history of GI problems, T'Nika had developed an arsenal of tricks to manage nausea, but morning sickness was a completely different beast. She had expected to throw up. What she hadn't expected was a strange salivating sensation, in which spit welled up in her mouth and tingled at the back of her jaw. It would have been annoying under any circumstances but was particularly difficult to manage while at work. Because of Covid-19 protocols, T'Nika had to wear an N95 mask at all times during her twelve-and-a-half-hour shifts. Whenever she needed to spit, she had to completely exit the facility, speed-walk down the hallway to the building's back door, and spend five to ten minutes in the parking lot, hocking into the night. She'd also noticed that mild physical exertion, like walking down a hallway, elevated her heart rate in a way it hadn't before she was pregnant. Between holding water and spitting, T'Nika joked that she felt like a camel.

Fetuses do not grow in isolation in the uterus. Pregnant people's entire bodies, from their hair to their toes, are affected in bizarre and unanticipated ways. They can become unwieldy, unrecognizable, and ungovernable. Certain symptoms or ailments, like nausea, heartburn, and back pain, are pretty much universal. Others are a mystery grab bag. Feet grow. Hair sprouts. Pelvic bones move. Hemorrhoids swell. Discharge discharges. There's no way to know ahead of time how someone's body will react to the towering swings in hormone levels, to the growth of a new organ, to carrying a baby for the better part of a year until it weighs as much as a bowling ball. And other than whispers from people who have been pregnant before, much of these afflictions and indignities remain unspoken. "Pregnancy makes weird vaginal secretions," wrote Lyz Lenz in her book *Belabored*. "A primordial soup of crotch slime—dissected and analyzed only on the deepest, darkest pregnancy message boards, where women post pictures and chime in on the 'normal or not normal' debate. Doctors don't tell you about the crotch slime. Nor do pregnancy books, I never read about it in even the most candid advice columns."

Certainly, some people glide through their pregnancies with minimal pain and suffering, but to become pregnant is to expose oneself to an array of possible effects that there's no way to anticipate. To T'Nika, being pregnant felt a little like her body was betraying her. The sci-fi and fantasy stories she loved seemed to best capture what it felt like to navigate this experience—unsettling, strange, parasitic, and alien. And, like many women, she found herself in the frustrating position of having to reconcile this new body with her existing life and obligations.

As a nurse, T'Nika had to be on her feet for over twelve hours without much time to rest or eat or drink water. She had always had abundant energy and a strong work ethic and could usually last an entire shift without going to the bathroom. A nocturnal schedule had suited her since nursing school; she could function on only five hours of sleep if needed and rarely had a problem staying awake. She'd drink yerba maté at midnight and go into "party mode." Between 2:00 a.m. and 4:00 a.m. was when exhaustion crept in, but once T'Nika made it through those vampire hours, the rest of the shift was easy. And when she got home, she and Daniel would often go on walks or runs; one summer, she even took a part-time job lifeguarding during the day. Sometimes she used the downtime to relax and watch TV, talk to her mom on the phone, hang out with her cats, read, practice the viola, or play video games. The key, she found, was to control her nap schedule—not too many naps, but not too few either. Now that she was pregnant, though, she couldn't sustain the same level of energy or push her body in the same way.

One day after work, T'Nika noticed that her pee was cloudy and concentrated, which made her worry that she had a urinary tract infection. So, she did what many pregnant women do before seeking medical help and consulted the internet. She was already a regular visitor to the NCBI website, the National Center for Biotechnology Information, run by the National Institutes of Health (NIH), and enjoyed perusing medical journals and reading academic papers and articles whenever there was a question about pregnancy or a medical condition she encountered at work or on TV. Now, she read that UTIs could be more common during pregnancy because of hormonal changes and that symptoms didn't necessarily show up in the same way as "regular" UTIs.

She wondered if maybe an infection was the reason why her heart rate sometimes felt faster than normal. She texted Marilyn to ask, hoping that if there was a problem, there might be a non-pharmacological solution. When seeing the sequence of GI specialists years before, she had felt like prescription after prescription was written at every turn, creating new problems that then had to be treated with more prescriptions, instead of taking the time to figure out the root cause. As a nurse, T'Nika believed in the importance of evidence-based practices and the value of allopathic medicine, but she valued naturopathic and holistic approaches as well. It was another reason she'd been drawn to using midwives. Because midwifery is oriented around the idea that birth is not, or at least not exclusively, a medical event, there is a current of skepticism regarding Western medicine's perceived tendency to over-pathologize and prescribe. There is also overlap between communities who embrace out-of-hospital birth and those who avoid the medical system in other ways, such as by forgoing vaccinations. Plant medicine is a core part of many birthing traditions, and midwives often employ homeopathic, herbal, or folk remedies—ranging from raspberry-leaf tea and dates to shorten labor to "midwives brew," a concoction to kick-start contractions. Some of the Andaluz midwives incorporated essential oils into their practices, and T'Nika enjoyed learning about those techniques and trying them out, such as Marilyn's suggestion she try peppermint oil on the back of her neck when she got a headache.

With the UTI query, Marilyn responded quickly, recommending a supplement called D-mannose and reminding her to stay hydrated. T'Nika bought a big new water bottle and made more of an effort to drink water consistently and go to the bathroom at work. Those measures were simple, but they had a tangible impact. She was figuring things out as she went, and for better or for worse, every day brought something new.

CHAPTER 13
Jillian

For her own prenatals, Jillian always scheduled herself for the last appointment of the day. That way, she didn't need someone to cover the front desk, and Chad, who was a manager at a cabinet manufacturing company, had the time to drive up after work. Chad enjoyed the appointments as an opportunity to participate and ask questions, and the Andaluz midwives enjoyed becoming better acquainted with their colleagues' spouse. "I've primed my husband for years about all this stuff," Jillian told them. "He's probably overly educated about birth."

Their love story had begun like so many these days: on Tinder. At the time, Jillian had been living in Portland for six months and wasn't looking for a serious relationship, but all her friends were aspiring midwives and every time they hung out, all they talked about was midwifery. She wanted to dress up, go to dinner, and talk about anything other than contractions and mucus plugs. She figured she'd go on a few casual dates, engage in some lighthearted chitchat, and, at the very least, make friends who were not involved in birth work. Then, in November 2015, she'd met Chad at a sushi restaurant called Daruma. He had kind brown eyes and a red-tinged beard. He made her laugh, and he was courteous, smart, and interesting. He told her how he bow-hunted for elk, had previously worked as a wilderness firefighter, and cultivated bonsai trees. He also drove a 1967 blue Ford Mustang, which he'd named Sybil. Jillian had actually noticed the car parked outside when she approached the restaurant, and when Chad walked up to it after dinner and opened the door, she knew she was done for. After the date, she thought, *I'm totally going to marry this guy.*

A few dates later, a random stranger told Chad and Jillian they were "twin souls." When Jillian's mom, Joyce, flew out from Missouri for a visit, Chad said he wanted to meet her, even though they hadn't been dating long, and insisted on paying for the meal. Joyce said he was a keeper. Four years later, Chad proposed to Jillian on a drive to the Dee Wright Observatory, an open stone structure amid a lava flow with epic views of the Cascade Mountains, with a ring containing a stone that had belonged to his grandmother.

Now, well into her second trimester, it was a little surreal to have Chad with her at Andaluz, talking to the midwives about symptoms and birth plans. Because of her midwifery background, Jillian didn't have many questions to ask her midwives at these appointments. She went through the standard list of medical updates with them—Was she having headaches? Nausea? Unusual swelling?—and did the requisite tests, checks, and scans—blood pressure, pulse, weight—but otherwise the hours were filled with casual conversation and chat from around the birth center. Eventually, she came to think of the sessions as less of a physical check-in and more of an opportunity to reflect on where she was in her pregnancy and how much further she had to go.

Those hours put everyone, especially Marilyn, in a good mood. Jillian's birth might be one of the last ones she attended before retirement. The prospect that one of her final births would be with someone she helped train—someone who was helping to carry on the legacy of midwifery—seemed like a meaningful note to end her career on. A passing of the torch.

Jillian still wasn't sure who she wanted to be her primary midwife:

Marilyn or Carrie. She had attended births with them both and had a good sense of what to expect from each. Marilyn was more of the traditional midwife archetype, oozing maternal vibes and generally hands-off unless you needed her. She had a well-stocked supply of midwifery stories, and for every question or concern a client raised, there was an anecdote to share, connecting with them by talking about subjects other than just pregnancy and babies. During appointments, she was known for digressions about pets, favorite spots to swim in the river, tattoos, which flowers were blooming, or new cars. She also loved when family members came to appointments—husbands, kids, moms, sisters—so she could draw them into the conversation. Carrie, who was in her early forties, dressed like the cool front woman in a rock band and was known to refer to the uterus as the "yute." She had given birth to her first baby at nineteen while living in a converted schoolbus, an experience that had inspired her to go to midwifery school. She matriculated at Birthingway in 2001, started working at Andaluz as a student that same year, and had been there ever since. She was straightforward, confident, and down-to-business with her clients, offering encouragement but also tough love to get the job done. Jillian thought of her as having more of a badass, empowering vibe.

Location was another factor to consider. Jillian was planning to give birth at her home in Carlton, which was about a one-hour-and-fifteen-minute drive away from Portland, where Carrie lived, and farther from Marilyn's home in Washington. Both drives were even longer with traffic. Jillian figured that she still had time before she had to decide. The decision might end up being made for her anyway—if one of the midwives was called to another birth first, she'd have to go with whoever was free.

In the meantime, the most pressing milestone she faced was the twenty-week anatomy scan. At that point, the fetus would be roughly the size of a bell pepper, and an advanced ultrasound would be used to make sure everything was developing normally—the organs, the curve of the spine, the face, and the limbs. It also was an opportunity to learn the sex of the baby, if parents wanted that information. Early on, Jillian and Chad had agreed to wait. People had already asked her if she had a sense of the sex, but she really didn't, and that was okay with her. She didn't want a preconceived notion about who the baby was or who they would be as a person until after they were born. If it was a boy, they wanted to name him Sydney, after Chad's grandfather. She also liked the name Silas, after the third baby she'd caught as a student (for whatever reason, the name had stuck with her). Those were the only two boy names they could agree on, as Chad disliked Jillian's suggestions—Wyatt, Forest, or Everett—and Jillian disliked Chad's favorite—Ripley—right back. If it was a girl, they thought maybe they'd name her Claire or Lola, after one of Jillian's grandmothers. Regardless of the sex, they knew the baby's middle name would be Stamper, which came from Chad's favorite book, *Sometimes a Great Notion* by Ken Kesey.

The anatomy scan can be simultaneously thrilling and terrifying—thrilling because it's the clearest, most vivid image that most parents-to-be have seen at that point in the pregnancy, and the fetus looks like an actual human baby; terrifying because what if something is wrong? Fetal abnormalities are sometimes presented as statistics, and parents must decide what to do with that information. Depending on what they learn, more advanced testing might be requested or difficult conversations may have to begin about whether to end the pregnancy. With drastic rollbacks and limits to abortion rights, there are even more barriers to accessing this type of necessary medical care, barriers that put people's lives at risk and put them through undue expense, stress, and trauma.

Luckily, the twenty-week anatomy scan went smoothly for Jillian, and it was news that she did not take for granted. The only hitch was that her placenta was anterior, meaning it had implanted on the front of the uterus instead of on the back. It wasn't a problem, but it could make it more difficult to capture an image of the baby and for Jillian to feel movement.

By this point in her pregnancy, Jillian was no longer plagued by nausea, but exhaustion lingered. On walks with the dogs—she and Chad had added a lovable cattle dog named Paisley to their family—Jillian had realized she was moving slower and would lose her breath more quickly. If she sat for a long period of time, or in a chair or stool without back support, her back ached. Getting up and down frequently throughout the day—letting clients into the birth center, refilling her water bottle, walking up and down stairs to restock supplies, popping into appointments to lend a hand—was becoming more and more of a challenge, as was sitting on her living room couch at home, which was low and squishy and had started to strain Jillian's back, making her feel like an upside-down turtle. She had reached the point where she moved through the world like a pregnant person.

It would be strange for her family members to see her this way when she went back to Missouri for her baby shower. It would be the first time she was visiting her family since becoming pregnant, and unlike Chad or Alysa or her coworkers at Andaluz, they hadn't seen her belly growing gradually. Chad wasn't joining her on the trip because he couldn't take time off work, so Jillian regaled him and Marilyn with the plans for the shower as her prenatal appointment hour drew to a close.

Jillian's baby shower was held in a neighborhood clubhouse in St. Louis and featured an outdoorsy theme (in line with a hiking boot baby announcement she had made), complete with buffalo plaid décor and woodland creature cutouts. Because of Covid, in-person attendance was limited to about ten guests, and others joined remotely on Zoom. They ate, played a few games, and Jillian opened baby presents. Jillian enjoyed being surrounded by people who had known her since she was a child, and something about attending her own baby shower made the gravity of the situation sink in. She didn't have much time left before her baby would be born.

"I can't believe I'm going to be someone's mother," Jillian said to her own mother as the party died down and they began cleaning things up. Joyce chuckled and told her she could relate. After giving birth to Jillian, one of her first thoughts had been *Holy shit. I'm somebody's mother and they expect me to know all these things!* She told Jillian it was a near guarantee she would freak out—no one quite knows what they are doing at first—but then she would figure it out.

After the weekend was over, Joyce drove Jillian to the airport for her flight back to Oregon. Jillian had flown in and out of Lambert countless times throughout her life, but as she hugged her mother goodbye at the security line and made her way to the gate, her mood shifted. For the first time in days, she was alone. She had said goodbye to her family and was still hours away from seeing Chad. It hit her that she was on her own and her time was hers. She could grab a bite to eat, read a magazine, listen to music. Nobody needed her attention in that moment. No one was depending on her. She would never be so unencumbered again. The liminal space of the airport seemed to mirror the liminal space she was in with pregnancy—not yet a mother, but not a person of unfettered childlessness either.

She was able to keep it together as she boarded the plane and found her seat, but as soon as the plane taxied toward the runway, Jillian burst into tears. Flying away from the city, the landscape, and the airport filled with nostalgia from her childhood felt too big to handle, more so than when she'd departed for midwifery school. This was more final. This was irreparable change.

Jillian's dad had given her a stuffed fox as a gift for the baby, and she hadn't had room to pack it in her carry-on bag, so she held it at her seat. Jillian had the whole row to herself and let herself bawl as she hugged the toy, like a kid clutching her "stuffie" for comfort. She felt pummeled by the enormity of what lay before her. It was overwhelming, but in a good way. The next time she saw this scenery—the next time she saw her family—everything would be different. Her mother wouldn't just be her mother; she'd be a grandmother. And Jillian wouldn't just be a daughter. There would never be another trip home to visit where it was just her. She'd be a mother herself.

CHAPTER 14
T'Nika

For a brief and glorious moment in the fall, T'Nika started to feel better. It was like the sun breaking through the clouds. The constipation and migraines had improved, and she had finally reined in her nausea. She had energy again. Even her coworkers had noticed a lift in her mood, and some noted it was the first time they'd seen her smile in weeks. Things were looking up as the second trimester began.

Unfortunately, it didn't last for long.

In October, she experienced intense ligament pain that caused every movement to hurt. The pain had been building gradually, localized in her hip and groin region, compounded by her exhausting work shifts. Before long, her whole body started to ache and simply getting out of bed was uncomfortable. T'Nika bought a belly band and tried wearing it for extra support (even though she didn't quite have a belly yet), but it didn't make a difference.

The new pain also made it harder—harder than it already was—for T'Nika to exercise. She knew it was good for her health, but pregnancy fundamentally changed how it felt to be in her body. If she overexerted herself, she felt a shooting pain in her cervix. Her pubic bone hurt. She was still getting frequent headaches and taking Tylenol three to four times a week. Sometimes in the mornings, her vision pulsed. She had stopped going for runs early in her first trimester because she often felt too tired, but she tried to walk six thousand steps a day when she could, tracking her movements on the smart watch she got for her birthday. But now, even the lowest-impact walks caused her heart to pound—usually at 160 beats per minute, which seemed high to her. Her blood pressure was also low—in the 80s over 50. One day, she went to a water aerobics class, figuring it would be difficult to get too worked up. As she stepped into the water, she realized she was the only participant there under retirement age. She tried to hold her own as the lone youthful person in the pool, but it was a struggle.

Determined to find answers, she returned to the internet, digging around in medical literature for more information about exercising while pregnant. She found that for the most part, elevated pulse or heart rate wasn't a problem unless it surpassed a certain threshold—if she could still catch her breath and talk through what she was doing, the activity was probably okay. It was sometimes hard to distinguish, though, what was cause for alarm and what wasn't. T'Nika had always thought she wanted four or maybe even five kids, like her own family and Daniel's. But as she arrived at Andaluz for her twenty-week anatomy scan, she wasn't sure how many more times she could put herself through this experience.

The appointment was set for the Brisa room with Dr. Seth, a naturopathic doctor who performed ultrasounds at Andaluz every week. The room was narrow and dark, with the curtains drawn, which made it easier to see what was showing up on the screen. T'Nika lay on the bed while Daniel took a seat on the other side of the room, until she called him over to sit closer and hold her hand during the scan. She had looked forward to this moment since the earliest days, eager to see how the amorphous goo and spawning clump of cells were taking shape into recognizable body parts of a baby. Her baby.

As Dr. Seth got his bearings with the scan, T'Nika's excitement grew. She could see the outlines of a humanlike shape on-screen. Head. Nose.

Arms. Legs. *There it is,* she thought. She caught a glimpse of what were maybe the baby's genitals—*I feel like that's a vagina,* she thought—but she wasn't sure. Meanwhile, Dr. Seth maneuvered the probe and pointed out body parts.

"Everything looks good," he said.

T'Nika paused, waiting for him to continue. She was hoping for insight beyond "good." She was pleased to learn the baby was healthy but craved more information because she still had the sense that anything could happen, that there was never really a point of being "in the clear." She had held her breath at each viability checkpoint, mentally ticking them off like mile markers on a highway. It was a positive, anticipatory kind of nervousness, and now that she was about halfway through her pregnancy, she wanted to linger in these moments and savor them. She wanted details. She prompted Dr. Seth to say more, asking him questions that required more clinical and scientific answers.

One of T'Nika's coworkers had a baby with a heart condition—was that possible here?

No, he answered, explaining more about the condition and showing her on the screen how he could tell that all was well.

And the umbilical cord—it had three blood vessels, right? One vein and two arteries?

Yes, he said, pointing out how the oxygen was moving in and out.

Then the doctor asked if they wanted to learn the sex of the baby.

T'Nika had never had any kind of intuition about whether she was having a boy or a girl, other than the brief glimmer at the beginning of the scan, but she and Daniel had agreed ahead of time that they wanted to know.

"It's a girl."

"Yaaay," T'Nika said, unsurprised and yet amazed all at once.

She and Daniel were delighted to be having a girl. They'd had a name picked out since before they were married, and T'Nika, a firstborn daughter, would now have a firstborn daughter herself. She looked down at her stomach, and then back at the ultrasound screen, and smiled.

Pregnancy can entail swings between extremes. One moment, feeling peaceful, strong, powerful, glowing—a creator of life—and the next feeling like crap, like a whale decaying on a seashore. The wonderment of growing a baby wasn't lost on T'Nika, but as the final weeks of the year approached, she wished she felt a bit more of the glow and less of the cetacean. It was weird to feel so horrible, and yet have nothing really be wrong.

The midwives at Andaluz had screened her carefully for complications and risk factors, and no red flags had popped up. T'Nika trusted them, but aside from some peace of mind, their reassurances didn't make her suffering easier to bear. The muscular and round ligament pain lingered on and on, at one point localizing in her left flank. She worried that something was wrong with her kidneys, but a test confirmed that there wasn't. An appointment with a chiropractor helped reduce the ligament pain and a visit to the optometrist improved her vision problems, and between those fixes, along with daily stretching and wearing her glasses more often, her migraines improved. But it was always push and pull with progress, like trying to keep an invasive plant at bay.

Starting in October, she began to experience unusual vaginal symptoms—things got itchy and burned down there. She managed the situation by changing her soap, keeping her nether regions dry, and wearing pads, but those measures went only so far. At work shifts, she had to change the pad halfway through. The issue remained through December, when at twenty-five weeks, T'Nika had her first appointment with a midwife named Megan. Megan had worked at Andaluz since 2013 and was slim and athletic, with long brown hair—she reminded T'Nika of a younger Marilyn. She told Megan that her labia were swollen and painful and she was experiencing burning and itching and weird discharge; the only time she felt any relief was in the shower. Megan ran a yeast infection culture, which turned up negative, and suggested herbal remedies.

By Christmas, it got so bad that T'Nika went to urgent care. Again, every test showed up negative, and so the doctor suggested she go to a primary care doctor to check for hormonal issues. Her PCP ordered another panel for a yeast infection, checked her hormones, and tested for bacterial vaginosis and trichomoniasis and STIs and other common vaginal infections. All negative. At that point, her doctor advised a visit to an OB/GYN specialist, and T'Nika made an appointment for January at a hospital practice. A nurse-midwife ran various panels, and once again, all the tests came back negative. The last thing the midwife could think to test for, she told T'Nika, was an autoimmune condition called lichen sclerosus (LS), which could mimic symptoms of yeast infections.

If LS goes untreated, it can cause the genital skin tissue to fuse. The only catch was that testing for the condition entailed a skin biopsy, which the midwife said was not advisable to do on pregnant women because the biopsy would take time to heal and could complicate a vaginal delivery. She advised T'Nika to have the skin biopsied after she gave birth, when the tissue down in her vaginal area would already be in a state of disarray. In the meantime, she could prescribe an antifungal steroid cream to use twice a day. T'Nika understood the recommendation but also found it frustrating. She was tired of living without concrete answers, shuttling between doctor's offices, and feeling like a medical mystery. She was also nervous about using the cream too frequently—steroids cause skin to thin, which prompted a new concern that if the skin thinned too much, she would be more likely to tear during labor.

Fortunately, the cream worked, and after some use, T'Nika was able to reduce the application to once or twice a week, and then only when she had a flare-up. She was grateful that the hospital had remedied the situation, but the experience only further solidified her commitment to the birth center. The medical problem had required a medical solution, but that wasn't how she was wanted to think about her birth. She preferred drinking tea on a queen-size bed to traversing the labyrinth of hospital parking garages and hallways and units and elevators, filling out stacks of forms, and waiting in exam rooms. It gave her flashbacks to all the time spent in hospitals in Boston, and all she could think as she faced it was: *Take me back to my birth center.*

In January, T'Nika was scheduled to take a gestational diabetes test, which pregnant people are screened for around twenty-eight weeks. Given all her ailments, T'Nika doubted that the test would go her way. *Screw it,* she thought. *I might as well enjoy myself when I don't yet know.* She baked up a storm during the holiday season, eating all the rich food and desserts she wanted. In what felt like a miraculous turn of events, she tested negative, which was one less thing to worry about. But as T'Nika entered the final weeks of her second trimester, she started to worry more about preeclampsia, a blood pressure condition that usually begins after twenty weeks and is a serious, even fatal, complication of pregnancy. Headaches—which had improved for T'Nika, but hadn't gone away entirely—can be a sign of the disorder. That made her nervous, particularly as an African American woman.

Preeclampsia is one of the top three pregnancy complications that lead to maternal mortality; rates of it among Black women run 60 percent higher than white women, and they are more likely to experience poor outcomes from the condition. Among women diagnosed with pregnancy-induced hypertension (eclampsia and preeclampsia), African American and Latina women were 9.9 and 7.9 times, respectively, more likely to die than white women with the same complications. T'Nika knew that to mitigate the risks, she should strive to keep her stress and tension levels down, as those could contribute to high blood pressure. It wasn't always easy though. Even when everything was going well—she had a stable income and comfortable home; she and Daniel were happy together, as they had always been; they had a strong support network and close relationships with family and friends—there was the underlying racial stress of being Black in America.

That summer, George Floyd's and Breonna Taylor's names had dominated headlines after they were murdered by police. The Covid-19 pandemic was disproportionately decimating Black and brown communities, and a band of marauders had recently stormed the US Capitol in an effort to overturn the 2020 election. Portland had been roiled by ongoing protests against police violence and white supremacy, and counterprotests were led by caravans of far-right extremists who rolled into town in pickup trucks waving American flags and guns. The city felt like a tinderbox. (Literally: there were also the widespread wildfires.) And through it all, there were the moments of everyday racism that sometimes seemed inescapable—like a neighbor who had yelled at T'Nika while she was checking her mailbox.

She wasn't alone. Studies have shown that Black and Native women report the highest number of stressful life events in the year before birth. "It's chronic stress that just happens all the time—there is never a period where there's rest from it, it's everywhere, it's in the air, it's just affecting everything," said Dr. Fleda Mask Jackson, an Atlanta researcher and member of the Black Mamas Matter Alliance. Anytime a person has to work harder for equal pay and respect, anytime they are mistreated by a boss or followed around a store while shopping or see another story in the news about police violence, the body has a physical reaction. As the journalist Linda Villarosa wrote in a *New York Times* article about Black maternal and infant mortality: "For black women in America, an inescapable atmosphere of societal and systemic racism can create a kind of toxic physiological stress, resulting in conditions—including hypertension and pre-eclampsia—that lead directly to higher rates of infant and maternal death. And that societal racism is further expressed in a pervasive, longstanding racial bias in health care—including the dismissal of legitimate concerns and symptoms—that can help explain poor birth outcomes even in the case of black women with the most advantages."

The physiological term for the impact of this chronic stress is "weathering," coined by a professor and researcher named Arline Geronimus at the University of Michigan. When under stress, a person's brain releases hormones including adrenaline and cortisol, which impact other bodily functions, like increasing blood pressure and quickening the heart rate. An allostatic load score aims to measure the impact of stress through "markers of physiological dysregulation"—the cumulative wear and tear on the body's systems. This "weathering" is a form of premature aging and increases the likelihood of developing chronic health conditions. Even when controlling for income and education, African American women have the highest allostatic load scores.

All of this, T'Nika knew, could have an impact on her birth experience. She had read extensively about racial inequities in health outcomes and knew that those inequities were driven by racism. That all-too-present understanding was why she had wanted to become a nurse in the first place, and why, as a pregnant patient, she felt safest at a birth center. Like Alison, she was glad to have access to higher-level medical care should she need it but hoped that she wouldn't. She didn't want to become another statistic.

The risk of dying from childbirth in the US is relatively low—23.8 deaths per 100,000 births—but the rate is one of the highest among high-income countries. Seven hundred to nine hundred people die in childbirth each year and many more almost die. Between 2003 and 2013, the US was one of eight countries in the world where maternal mortality was rising, a cohort that included Afghanistan and South Sudan.

Although most examples of maternal death in popular culture tend to occur during delivery, in reality half of the fatalities occur in the days and weeks after. In fact, a maternal or pregnancy-related death can happen anytime during pregnancy up until one year postbirth. Approximately one-third of maternal deaths happen during pregnancy, and 17 percent occur on the day of delivery. 52 percent of deaths occur after delivery or postpartum: 19 percent of all maternal deaths occur between one and six days postpartum; 21 percent of all maternal deaths are between one and six weeks postpartum; and 12 percent of all maternal deaths take place during the remaining portion of the year. For every maternal death, seventy to eighty cases of severe maternal illness occur. Sixty thousand mothers experience "severe maternal morbidity," or serious complications from pregnancy and delivery, in the US each year. The CDC estimates that rates of severe maternal morbidity are 3.2 times higher among Black mothers than white mothers and 2.3 higher among American Indian and Alaska Native mothers.

In 2014, WHO, UNICEF, UNFPA, the World Bank, and the UN Population Division jointly issued a report on maternal mortality around the world. The report found that between 1990 and 2013, the maternal mortality ratio (MMR) in the US had increased by 136 percent—from twelve to twenty-eight maternal deaths for every one hundred thousand live births, nearly double the rate of Saudi Arabia and more than triple that of the United Kingdom. Out of all the countries surveyed, the US had the highest annual increase in maternal deaths. In WHO rankings, the US has fallen to fifty-fifth in the world. As the Executive Director of Merck for Mothers put it: an American woman in 1990 had a better chance of surviving childbirth than her own daughter does today.*

These statistics are heavily racialized. Although the MMR doesn't compare favorably across the board—even for white women in the US, maternal mortality ratios are higher than for women in twenty-four other industrialized countries—Black women are 243 percent more likely to die from pregnancy or childbirth-related causes, according to the CDC. Black women face similar rates of death to those of women delivering in Mexico and Uzbekistan, with rates of forty per one hundred thousand. In certain parts of the country, the rates are even higher. In Chicksaw County, Mississippi, for instance, the MMR for women of color (595 per 100,000 live births) is higher than rates in some countries in sub-Saharan Africa, including Kenya (400) and Rwanda (320).

The disparities are even greater for high-risk pregnancies, from which Black women are 5.6 times more likely to die than white women.

---

* There is also a steep financial toll. According to an investigation published by the Commonwealth Fund, the medical and nonmedical impact of morbidity conditions, on both mother and child, for all children born in 2019 through their fifth birthdays, is estimated to be at least $32.3 billion.

Morbidity has also soared, rising nearly 200 percent from 1993 to 2014, the last year for which statistics are available. A portion of these increases is attributable to changes in data collection and measurement, but not all.

The fact that the US has a perinatal morbidity and mortality problem, and that the severity of the problem is driven by racial inequities, is not new. In the twentieth-century interwar period, various governmental bodies conducted research and published reports on maternal and infant mortality, finding that rates in the US were both higher than they should be and compared unfavorably to peer countries in Europe. Those reports led to changes, such as standardizing medical education and the implementation of antiseptic protocols, which caused the mortality rates to drop. However, the rate of decline was much faster among white women than Black women, and though the overall rates went down, the gaps in outcomes persisted. The disparities have not budged. In fact, by some measurements and metrics, the chasm has gotten worse.

Take preterm birth and infant mortality. Black and American Indian and Alaska Native women are 60 percent more likely to give birth preterm than white women, according to March of Dimes, and each year in the US, approximately twenty-one thousand infants die before their first birthday. Black infants in America are more than twice as likely to die as white infants, at a rate of 11.3 per 1,000 as compared to 4.9 per 1,000, respectively. As Villarosa noted in the *Times*, the disparity is actually wider than it was in 1850—fifteen years before the end of slavery.

The severity, stickiness, and scope of these problems lead to the question of *why*. An oft-cited explanation used to be that the childbearing population got "older, fatter, and sicker," but other countries that have seen similar rises in those risk factors have not seen their maternal mortality rates increase. "It is hard to imagine some other scenario in which patients are dying in hospitals from complications of routine procedures—appendectomies, say—and instead of studying the care the patients received leading up to their deaths, review panels focus on the patients' lifestyles in the year before their procedure," said the writer Kim Brooks in an op-ed.

Another common yet unsatisfactory explanation is that it's not racial inequities, but socioeconomic ones, that are the root of the problem. Black Americans are two and a half times more likely than white Americans to live below the poverty line. Despite high workforce participation rates, Black women are paid 63 percent of what white men are paid. The median white household had ten times the wealth of the median Black household—$171,000 as opposed to $17,150—in 2016. Due to histories of redlining, gentrification, and white flight, as well as pay disparities, Black women are more likely to live in low-income areas. Women living in low-income areas across the US are twice as likely to suffer a maternal death as women in high-income areas. The more segregated the city, the greater the birth disparities.

This is, in part, due to the greater incidence of environmental stressors in historically underserved communities. According to the Maternal Vulnerability Index, which looks at forty-three indicators associated with maternal health outcomes, Black women and American Indian and Alaska Native women are 1.6 times and 2.6 times, respectively, as likely as white women to live under conditions that create problems during and after pregnancy.

Black women are more likely to live in housing facilities that do not meet health safety regulations; Black communities at large are faced with air pollution levels 1.54 times higher than that of the average American population; and as showcased in Flint and Newark, unsafe drinking water is a prevalent problem. Black women are also more likely to live in "heat islands," areas that, due to denser buildings and less greenery, experience higher temperatures. (Heat has been linked with an increased chance of developing preeclampsia and a higher risk of preterm delivery.) Food deserts, areas in which affordable, fresh, healthy foods are hard to come by, are an issue as well. These externalities contribute to higher rates of chronic health conditions like diabetes, hypertension, and cardiovascular disease, which can lead to pregnancy complications and make giving birth more dangerous.

The higher likelihood of environmental stressors is met by a lower likelihood of access to quality health coverage. Black women are more likely to be uninsured than white women, which can make it prohibitively expensive to access preventative care and treatment, and they are less likely to go into pregnancy in good health. In addition to gaps in insurance coverage, prenatal care may also be delayed due to mistrust of the medical profession and concerns about discrimination, as well as logistical barriers, like difficulty taking time off work, securing childcare, and finding transportation to appointments. Native American and Alaska Native women are 3.6 times, African American women 2.6 times, and Latina women 2.5 times as likely as white women to receive late or no prenatal care.

And then there's the quality of hospitals where Black women are most likely to give birth. Three-quarters of Black mothers deliver in about a quarter of the country's hospitals. These "Black-serving hospitals"—healthcare institutions in predominantly Black communities or that predominately serve Black folks—are disadvantaged by historical segregation and generally have fewer resources. In the *Birth Settings in America* report, the National Academies of Sciences, Engineering, and Medicine researchers found that the reality of facility-based care for Black women includes lack of access, segregated wards, denial or delays in receiving care, biased treatment, and substandard care. This means that the women most likely to have serious complications like preeclampsia, hemorrhage, infection, and embolism are accessing care in the places least equipped to deftly manage them. In an analysis of two years of hospital inpatient discharge data from New York, Illinois, and Florida, *ProPublica* found that women who hemorrhage at disproportionately Black-serving hospitals are far more likely to wind up with severe complications, like a hysterectomy. The pattern persisted when splicing the data for only the healthiest women and for white women at those hospitals. "While a handful of low black-serving hospitals had high complication rates, our analysis found that, on average, outcomes at hospitals that served a high number of black patients were far worse," the article said.

In research conducted of New York City hospitals, Dr. Elizabeth

Howell, chair of obstetrics and gynecology at Penn Medicine, found that Black mothers were twice as likely to suffer harm when delivering babies as white mothers, even after adjusting for patients' differing characteristics, suggesting that some of the outcome disparities may be due to hospital quality. In a separate study, she estimated that the rate of harm for Black women would fall by nearly 50 percent if they gave birth at the same hospitals as white women.

In another survey from New York City, women of color reported receiving poor communication, dehumanizing care, verbal abuse, abandonment, and rough treatment. Many patients felt ignored by providers and devalued during their maternity care. In California, the people interviewed by the collective Black Women Birthing Justice spoke of birth as a battle: "This study reveals that the relationships between pregnant black individuals and their health-care providers are often a source of stress, anger and distress during a vulnerable time," the researchers wrote in a book about their findings. These dynamics can make it more difficult for Black women to advocate for themselves, or for their support network to advocate for them, as their attempts at self-advocacy may be interpreted as argumentative, aggressive, and a threat to the order of the hospital. Sometimes, the mistreatment and bias are explicit, but they can also manifest in more subtle ways that are harder to pinpoint but are equally pernicious and detrimental. "If doctors and nurses give dismissive looks or make a woman feel unworthy, that also constitutes a repertoire of racism," wrote the anthropologist Dr. Dána-Ain Davis. "It may involve stereotyping a patient, which can lead to a misdiagnosis, or setting aside a woman's concerns about the fears she has for her health, her newborn's health, or the treatment of her partner."

Higher socioeconomic status, safer neighborhoods, more education, or even better hospitals do not mitigate the negative impact of racism and discrimination. A Black woman with a college degree is 60 percent more likely to have a maternal death than a white woman with less than a high school education. Even Black women with all the resources in the world—celebrities like Beyoncé and Serena Williams—are not protected.

In 2018, Beyoncé wrote an article for *Vogue* detailing her experience developing preeclampsia while giving birth to her twins, which resulted in bed rest, an emergency C-section, and a NICU stay for the children. That same year, Serena Williams shared her birth story about how she almost died after giving birth to her daughter, Olympia, who was also born by emergency C-section; Williams developed a life-threatening pulmonary embolism after surgery, and when she explained the symptoms to the doctors, she was dismissed as being confused because of her medication. And then there's the story of Shalon Irving, a thirty-six-year-old epidemiologist at the CDC whose actual job was working to eradicate disparities in health access and outcomes. As detailed in a *ProPublica* investigation, Irving had two master's degrees and a dual-subject PhD, "gold-plated insurance," and a "rock-solid support system." Those protective factors did not ensure that she would survive childbirth, and she died after giving birth to her daughter, Soleil.

In short, it's not race that's the risk factor—it's the experience of being Black in America. "There is no magic Black gene for increased risk," Dr. Joia Crear-Perry, the founder and president of the National Birth Equity Collaborative, said in an interview with *Reveal News*. "That's due to the impact of racism on my body, not that I was innately, inherently broken. . . . The thing that harms Black people is not our mere existence. It's all the policies and cultural beliefs that we are broken that harm Black people and our health."

The other demographic group with the starkest racial inequities in pregnancy and birth outcomes are Native and Indigenous women.* American Indian and Alaska Native (AIAN) women experience higher rates of ma-

---

* Despite also experiencing systemic obstacles to accessing healthcare, Latina women and infants fare similarly to their white counterparts on many measures of maternal and infant health. (Data is limited for Asian and Pacific Islander women because maternal and infant outcomes vary significantly among ethnic groups.)

ternal mortality and severe morbidity, including a preterm labor rate and an obstetrical hemorrhage rate that is more than twice that of white women. They are 1.4 times more likely than white women to be diagnosed with gestational hypertension and preeclampsia and 1.5 to 2 times more likely to be diagnosed with gestational diabetes. "Adverse maternal health outcomes are, in part, due to the historical trauma of systemic racism, colonization, genocide, forced migration, reproductive coercion and cultural erasure," said a report from the National Partnership for Women & Families.

As with Black women, these disparities are the result of unequal social conditions, medical racism, and the effects of weathering due to chronic stress and trauma. Native women are more likely than white women to experience high levels of poverty, live in hazardous conditions, experience food insecurity, and lack access to health insurance, as well as to experience sexual and interpersonal violence. They are three to four times more likely than white women to begin prenatal care in the third trimester and receive a lower quality of care than white women—care that is devoid of traditional cultural birth practices found in Indigenous communities.

Furthermore, the history of forced sterilization and infant separation policies has led to distrust between AIAN women and mainstream healthcare providers. Native American mothers are more likely than white women to experience discrimination and delays in care and to see a different provider each time they attempt to access prenatal care. 25 percent of AIAN women report experiencing discrimination when going to the doctor or a clinic.

Although race is a salient factor, there are many others that also contribute to disparate health outcomes. High among them is living in a rural location, where higher-level and emergency healthcare is often farther away. Making matters worse is the fact that rural hospitals are closing in droves. As many as five million women live in maternity care deserts, meaning counties with neither an OB/GYN, a nurse-midwife, nor a hospital with a maternity unit. An additional ten million live in areas with limited access to maternity care. Mortality rates for both infants and mothers decrease as urbanization increases.

Another factor is state policy. Many of the states with the most egregious maternal and infant mortality rates have refused to expand and extend Medicaid eligibility coverage, which would be a key step toward improving outcomes. They have also passed some of the country's strictest abortion laws. Giving birth is exponentially more dangerous than abortion, and yet politicians who oppose abortion for the purported harm it does to women and babies often fail to advocate for simple measures that would improve their health and well-being, like extending Medicaid coverage to a year postpartum and mandatory paid leave. Following the overturning of *Roe v. Wade* in 2022, researchers estimated that abortion bans will result in a 24 percent increase in maternal deaths each year. That's hundreds of additional deaths, with the greatest increase among Black women.

Each and every maternal and infant morbidity and death is a tragedy with a ripple effect, consequences that can last for generations (known as the "aftershock"). Meanwhile, the CDC estimates that more than 80 percent of current maternal deaths in the United States are preventable. Improvement is desperately needed from the top down and the bottom up. The flaws and inequities endemic in the system are a feature, not a bug. "These experiences collectively taught me that a bad system will beat a good person every time," said Dr. Neel Shah of Harvard. "And that every system is perfectly designed to get the results that it gets. The inequity we see is because the system itself is racist, misogynist & must be intentionally redesigned."

CHAPTER 15
Jillian

When Jillian returned from Missouri, the birth center was busy. Really busy. In early December, it was hit by a "birth storm"—eight births in less than a week. A family arrived at the birth center at 5:00 a.m. on a Wednesday morning, had the baby at 11:00 a.m., and checked out on Thursday. Another showed up on Thursday and gave birth late that evening. While that family was discharging from the birth center on Friday, another came in, followed by two other people in labor. Someone also gave birth at the cottage on Friday, and someone else arrived at the Portland center on Saturday. And then more on Sunday. Every single birthing suite at Andaluz and the cottage was occupied.

Birth storms of that magnitude were relatively rare at Andaluz—a combination of families who went past their November due dates, plus a few December moms who went into labor early—but when they happened, it was all hands on deck, because not only were the births happening, but routine prenatal and postpartum appointments were scheduled as well. Marilyn was set to attend five of the births, Carrie two, and a midwife named Patricia was set for the birth at the cottage, leaving Jillian scrambling to reschedule prenatal appointments and find other midwives to cover the others.

Andaluz's protocol was to have three people at every birth—the main midwife and two students, a primary and a secondary, who arrived at births before the midwife to set up. During labor, the primary student helped with tasks like checking the baby's heartbeat, which they did periodically throughout the labor (and more frequently toward the end), and the mom's pulse. They also helped organize supplies and made sure the midwife had the instruments she needed on hand, like surgical gloves and a clamp and scissors for cutting the umbilical cord.

The secondary student's main task was charting—inputting all the data around the fetal heartbeat, pulse, and other vitals into medical records, in part to facilitate a smoother transfer to the hospital in the event that it was needed. The trio of midwives and students also kept one another company because labors tended to involve a lot of waiting and downtime. Several Andaluz apprentices were out of town in December because of the holidays, and Jennifer asked Jillian to cover the secondary-student role for two births at the cottage. She was looking forward to it, since she hadn't been staffed on a birth for about a year and missed the excitement and sense of purpose.

The cottage was a small two-room stone house on the sprawling property where Jennifer and her family lived in Dundee, a pastoral hive of activity, featuring a spacious pen where a handful of horses milled around, nibbling on grass or standing in the shade of the apple trees. Every time a car pulled into the driveway, the Gallardo dogs, Mellie and Luna, trotted out to greet it and sidled up to the driver's-side door in the hope of being petted. Out in front of the main house was a grassy yard with hammocks, an aboveground pool, a trampoline, and a treehouse perched near the fence; past the yard were coops for the chickens and rabbits, as well as a stable. There were vegetable boxes off to the side of the house and a wide porch with children constantly coming and going, yelling about a brother stealing the TV remote, crying because Mellie stole a bowl of spaghetti off the counter, or asking Jennifer if they could have $10 to buy a new pair of sandals. The birth cottage was separate from the main house, its own island in the middle of the hullabaloo, but the boundaries were fluid, with midwives running into Jennifer's house in between appointments to grab a snack, ask her a question, or hang out.

The cottage itself was cozy and opened into a living room, with red leather couches and armchairs and a large stone fireplace and chimney. A staircase led up to a loft, which had supply storage and toys for kids to play with, along with a bed where midwives or students could crash. Straight ahead from the entrance, through the seating area, was a roomy bathroom painted in a maroon color with a birth tub and a shower.

Next to the seating area in the cottage was a small kitchenette lined with full bookshelves, and stocked with snacks, a sink and microwave, and a dining table for four. To the left of the kitchen was a bedroom, bright, sunny, and dominated by a large bed and an assortment of stools and chairs, where prenatal appointments were held.

Jillian was assigned to be on call just before Christmas for the birth of a mother named Martina, who had also had older children at Andaluz. A member of a large Latinx family, Martina chose to give birth outside the hospital in part so her husband, mother, kids, and sisters could be present. It was also less stressful for her husband, a combat veteran who found hospital environments triggering.

Jillian was at home watching a movie with Chad the Monday before Christmas when she received a text from Patricia.

"*Hey, Martina is having some light action and it could be tonight.*"

Jillian had already laid out clothes that were comfortable and easy to move in. Her go-to outfit was a short-sleeve T-shirt that enabled her to stick her arm in and out of a birth tub (and other places) and listen to the baby's heartbeat without getting her clothes wet, with a warm cardigan with roomy pockets that could quickly come on and off.

After a few minutes, Patricia sent another text: "*Things are picking up fast, so let's meet at the cottage in thirty minutes.*"

Jillian changed out of her pajamas and hustled over.

When she arrived, Patricia, Martina, and Martina's sisters were already in the bathroom around the tub. Everything was moving smoothly, so Jillian charted out in the common room on the couches. Within two hours, Martina's baby was born, her first son.

Then, she started to bleed heavily.

Patricia had Martina get out of the tub and lay on the bathroom floor on a soft blanket, while the midwives initiated their hemorrhage protocol. Jillian helped draw up an injection of Pitocin (while midwives in community settings don't use Pitocin to induce or supplement labor, they can use the drug as an antihemorrhagic agent because it causes the uterus to contract), which brought the situation under control. After things settled, Martina was able to stay at the cottage, snuggled in bed with her baby, instead of transferring to the hospital.

Jillian drove back home, exhilarated, exhausted, and fulfilled. She had forgotten how much she loved being at births, even when it meant being on call at all hours. Situations like that were why she and her colleagues trained, why they had the skills they did. What she had just participated in made any interruptions to her life worthwhile. Nothing beat the adrenaline rush.

Mentally, Jillian was all for doing more of it—but physically, not so much. Due to the pregnancy, staying up later or getting out of bed earlier than she normally would was tough, as was not being able to eat every couple of hours. At the cottage, it had been harder for her to sit for long periods of time and deny her own needs. She had really had to pee during Martina's birth, but Martina had been pushing fast and Jillian couldn't leave her post. Then the hemorrhage happened. By the time Martina was stabilized and Jillian could go to the bathroom, forty minutes had passed.

She also hadn't anticipated the effect that being present at births would have on her hormonally. When mothers were pushing during the births she attended, Jillian swore that she could feel her baby "vibing" on their oxytocin, also known as the "love hormone." It was as if he or she could pick up on what was happening.

All of this gave her a growing sense of anticipation around her own birth—how it would go, how she would handle it. She also felt twinges of sadness. Those were the last births she would attend for a long time. Once her baby came, she had no idea how long it would take to return to a life that resembled the one she was living now, where she could jump in the car and drive to a birth at a moment's notice. Or if she ever would.

CHAPTER 16
Alison

One of Alison's friends had told her that pregnancy could be divided into distinct phases: the first trimester was all feeling exhausted and ill and the third was feeling elephantine and aching all over. The second, though, it was possible to enjoy. To feel "normal," even. As she reached fourteen weeks, Alison was skeptical. She still had morning sickness, her pants had stopped fitting, and her breasts were swollen and sore. She wasn't even halfway there, and though she was excited about her emerging baby bump, she already was feeling an undercurrent of consternation. One night, when Alison and Steve walked to their favorite burrito place for dinner, there was a woman ahead of them in line. A very pregnant woman. A very, *very* pregnant woman. She appeared about to pop. Alison and Steve stared at her with wide eyes, and then at each other. Alison could not imagine being that big. She started thinking of that woman as the "burrito mom" with a sense of foreboding. That was what was coming.

In the meantime, though, she came to see what her friend meant about the second trimester. Her nausea dissipated after fifteen weeks, and she got a burst of energy. She wasn't necessarily motivated to go running, but on one sunny Sunday, she spent four hours tidying the yard. Caught up in her routine of teaching and school and friends, she felt like her usual, nonpregnant self, doing her usual thing. She could almost forget that she was pregnant at times, until another benchmark reminded her.

At first, she felt just a flutter. Maybe it was nothing, she told herself. Anything could feel like a flutter—gas or her stomach rumbling.

Then one day in October, around twenty weeks, she and Steve were lying in bed and she felt it. An indisputable, undeniable *kick*.

She froze for a moment, taut with anticipation to see if it would happen again. She tried to stay perfectly still, so she wouldn't miss it if she did. After a few moments, it happened again. Alison told Steve to put his hand on her belly, rushing out the words in case he'd miss his chance. He felt it too. *Wow,* Alison thought, almost floating outside herself. *It's really happening.* Intellectually she had known a baby was growing inside her. But to *feel* it? That was a new and indescribable sensation, a form of communication and closeness she'd never felt before. Now it felt like she and the baby—she and Theo—were in this together. For someone who had been so nervous about pregnancy loss, that development meant everything. On her own, without the aid of an ultrasound or midwife, Alison could know at any moment that he was doing okay. Before, the multiweek gaps between appointments had felt like radio silence. If something went wrong, she wouldn't know until the next prenatal, and so part of her braced for bad news every time she walked into the birth center. Now, the kicks and punches and flutters were like check-ins, little missives from the beyond that said: "I'm here and doing just fine."

In November, she went in for a second attempt at her anatomy scan. A month earlier, it had been difficult to get a good image of Theo; parts of the fetus had been "suboptimally visualized," meaning he wasn't in a good position for the scan and needed to be reevaluated. This time, fortunately, the baby was in a better spot, moving around the screen. He looked like he was sucking his thumb.

These were Alison's favorite kinds of appointments—tangible things were being checked and measured. The more she knew, the more she felt secure in the fact that she was healthy and her pregnancy was low-risk.

There was a system in place to keep it that way, which made it easier to face all the other things she felt she had to do before Theo arrived.

Alison was an overachiever and a planner, the type of person who started writing a packing list two weeks before a trip. Her nerves about birth and all the roiling uncertainty that it involved meant that a part of her wanted to do all the things—read the books, peruse the apps, hire the doula, buy the birth ball. They felt important because they were her first choices as a parent. She wanted to be strategic and deliberate, but each item or pregnancy question required a fair amount of research.

One of these choices was whether to get a doula. She liked the idea of having a dedicated support person who would know what to expect during birth. Who wouldn't? But it was yet another expense. Doulas were pricey and would likely cost $1,000 to $1,500. Even though Alison's health insurance covered the Midwifery Birth Center, she'd still have to pay some amount out-of-pocket.* The miscarriage had been expensive, and she wasn't sure how much more money she wanted to throw into the Charybdis of pregnancy care. Her gut reaction was *Do I have to?* Did she really need a doula? She'd already done so much legwork to choose a birth center and was not keen on undergoing the whole research-interview-decision process again. Sometimes it felt like the more she learned, the more questions she had, like there was no end to the decisions to be made and the information to absorb. In the beginning of her pregnancy, each decision had elicited a frisson of excitement and anticipation. Now, it was all starting to feel like a grind.

During one prenatal visit at around the six-month mark, a WHA midwife named Gina mentioned that all patients were asked to watch two birthing class videos online at around thirty-two weeks and sign a

* Oregon is one of just a few states that provides Medicaid reimbursement for doula care, although the reimbursement rates are low. Some hospitals and healthcare systems have also started to introduce their own doula programs, in which interested patients are assigned a doula when they are admitted in labor.

form saying they watched them. Alison didn't want to wait that long. She was teaching full-time and attending school two nights a week at Washington State University, working toward a graduate degree in school administration. The baby was due right around the spring midterms. One of Alison's professors said she was willing to be flexible on assignment deadlines and that Alison could accept an "Incomplete" mark if she needed to and finish the class at a later date. It was a generous option, but one Alison preferred not to fall back on. She wanted to complete as many of her academic and professional duties at school as possible before going on maternity leave.

Even the prospect of creating a registry for their baby shower, which Alison had previously been enthused about, was unappealing because it spawned so many other decisions. Where would the baby sleep? How would they transport him around? What kind of diapers would they use? How would they feed him? It wasn't just building a registry—it was figuring out her entire parenting philosophy. Surely, Alison thought, plenty of people gave birth and raised children without so much "stuff." She knew she was privileged to have access to resources, but a lot of the "stuff" seemed like bullshit to her—consumerist solutions advertised to meet manufactured needs. She wanted to be prepared, but the pressure to be prepared was exhausting. Decision fatigue descended, but she didn't know how to exist as a pregnant person without feeling compelled to vigilance.

She wondered if hiring a doula would help her relax because there would be someone else with expertise to rely on. She continued to go back and forth over the decision, polling the people around her for their thoughts, including Gina. "A lot of people do," the midwife replied when Alison asked, "but a lot of people don't. It can be worthwhile, but it's up to you whether you want to incur that cost." That wasn't particularly clarifying. Alison tried a more specific question. Out of every ten people at the birth center, she asked, how many hired a doula? Gina estimated around eight.

Great, Alison thought. *I guess I need a doula.*

The word "doula" comes from ancient Greek and roughly translates to "a woman who serves." Today, the term refers to a professional who provides emotional, physical, and informational support to people throughout the pregnancy, birth, and early postpartum period. Unlike midwives, who are trained to help deliver babies, doulas do not provide medical care—an oversimplification, albeit a helpful one, is that doulas deal with matters above the waist and midwives deal below.

The concept of the modern doula first emerged in the late 1960s, when the anthropologist Dana Raphael, who studied with Margaret Mead and was a co-founder of the Human Lactation Center, wrote a paper in 1969 advocating for female attendants who could help new mothers during and after birth with things like breastfeeding, referring to them as "doulas." Around the same time, a neonatologist at Stanford, Dr. Marshall Klaus, and a pediatrician in the neonatal unit of Case Western Reserve University Hospital, Dr. John Kennell, were studying infant-mother bonding. In 1973, they traveled to Guatemala for research and noticed that when a female student stayed with a laboring mother, her labor was shorter. They, too, adopted the term "doula" to explain the role, and went on to conduct formal studies about the impact that "continuous emotional and physical support from another woman" had on women in labor, finding that with doula support, a woman's labor was shorter, discomfort and the need for cesareans decreased, and maternal bonding increased. In 1992, Klaus and his wife, Phyllis; Kennell; and fellow maternal health experts Penny Simkin and Annie Kennedy formed Doulas of North America (DONA) to train and certify doulas, hoping to formalize, legitimize, and mainstream the profession.

One of the reasons people hire doulas is because they believe that having a trained person in the room who is well-versed on their preferences increases the likelihood that those preferences will be respected. Pregnancy in no way undermines or qualifies the fundamental right that people have to bodily autonomy. A long history of judicial (and ethical) precedent states that all patients, including pregnant people, have the right to refuse treatment, but refusing a procedure as a pregnant person can be a fraught endeavor. There are abundant examples of women who had forced episiotomies or court-ordered cesarean sections or were threatened with calls to Child Protective Services if they didn't comply with a doctor's directive, but the coercion is not always so explicit. Pressure may be couched in solicitude—"You'll feel so much better with an epidural. Why would you want to suffer?"—but by the eighth or tenth or twelfth "offer," it takes on a new tone. In some cases, mothers may feel like the hospital staff did not accurately represent a situation to them or lay out a real spectrum of options.

Labor is a profoundly vulnerable state, and many people struggle to advocate for themselves under those circumstances, especially when surrounded by medical professionals who are figures of authority. 15 percent of mothers report feeling pressure from health professionals to accept inductions, epidurals, and cesareans. One in six women experience at least one form of mistreatment during labor, which can include being shouted at; scolded or threatened; and having requests for help ignored or refused. Among women of color, that number is consistently and significantly higher at a rate of one in three. Around one in three people describe their births as traumatic, and nearly a quarter of women who give birth report having some PTSD symptoms afterward. The physical experience of birth can be traumatic even when there is no coercion or mistreatment, but in many cases, the trauma stems from feelings of violation and powerlessness, from feeling dismissed, ignored, or disregarded, from having agency stripped away, from lacking or losing control.

Like women of color, members of the LGBTQ community face particular vulnerabilities, as they are routinely "misgendered, mistreated, and denied health care outright" when seeking healthcare in general, and pregnancy-related care specifically. A study from the Center for American Progress revealed that 29 percent of transgender people said a healthcare provider refused to see them, 23 percent said a provider intentionally misgendered them or used the wrong name, 21 percent said they received harsh or abusive language, and 29 percent experienced unwanted physical contact, with higher rates for people of color and people with disabilities. The presence of a doula can help people feel like they have an ally in the room, someone who is watching what's going on and has their interests in mind. Doulas can nudge clients to ask questions, help them make sense of information, encourage them to speak up, or simply request a moment to think things through when faced with a decision.

Medicine runs on the principle of informed consent, which means that healthcare providers have an obligation to fully and accurately inform patients of the risks and benefits of courses of action and to obtain their consent to pursue those actions. Patients sign all kinds of consent forms when they enter a hospital, but that doesn't mean they are agreeing to having procedures performed against their will or without their knowledge. It's not consent if someone doesn't have the capacity to refuse.

In recent years, advocates in the US have adopted the term "obstetric violence," which was first coined in 2008 in Venezuela, to describe violations of human rights involving informed consent and bodily autonomy in maternal healthcare. Using the word "violence" aims to position obstetric violence within the broader landscape of gender-based violence and emphasizes the transgression of personal boundaries and civil liberties. "Part of what makes obstetric violence so troubling is that it challenges the trust that most people have in their physicians and other health care providers," wrote the legal scholar Elizabeth Kukura. "Doctors care for patients in their weak and vulnerable moments, and patients trust their doctors to look out for their best interests and help them heal. This deep level of trust in health care providers makes mistreatment during childbirth feel like a betrayal and may make it harder for family, friends, and the broader public to acknowledge and grapple with this problem."

Awareness of coercive dynamics in the delivery room has exploded in recent years—on social media, online pregnancy/parenting forums, and through organizations like the National Advocates for Pregnant Women, the Black Mamas Matter Alliance, Birth Monopoly, and ImprovingBirth, people are sharing stories of birth trauma and having their experiences validated. There is growing recognition of the "mismatch" between the care people expect to receive and the care they do receive. This has led to louder calls for more humane, ethical treatment and greater interest in professionals, like doulas, who can help people go into labor feeling buttressed, regardless of what their expectations or plans for birth are. As the doula pioneer Penny Simkin put it, "It's not how you give birth. It's how you're cared for that matters."

On occasion, doula support has been cast as a thing privileged women shell out for to have the "perfect birth." Certainly, there is some truth to that—doula care can be expensive and almost always paid for out-of-pocket. However, a growing number of organizations, like Shafia Monroe's International Center for Traditional Childbearing (ICTC), Uzazi Village in St. Louis, and Chanel Porchia-Albert's Ancient Song in Brooklyn, have implemented "village" or community models to make doula care and doula training accessible, affordable, and culturally congruent.

A good doula strengthens people's capacity to be actively engaged in maternity care decisions, boosts their confidence, and, when required, may interrupt harm across provider types and environments, which manifests in improved outcomes. A review of forty-one birth practices published in the *American Journal of Obstetrics & Gynecology* found that continuous labor support was among the most effective of all the practices reviewed, and one of only three practices to receive an "A" grade. In 2017, it also released a statement noting that "evidence suggests that, in addition to regular nursing care, continuous one-to-one emotional support provided by support personnel, such as a doula, is associated with improved outcomes for women in labor."

A Cochrane meta-analysis spanning twenty-two studies involving 15,288 subjects found that continuous labor support contributes to several positive outcomes, including increased spontaneous vaginal birth, shorter labors, a lower C-section rate, and babies who were healthier at birth. The authors concluded that the benefits were so substantial that "all women should have continuous support throughout labour and birth." Other studies have shown that doula support has helped decrease the overall cesarean rate by half, the length of labor by a quarter, and requests for an epidural—among Medicaid enrollees, the C-section rate is 22.3 percent with doulas and 31.5 percent without. After birth, it can increase rates of breastfeeding and decrease postpartum depression. And because doulas increase the likelihood of vaginal birth, they help contribute to lowering the costs of maternity care. In one study, doula support in the United States was associated with Medicaid expenditure savings averaging around $1,000 per birth.

Alison knew she couldn't control or micromanage how her birth would go, but she could control some things, and hiring a doula felt like one of them. If she ended up going to the hospital to give birth, for whatever reason, she was worried the money spent on the doula would be a waste, but then she realized that her fear of going to the hospital might be the best reason to invest in one. In the event she had to transfer, a doula would be one more person there to support her and help her navigate the new environment. That support would be invaluable.

Once the decision was made, WHA recommended an agency called Doula Love, which has a roster of around fifteen doulas. To ensure a good fit, the agency provided "matchmaking" services, in which each client filled out a form about their preferences and received a short list of doulas who aligned with those needs. The agency required its doulas to have attended a minimum of ten births, but also had a student program and offered their services on a sliding scale or for free for clients who qualified. "I really feel like my job as a doula is to help educate people in the way they want to be educated and help them make the choices that are the right choices for them," Wendy Scharp, the agency's owner, explained. "The goal is that people feel supported and provided with good information."

At twenty-six weeks pregnant, Alison filled out their intake form and received the bios of two doulas who matched her requests. (She appreciated that she hadn't had to do the vetting herself.) When it came to doulas, Alison wasn't sure what she was supposed to look for beyond "experienced" and "nice," so she found a list of interview questions online and cherry-picked the ones she found relevant. She decided to interview Katherine, who was the older of the two options and had attended over one hundred births. That evening, Alison made pasta with mushrooms and brown butter sauce for dinner, before sitting down with Steve in front of a laptop on the dining room table. The interview was casual, with Katherine's five-year-old popping in and out of the screen, and Alison liked her "mom vibe." When Alison asked what was included in the scope of the doula service, Katherine walked her through each step. Once Alison was in early labor, she explained, Katherine would come to their house, help her determine when it was time to go to the birth center, and accompany them there. During birth, she'd provide whatever additional support was needed, whether that was making a cold compress, texting family members updates, or asking for clarification on medical terms. Alison asked if it was okay to email or text or call her with questions before she was in labor, and Katherine encouraged her to do so. After the call, Alison and Steve discussed their options. Ultimately, they both felt it was good to have as much support as they could, and Katherine could help with that. They decided to hire her. A doula was now part of their birth plan.

The weekend before Thanksgiving, Alison and Steve settled into their living room, a wide-open room with a white shag rug, a gray couch, and shelves filled with sound equipment and records, to watch the Midwifery Birth Center's birth videos. Before pressing play, they opened a bag of chips and cracked open beers (nonalcoholic for Alison, regular for Steve), ready to receive an education.

The first video covered the what-ifs of giving birth and went through various scenarios in which someone would not be able to give birth at the birth center, like if the baby came prematurely or hadn't come by forty-two weeks, if the baby was breech, or if the mother's blood pressure was out of the safe range. The video also reviewed potential complications and the most common reasons for transfers—usually because labor was taking a long time and the mother needed rest that only an epidural or narcotics could provide.

The second video focused on mentally preparing for the birth, to the extent possible. It emphasized that it was important to have a "choice" rather than an "avoidance" mentality in choosing to have an unmedicated birth at a birth center because when things got hard—too hard, impossibly hard—it was helpful to have a rooted sense of the "why." It also touched on the importance of being adaptable if (or when) things didn't go according to plan.

Alison was struck by the video's advice. Until that moment, she had been more focused on the "what"—what she could do, what she could buy, what she could expect and prepare—than on the "how"—how she would prepare herself, mentally and emotionally, for labor, which would probably entail the most pain she'd ever felt in her life. She wasn't someone who coped well with unknowns and therefore had focused on how she could exert control over the situation rather than coming to terms with her lack of control. Maybe the best thing she could do to prepare for childbirth, she realized, was to work on making peace with the unpredictability. Once labor started, she wouldn't be able to stop it. She would be on that voyage, wherever and however it went. What if she let go of the idea that everything had to go according to plan for it to be "okay"? Instead of dwelling on all that could go wrong, she could make the choice to concentrate on what could go right. Instead of catastrophizing, she could remind herself that everything she was experiencing was normal. Lots of people had babies, and in the grand scheme of things, birth was routine. She could expect the best and prepare for the worst and convince herself that everything would happen the way it needed to. Easier said than done, to be sure, but it was an important shift in thinking for her and for Steve.

As they talked through it all after the videos were done, Alison recalled a nature documentary she'd seen as a kid in which a sheep gave birth and remained perfectly calm throughout. Alison resolved to do her best to channel that energy—she would try to be like the sheep. "Be like a sheep" became her new mantra.

CHAPTER 17
T'Nika

After graduating from her RN program in August, T'Nika continued to press forward with her career goals. She was preparing to take the National Council Licensure Examination, or NCLEX, which nurses must pass in order to practice, at the end of October, and at the same time, she and Daniel were in the process of moving from an apartment in Southwest Portland to a house in Southeast with a yard and room for a nursery. That kind of change, combined with studying for the exam and pregnancy and work, was a lot to shoulder at once, but T'Nika passed the NCLEX exam on her first try. She was elated, proud of herself and of what the accomplishment meant for her future. She knew she had the job at the long-term-care facility as an LPN as long as she needed, but she was ready to move onward and upward. What she was most interested in pursuing was an RN residency, which would both leverage her new credentials and provide more experience and training.

In applying for a residency, T'Nika had focused her application efforts toward one of the major hospital systems in Portland, which operated multiple hospitals and outpatient facilities in the area, but she had never gotten past the initial screening for any of those positions, receiving responses that she didn't qualify or receiving none at all. *What am I doing wrong?* she wondered, as yet another rejection came through. Was it because she had graduated from Concordia University, which had recently announced it was closing? Was she missing the mark on some of the application questions? Was the apostrophe in her name confusing the online application system? Was something off about her résumé? It was frustrating to have no idea what the problem was, and the closer it got to her due date, the more nerve-wracking it became.

T'Nika wasn't alone with that concern. Getting and keeping a job while pregnant can be a struggle. A 2020 study from Baylor University published in the *Journal of Applied Psychology* surveyed pregnant employees about perceived pregnancy discrimination, perceived stress, demographics, and postpartum depressive symptoms, as well as the babies' health indicators, such as gestational age, Apgar score, and birth weight. The results showed that pregnancy discrimination has a negative impact on the health of mothers and babies, linked to increased levels of postpartum depressive symptoms, lower birth weights, lower gestational ages, and increased numbers of doctor visits for babies. Approximately 250,000 pregnant workers are denied requests for accommodations during their pregnancies each year, and many women don't make the request at all, fearing retaliation from employers. Between 2010 and 2020, fifty thousand pregnancy discrimination claims were filed with the Equal Employment Opportunity Commission and Fair Employment Practices Agencies in the United States—28.6 percent of which were filed by Black women, who are disproportionately impacted, despite making up 14.3 percent of the female workforce.

Like pregnancy discrimination, insufficient maternity leave also has a negative impact on both parents and babies. Taking time off after birth helps people manage the physiological and psychological demands of new parenthood. It provides short-term and long-term physical and mental health benefits. People who take longer than twelve weeks' maternity leave report fewer depressive symptoms, a reduction in severe depression, and improvement in their overall mental health. It also enables critical time for bonding with the new baby and development. Research from the Infant Studies of Language and Neurocognitive Development Lab at New York University found that infants with mothers who had three months of paid parental leave experienced more advanced neurological development than those whose mothers had access to only unpaid leave during the same period of time. The Family and Medical Leave Act provides unpaid leave, but only about 60 percent of private-sector workers are eligible. Of that 60 percent, 46 percent struggle to afford the time off.

Whether it's a pregnant fast-food worker who is unable to sit down during her shift or a lawyer at a white-shoe law firm hoping to make partner, having a child affects their employment prospects in a way that it just doesn't for non-childbearing partners. According to research from professors Michelle Budig and Paula England, working mothers face a penalty of losing 15 percent of income per child under the age of five. At 20 percent, the penalty for Black and Native American women is twice that of white women, while for Latinx and Asian women, it's 18 percent and 13 percent, respectively. Experts call it the Motherhood Tax. The penalty is the greatest for low-income women, while men actually get a pay bump for having children, known as the Fatherhood Bonus, with the biggest bump going to high-income men.

T'Nika worried that the longer it took her to find a job, the narrower her prospects would be. Who would hire someone, only to have them go on maternity leave a month later? Looking for advice, T'Nika reached out to an old friend from the Black Student Union at the University of Oregon, Danielle, who had recently been hired for a nursing job on the medical surgical floor at one of the hospitals where T'Nika was applying.

Danielle offered to help by connecting T'Nika with her manager, who in turn said that, thanks to Danielle's praise, she would ensure T'Nika's application made it to the next round. (Around the same time, T'Nika was finally asked to interview for another position, but after mentioning she was pregnant, she never heard back.) The interview for the job on Danielle's unit went well, and the manager told T'Nika that when a position opened up, she was hired. T'Nika wasn't ready to celebrate yet, since a specific job hadn't been offered and the timeline was unclear, but at least she had a solid lead.

Just after Christmas, on December 28, the good news arrived: a residency position on the medical surgical floor was hers. She was hired as a night shift nurse and would see a broad spectrum of patients, helping prepare them for surgical procedures and caring for them as they recovered. Her start date was January 18, two months before her due date.

T'Nika was glad to have found a job, and one she was interested in, but she remained skeptical it would work out. After all the struggle involved in applying, it was hard to trust that things wouldn't fall through. Even though she knew the pregnancy wasn't a strike against her, she felt a little self-conscious about showing up to a new job while visibly pregnant. It was also draining. The training shifts started at 7:30 a.m., when all the patients received their medications and the doctors and nurses made rounds and performed assessments. Those early hours were a hustle because if the routine tasks weren't completed in a timely manner, it could throw off the rest of the day. T'Nika was supposed to have two fifteen-minute breaks and a thirty-minute lunch break, but those didn't always happen. She wanted to prove herself and didn't like asking for help or requesting special accommodations, but her feet were swelling, a lot, despite her compression socks. By the end of the shift, her flat feet looked like sausages. She wanted to make a good impression as a diligent worker and a reliable coworker—not someone who needed to take frequent breaks—but it was a challenge to sink her teeth into the new job and work environment when she was so uncomfortable all the time. When she mentioned the feet swelling during a prenatal appointment at Andaluz, Marilyn advised her to take a ten-minute break to put her feet up every two hours. T'Nika knew her preceptor would agree to that break schedule, but she asked Marilyn to write her an official request anyway. The note helped her feel more secure asserting that need and claiming the time to sit down.

There was also the awkwardness of working at a hospital but planning to give birth outside of one. When colleagues inquired and T'Nika told them her plan was a birth center, she noticed the looks of surprise or confusion. Why would someone who worked in a hospital not want to give birth there? To lighten the conversation, T'Nika always emphasized that she was going to a water birth center with big tubs. The emphasis on water seemed to mitigate some of the disbelief, as if that reason was easier to digest than a deeper skepticism with hospital-based maternity care.

It wasn't until her first week of classes—sitting in a classroom at the hospital with other residents—that she finally began to feel secure in her new job. And to her surprise, her pregnancy, which she had worried was a liability, was the norm. At least four other nurses on her floor were pregnant, too, one of them with a due date five days after T'Nika's, and there were active lines of communication for discussing workplace accommodations and leave schedules. During her initial weeks on the job, she was told that in terms of maternity leave, she could either take two weeks off before or work right up until her due date. (Daniel was planning to take five weeks of leave, but his job was remote, so even once he went back to work, he would still be home.) T'Nika had been nervous to broach the subject, but her boss had been encouraging, which in turn gave her the confidence to do what she wanted. She decided to stop working two weeks before her due date. Those weeks were unpaid, and of course she would miss the income, but she and Daniel would be okay without it. The thought of trundling around the hospital floor at forty weeks pregnant was just not appealing.

To get approved for leave, T'Nika contacted the company that managed benefits for the hospital. It took some time to get connected with the right person and for T'Nika to figure out what benefits she qualified for as a brand-new employee, but after some back-and-forth, they worked out a plan. T'Nika would complete the first four weeks of her training and then work two weeks of regular night shifts before going on maternity leave, which would start on March 6. Once the baby was born, she would get six weeks of short-term disability leave paid at 65 percent of her salary. After that, she could get another six weeks, also paid at 65 percent, that could be split up throughout the first year. When she returned to work, she would finish up the final four weeks of the training and then start on regular night shifts. In total, T'Nika planned to take ten weeks of leave after birth and then two more weeks over the summer, an arrangement that felt generous compared to many people she knew.

For months, T'Nika had focused much of her energy on figuring out her job and leave situation. With those things sorted, her mind turned to specific fears she had around staying healthy. T'Nika's blood pressure had remained in a normal range as her pregnancy progressed, but concerns about preeclampsia lingered, especially after talking to a close family friend named Kayla.

When Kayla had given birth to her twins years before, it was a difficult delivery. T'Nika knew she'd faced complications and her babies spent time in the NICU, but the details, as shared at the time, were vague and passed on secondhand. Kayla was a private person and hadn't wanted to talk openly about what she'd been through. T'Nika had tried to ask her before, but Kayla always shut down that line of questioning. Now that she was pregnant herself, though, T'Nika was even more curious. She resolved to ask Kayla directly what happened the next time they saw each other, at a family event scheduled near the end of T'Nika's second trimester. T'Nika reasoned that being pregnant herself was justification for prying into what she knew was a sensitive, personal matter. At the party, she asked Kayla if she'd share more information about the "serious stuff" she'd been through.

"I didn't say anything," Kayla said, "because I didn't want to traumatize you," explaining that when she was pregnant, she hadn't liked when people shared their traumatic birth stories. They scared her, and she wanted to protect T'Nika from that. But if T'Nika wanted to know, she would tell her.

Twins can involve more complicated births, and they are more likely to be premature. Kayla's pregnancy had proceeded without complication, but in her third trimester, she developed preeclampsia. Her labor and delivery required urgent intervention, and both her life and the lives of her babies were at risk. The story she shared was terrifying, and it underscored for T'Nika what was at stake—the potential loss of everything that mattered to her, the loss of her own life and future, the loss of her child. Thankfully, Kayla's healthcare team knew what they were doing, and Kayla and her twins pulled through, but it felt like a close call, one that left the whole family feeling scared and shaken.

Like T'Nika, Kayla was someone with resources and a solid support system, and even that hadn't prevented a crisis from happening. The story reminded her that if it could happen to Kayla, it could happen to her, too, even though she wasn't having twins, because they were both Black women giving birth in America. In some ways, the conversation was a reality check, and T'Nika started to worry more than she had before about getting "risked out" of the birth center.

Since birth centers only serve "low-risk clients," people with particular risk factors or complications (like preeclampsia) are not eligible to give birth in them and are usually referred to a hospital. While those guidelines are in place to protect health and safety, they can also be a barrier to out-of-hospital birth and midwifery care, particularly for groups that experience certain conditions—like cardiovascular disease, diabetes, or high blood pressure—at higher rates. "Several of our participants shared that they felt forced into having a hospital birth because of their high-risk status," the authors of *Battling Over Birth* wrote about their findings.

T'Nika had no problem transferring to an OB or a hospital if she needed to, but she really, really hoped she wouldn't need to. With every prenatal appointment, she felt more comfortable at Andaluz. The reminder that she might not be able to give birth there was disheartening, but she was still grateful to Kayla for opening up. She knew the subject wasn't easy to talk about, but it felt important to share in moments of both pain and celebration. T'Nika did not want to approach her pregnancy from a place of fear, but she also did not want to be naive to the risks. That tension can be tricky to navigate for women and their care providers, and especially for Black women.

The racial inequities in maternal outcomes are real, stark, and unjust. They are a national disgrace and merit recognition, attention, and action. While all the attention the media has started to pay to maternal inequities is positive because it has helped spur activism and political change, the midwife Shafia Monroe said that it has also added to the climate of stress and fear. "Birth is very different for white America," said Monroe. "It's this wonderful experience about finding yourself and changing your life, but for us, it's about survival and reclaiming our rights as Black women in this country."

Monroe believed that expanding access to midwifery and community birth could help address these imbalances—helping families of color get out of a system that was harming them; reducing racial inequities; and reclaiming birth as a joyful, meaningful rite, rather than an ordeal to survive—and there was a growing consensus around this belief. A 2020 report from the Center for American Progress argued that "expanding access to midwives and doulas, especially those who are part of the communities they support, can significantly improve the health and birthing outcomes and experiences of people of color and LGBTQ people. . . . Community-based birth workers have the unique capacity to challenge bias in the medicalized birth system and undo the exclusion of traditional, community-centered practices around pregnancy and birth."

However, as the report (and Monroe) have noted, it's not enough to change the birth setting or provider type. Tackling the underlying reasons for health disparities so fewer people are risked out is necessary to making midwifery care more accessible, as is diversifying the maternal healthcare workforce. People of color may not feel comfortable at a birth center, or in a hospital unit, where all the care providers are white. "We have to go beyond just talking about giving people, especially low-income people, access to care," said Angela Doyinsola Aina, executive director of the Black Mamas Matter Alliance, at an American Public Health Association conference. "We also need to ask whether that care is high quality and culturally relevant."

Studies have shown that outcomes are better for Black infants when they are cared for by Black physicians. When researchers from George Mason University analyzed 1.8 million hospital births in Florida between 1992 and 2015, the data suggested that newborn-physician race concordance was associated with a significant improvement in mortality, particularly during more challenging births and in Black-serving hospitals. While that study focused on physicians, a more diverse maternal healthcare workforce—including nurses, midwives, and doulas—is a key part of building a more equitable system overall.

That was part of why T'Nika was so committed to becoming a nurse. Whether she worked in a hospital or a birth center, she wanted to be a familiar, friendly face in the room who let people know she had their back. Her desire to give birth at Andaluz, her interest in nursing in a hospital L&D unit, and her goal of becoming a nurse-midwife were all part of the same calculations. They were motivated by a commitment to ensuring that patients like her—and Kayla and her children—felt safe, seen, and cared for, wherever they gave birth, and that they had a range of options.

That should be a given, but she knew it wasn't.

CHAPTER 18
Jillian

Until they reached twenty-eight weeks of pregnancy, Andaluz clients had prenatal appointments once a month, at which point they switched to one every two weeks. From thirty-six weeks on, clients saw a midwife once a week until they went into labor. That schedule, which involves a total of twelve to fourteen visits, is the standard among OB practices as well. It was introduced in the 1930s by the Children's Bureau and has remained essentially unchanged ever since, although there are now doctors, midwives, and public health researchers questioning whether all those appointments—which add up to roughly one full week of missed work or childcare—is appropriate for all patients, especially with improved screening technology and especially if they are low-risk.

Jillian, for one, didn't mind the increasing frequency of her appointments. She was at the birth center most days anyway, and she was finding them to be a great learning experience. Even as the client, she had her "midwife brain" switched on, which added a whole new layer to her education. She appreciated the opportunity to experience care from the other side, picking up practical tips from her team. For example, she had always been delicate and careful when palpating a client's stomach, but once she had felt the sensation herself, she realized she could be firmer with her touch.

Though there were distinct benefits to possessing more knowledge than most people preparing to give birth for the first time, there could be drawbacks too. She worried that she wouldn't be able to turn off her "midwife brain" when she needed to. Friction between her client side and midwife side escalated when it came time to test for gestational diabetes. The usual method at Andaluz (and elsewhere) for screening for gestational diabetes was simple: a client was given a glucose solution to drink and then the blood was tested to determine how effectively the body tolerated the sugar. Jillian thought the drink was gross and opted to test herself instead. She bought an at-home glucometer and pricked her finger after eating breakfast and dinner for ten days, putting the drop of blood on a strip each time and plugging it into an at-home machine that indicated sugar levels. Though she enjoyed the opportunity to learn more about her body and how it reacted to food, access to the information wasn't always helpful: sometimes, she'd see a number and think, *Oh, God. This is a really bad number. This is crazy. My sugar shouldn't be this high or low*. One day, she saw a result with what she interpreted as a problematic reading and showed it to Carrie, who was confused by the alarm over pretty standard numbers. Jillian's numbers were fine, she countered, and in the normal range. It was almost like, as the client instead of the midwife, Jillian couldn't interpret the data as clearly. It was easier to be calm and objective when the numbers pertained to someone else. (Ultimately, her gestational diabetes test came back negative.)

Jillian was in the unusual position of interacting with people having normal, uncomplicated pregnancies every day at the birth center and keeping a mental catalog of all the possible complications that could arise. So far, her own pregnancy had been uneventful. There was no reason to think that would change, but in the event it did, Jillian's greatest concern was having to contend with Covid.

Jillian's due date was a year into the pandemic (and before vaccines were widely available), which had unleashed a swarm of new things for people to grapple with when giving birth in a hospital. Hospitals were still figuring out how to limit the transmission of the disease while also ensuring people got the healthcare they needed. Regulations and policies around laboring women had changed repeatedly, and it was hard to keep track of which hospital had which rules. Jillian feared the possibility of going to the hospital without Chad, if she wasn't allowed a support person, and dreaded the prospect of having to wear a mask in labor. She was terrified that she'd be separated from her baby if she tested positive for Covid when she entered the hospital, or that she'd catch Covid while there. Jillian knew how to advocate for herself when it came to familiar labor and delivery issues, but no one knew how to prepare for childbirth in an unprecedented global pandemic.

For many families, Covid fundamentally changed the way they viewed risk when deciding where to give birth. The hospital no longer felt like the safest place to be, and some of the new rules, like no support people allowed, could be deal breakers. As a result, community birth started to attract interest from people who might not have considered it before, and early in the pandemic, midwives reported surges in inquiries. An analysis of CDC data showed that planned home births and births at birth centers increased by 20.2 percent and 9.2 percent, respectively, in 2020.

Jillian had always been set on home birth, but the pandemic did make her feel more nervous than she otherwise would have been about a hospital transfer. To her, it felt even more crucial to avoid the hospital if she could, which would entail a combination of luck, the know-how of her midwives, and her own mindset. As an apprentice, she had seen again and again how important it was for people to surrender and let go, and she'd heard stories from midwifery friends and colleagues about how challenging it could be to stop monitoring or analyzing what was happening and be present in the moment. She didn't want to get in her own way. Whenever these worries popped into her mind, she told herself, *I'll just have to cross that bridge when I come to it.*

In the meantime, there were so many other things to think about. The baby was about the size of an eggplant, and Jillian couldn't help but notice with shock how fast the weeks were flying by. Early in pregnancy, she felt like she had all the time in the world, but suddenly, in January, a few weeks into her third trimester, she seemed to be running out of it. All the tasks she wanted and needed to get done were piling up, and she felt the pressure of a deadline.

To start, their house was a fixer-upper still in the "fixer" stage. In February, Carrie and Marilyn were scheduled to conduct a home visit to get a sense of the space and review a supply checklist with Jillian. Ideally, the house wouldn't look like a work zone when they arrived. Jillian and Chad had already stripped the paint, repainted, ripped up the floors, and taken off all the doors in order to replace them, but they still needed the floors and doors done before the baby came.

She also needed to assemble her collection of birth supplies. One benefit of going to a hospital or birth center was that people could show up with a change of clothes, a toothbrush, a baby outfit, and that was it. To a home birth, midwives brought bags filled with essential medical supplies: a Doppler, cord clamp, gloves, sterile solution, stethoscope, thermometer, oxygen tank, and medications, like Pitocin. Jillian had her own well-stocked midwifery bag with gear and planned to borrow other items, like a blood pressure cuff and a peanut ball, from Andaluz. She also purchased a $65 home birth kit online from a company called Radiant Belly, which included alcohol prep pads, mesh briefs, lubricating jelly, perineal irrigation bottles, and plastic-backed sheets, which protected bedding from all the fluids. There were the supplies she'd need for after birth as well. She had received gifts at her baby shower, including a baby carrier and bassinet, and was borrowing other items from friends, but Jillian did not want to forget anything. She still had to set up the nursery, on top of the responsibilities she had to handle at Andaluz, which included training the person who was replacing her as office manager while she was away.

At thirty-one weeks, with all these other to-dos swirling around, Jillian was hammered with a wave of angst about her future. She had accepted the reality that she was deferring her midwifery career—first when she had taken the Andaluz office manager job, and then again when she had found out she was pregnant—and made peace with the prospect that she might not be able to apply for her NARM certification for another year. Or, at least, she thought she had. Suddenly, she couldn't stop thinking about how much harder it would be to get certified once the baby was born, and what that could mean for her professionally and personally. The process required compiling all her educational and apprenticeship materials and sending them into NARM, and she would then have to take a lengthy exam if accepted. Jillian didn't want to lose momentum. She considered that maybe thirty-one-weeks pregnant was the right time to go for it, since she was still going into the birth center every week, interacting with the midwives, keeping her skills and knowledge fresh, and able to hop in the car and run errands whenever she needed. Everything would be more difficult with a baby. What if it took her years to get all those materials organized? What if she waited so long, the births she logged during her apprenticeship expired and she had to do them all over again? What if with a new baby, she didn't have the energy or focus to study for the test? Or to attend births?

My due date is in nine weeks, she thought as she caught a glimpse of the calendar. *I have to do this now, or I possibly never will.*

Galvanized, she took the steps needed to initiate the application process, requesting her transcript from Birthingway and submitting the paperwork from her apprenticeship, which involved having her preceptors log and sign off on every birth she assisted. She also gathered documentation of five "continuity of care" clients, whom Jillian worked with throughout their prenatal, birth, newborn, and postpartum appointments. Completing the paperwork was time-consuming because the midwives were busy and could be tricky to pin down, but she hoped to put the envelope in the mail within a week or two. From there, the application would take a few weeks to process, and Jillian would have to schedule a date to take the NARM exam, which was not only exhaustive and theory-oriented, but also, at $900, expensive. Once the NARM certification was in hand, she would submit that information to Oregon to get a licensed direct-entry midwifery (LDM) license from the state. And then, at long last, whenever she was ready, she could start to practice as a full-fledged midwife.

It was a long road, and although Jillian had come far, she still had far to go. The scramble to get certified before the baby arrived was stressful and overwhelming, but it was stressful and overwhelming to continue postponing as well. Jillian didn't want everything she'd worked for to be lost. She didn't want to get derailed or sidetracked and struggle to follow through. Her life as she knew it was about to transform, but that didn't mean everything she'd previously worked toward or cared about had to evaporate. She was adamant about seeing this through.

CHAPTER 19
Alison

One weekend in early December, Alison was standing under the stream of warm water in the shower when, suddenly, she toppled backward. She shrieked as she went down onto her butt, the sound ricocheting around the enclosed space of the bathroom. She froze on the floor of the shower, shocked, dripping wet, and hesitant to move.

Steve came tearing down the stairs from his office up in the loft and burst through the bathroom door, pulling back the shower curtain.

"ARE YOU OKAY?" he gasped, his eyes wide.

"I think so," Alison replied, not entirely convinced. After a moment and a breath, she braced herself on the side of the shower and gingerly pulled herself up. Once vertical, she turned off the water and took a quick physical inventory. She rolled her neck and touched her belly and arms and legs. Everything seemed fine. The banshee shriek may have been rather dramatic, as it wasn't a hard fall and she hadn't injured herself, but still, she was rattled. It had happened so fast, and if she had fallen forward, she or the baby could have been hurt. It felt like a close call.

A few days later, while Steve was out of town for work, she fell again while taking the dog on a walk to a hillside park a mile and a half from their house, a walk she'd done countless times before. One moment she was standing upright, strolling down a gentle hill. The next moment, she wasn't. After it happened, she paused on the ground to get her bearings. When she didn't notice any pain, she hoisted herself up, dusted herself off, looked around to see if there were any witnesses, and continued the walk, slower now and more mindful of her steps.

Had it been just one fall, or had Alison not been pregnant, she wouldn't have been worried. She could be clumsy, and she'd played sports and skied for years—she was familiar with the ground. But two falls, while pregnant, out of the blue, for no reason, in such a short window seemed like a cause for concern.

She called the birth center to let them know what had happened. The receptionist who answered the phone asked a series of questions, including if she could still feel the baby moving. Alison said she wasn't sure; at this point in her pregnancy, the baby wasn't moving all the time. The receptionist said that everything was probably okay, but the "probably" sent Alison into an emotional spiral. Every fear and anxiety she'd worked hard to move past came rushing forward. Even over the phone, the receptionist could sense that Alison was upset and said she would have a midwife call her as soon as possible, but in the meantime, Alison should try to stay calm. Alison did her best to channel a sheep.

A midwife called around 6:00 p.m., fresh off attending a birth, and Alison told her the full story of the falls. Alison made it clear that she wasn't injured and tried to strike the right balance between expressing her concerns without seeming histrionic.

The midwife said that a minor fall, especially one that didn't directly impact the belly, was not necessarily a cause for alarm; given that Alison wasn't in pain and hadn't experienced any new symptoms after the falls, all signs indicated that she was okay. But, the midwife said, it was good that Alison had let them know—better to be safe than sorry—and of course she had felt scared and shed some tears. Her concern was understandable, especially for someone going through this for the first time. The midwife explained that the likely culprit was a changing center of gravity. As pregnancy advanced, it could be an adjustment, physically and emotionally, to maintain balance.

That explanation made sense to Alison, and prompted her to contemplate just how unfamiliar her body could feel at times and how complicated that could be. Though she mostly felt proud about her expanding belly, she was also feeling twinges of distress about the fact that her body was changing, particularly the weight gain. She had always endeavored to stay healthy and fit and had been the same size for most of her life. Now, seemingly overnight, the cute baby bump was becoming . . . less cute. She was at a point where she wasn't so big that she clearly looked pregnant under her winter coat, but big enough that it changed her silhouette. When she looked in a mirror or caught her reflection in a store window, she felt she looked bloated rather than pregnant, which in turn made her feel hyper visible and self-conscious, and then made her feel self-conscious and guilty about feeling self-conscious.

Weight gain during pregnancy can be a tricky thing. There are increased health risks if an expectant mother enters a pregnancy with a body mass index (BMI) under or over a certain threshold, or gains too little or too much weight during the nine months. According to a study from Northwestern, over half of women are classified as obese when they start their pregnancies and/or have high blood pressure or diabetes, which can lead to complications like preeclampsia. While those risks are real, weight bias in healthcare is a well-documented phenomenon. Many studies have shown that overweight and obese women face widespread discrimination in healthcare. A high BMI can cause care providers to either classify someone as high-risk based on their weight alone, regardless of other indicators, or do the opposite—overlook warning signs about pregnancy complications.

This becomes especially difficult to manage when faced with the opposing cultural messages that emerge about what defines health in pregnancy. After a lifetime of social pressure to keep weight off and stay trim, Alison was suddenly "supposed" to feel proud and maternal about weight gain, eating for two and indulging in cravings—but only until the baby was born. Then, there would be pressure to "get her body back." The reversals were jarring. Alison was aware of the myriad ways in which society fetishized thinness and stigmatized fatness and how those dynamics were toxic and harmful. She didn't think being thin was a virtue, and she knew her value and self-worth had nothing to do with the number on a scale or the size of her pants. But she was also a woman, born and raised in America, and the tendrils of expectation around her appearance were burrowed deep. Try as she might, she couldn't flip a switch and suddenly feel completely at peace with an additional twenty pounds. It took some getting used to.

At her next prenatal appointment in mid-December, Alison asked Gina to weigh her. The scale showed that she had gained exactly what was expected for her stage of pregnancy, or maybe even a little less. That assuaged her concerns, but it was somehow still hard to believe that it was normal for her body to change so much in such a short period of time. Then she remembered the "burrito mom" (the super-pregnant woman she and Steve had seen at the takeout spot). Alison still thought of her from time to time—a reminder that she wasn't done changing yet.

After weighing Alison and logging her vital stats, Gina asked if she had selected a pediatrician. It wasn't the first time Alison had been asked that question, and the truth was, she hadn't even started to look. It had been an innocent inquiry from Gina, a box to check on a list, but Alison got defensive. Being asked the question again, with no forward movement on her part, was making her feel like she was failing, like she hadn't done her homework. It also made her feel like she was being nagged. The baby wasn't due until March. Surely there was plenty of time. She didn't understand what the rush was, but she kept her protestations to herself. She promised Gina she'd look into it before the next appointment, and they moved on.

After a few more checks, it was time to listen to the baby. The midwifery student helping Gina with the prenatal exam was tasked with finding the baby's heartbeat, and Alison lay back in the seat, eager to hear the latest from Theo. For a few agonizing moments, the room was quiet as the student searched for the right spot to listen. Then, nervously, she mentioned that she was having a hard time picking up the sound. Alison tried not to freak out as her mind flashed back to her miscarriage. That loss was hard, but this would be so much worse. She was so much further along. With every silent millisecond that passed, she felt her chest getting tighter.

Then, the steady rhythm of the heartbeat filled the room.

Alison exhaled deeply, gratefully. Everyone was okay. It was time to go home. After the student cleaned up and Alison was cleared, she put on her coat and went to use the bathroom. When she returned to the exam room on the way out, though, the midwife stopped her, saying that they needed to give her a Tdap shot (tetanus, diphtheria, and pertussis). Alison was confused because she was pretty sure she'd received the Tdap at her last appointment. Since it was flu season, Alison had asked to get her flu shot earlier than WHA's schedule dictated, and because she was already getting one vaccine, it had made sense to give her the Tdap shot as well. Maybe it hadn't been logged in her chart? Everyone seemed a little flustered, and after some back-and-forth, Alison got the Tdap vaccine, just to be sure. Alison was annoyed that what seemed like a simple request—to get a shot a few weeks early—had seemed to throw the whole system off-kilter.

Alison knew it wasn't a big deal, but it felt like one thing too many for that particular day. She drove home that evening feeling irritable, anxious, and destabilized. She was supposed to pick a pediatrician sooner than made sense to her but had to wait longer than she wanted to get a flu shot. She was expected to get a doula and prepare for birth but wasn't supposed to watch the instructional birth videos before well into her third trimester. It was curious that what had drawn her to the birth center at the outset—the structure and adherence to well-defined protocols and plans—was now the thing she was chafing against.

She was tempted to call to discuss how the afternoon's events had affected her, but she also didn't want to be "that person," difficult and demanding and acting as if she were the sole patient to be attended to. She was normally positive, diplomatic, and easygoing, but now pregnancy was making her critical in a way that wasn't usual for her. She felt particularly bad about her vexation with the midwifery student—she herself had once been a student teacher, so she understood the importance of apprenticeships to professional development. But at the same time, the student's delay in finding the heartbeat had been triggering. And what if there was a student present when she was in labor who didn't notice something or know what to do?

When she got home, Alison cried to Steve, telling him that maybe she didn't want to have the baby at the birth center after all. But she also did not want to have the baby at the hospital or at home. The thought of changing the plan now, when they had already come so far, felt even more overwhelming. She felt like she had nowhere to go.

Steve—gently, with empathy, and not in so many words—said that changing course would be ridiculous, and that one "meh" appointment shouldn't throw off their birth plan. Alison knew he was right, but she felt trapped in her body and in her head, caught between swings of awe, terror, and ennui.

The next day, when she felt steadier, she called a few pediatricians in the Vancouver area from a list that the birth center had provided. One suggested she look through the doctors' pictures and bios on their website, as if she was online dating. Alison reluctantly settled in to read bios and compare reviews when it dawned on her: She didn't have to spend hours doing this. Any choice she made would be fine. She could spend twenty minutes on the project and move on. She could choose to relieve herself of some of this self-imposed pressure. She didn't have to give every single task her all, and if they didn't like the pediatrician, they could find a new one. *I can give myself a break,* she thought.

One aspect of preparing for the baby that Alison had been looking forward to was attending childbirth classes. So many movies that involved pregnancy included staple scenes of pregnant women sitting on birth balls practicing short panting breaths, and it always looked kind of fun to her. Along with Katherine's doula services, the package she'd purchased from Doula Love included access to three of their classes. Everyone was encouraged to take Birth 101, which addressed the anatomy and mechanics of birth. Then, they could select one class from two additional categories: "Getting the Baby Out" and another featuring various postpartum subjects. Alison signed up for a class on labor positions and one on breastfeeding, but the subject she was most interested in was anatomy.

Alison thought of herself as having a solid working knowledge of the female reproductive system, but there was a lot to learn, and as a first-time mother, she didn't have much of a frame of reference for how things worked or reacted during labor. It was like John Locke's philosophical problem of the pineapple—how could you know the taste of a pineapple without having ever tasted one? Words alone didn't convey the essence. She knew a contraction was a tightening of the muscles of the uterus, but that didn't mean she understood what it would or should feel like. How would she know if she was having a contraction? Would it be obvious? How did a contraction feel different than, say, a period cramp or a stomachache or the baby switching positions?

The same was true of labor pain. Alison knew and expected labor to be painful, but it was impossible to anticipate the specifics. Amid so many new sensations, would she know what was "normal" pain and what was pain signaling that something was wrong?

Birth 101 took place on a Sunday from 10:00 a.m. to 2:00 p.m. on Zoom, held virtually because of the pandemic. The news came as a bit of a letdown—Alison already spent her whole workday on Zoom and had hoped the class would be a place to make mom friends—but she was also reassured by the precaution. She wouldn't have been comfortable going to an indoor group class with the pandemic still at its height and Covid vaccines not yet available. The virtual option was more appealing to Steve as well, who was shy around new people.

To start, the doula and childbirth educator who led the class used a model of a pelvis and a baby doll to demonstrate how babies make their way down the birth canal, before discussing common interventions that happen during labor, such as what inductions entail and how epidurals are administered. Alison was surprised by how much of the information was new to her.

The next evening, she and Steve took the labor positions class, which lasted for two hours. The doula reviewed positions the baby might be in during labor and positions the birthing person could do during contractions—a squat, say, or getting on hands and knees. Then she had the couples practice the positions, including one where the person in labor drapes their arms over a partner's neck and sways, like a slow dance. Alison was proud of Steve for how actively he participated, given that he was a "Never-Dancer." (Part of the reason they'd held their wedding in the morning instead of at night was so Steve wouldn't be tortured by being forced to dance in front of a crowd.) They signed off feeling more prepared and informed. Later that week, they logged in to the breastfeeding class, which also lasted for two hours.

It was all interesting and relevant information, but after four hours on a weekend plus two hours on two nights after work, plus the birth center videos they'd already watched, Steve was pushed past his limit with birth-related content. Alison was getting there too. Her tipping point had come after watching an Instagram influencer video discussing babies and body temperature. The speaker explained how new parents often get freaked out about their baby's temperature when they are sleeping, and advised considering what the viewer, as the parent, was wearing—if they were comfortable in their clothing, the baby would likely be comfortable in similar clothing. Basically: don't put a baby in flannel pajamas and a sleep slack if it's 90 degrees. When the video was over, Alison stared at her phone, feeling slightly stunned. Did that type of advice *really* need to be spelled out in minute detail? she thought. It was hardly rocket science, and yet it was being treated almost as a hidden or unexpected piece of insight. Alison may not have had a huge reservoir of knowledge about babies, but she did have common sense and a basic understanding of how human bodies worked.

For so long, she had done everything she could to absorb tips and data and best practices, but watching the video was a reminder that she was a smart, capable person who could figure some things out on her own. She didn't need an "expert" or influencer to guide her every step of the way. She trusted her instincts and capabilities in other areas of her life, so why not in this one? She decided to unfollow the account. Maybe there was such a thing as too much information.

CHAPTER 20
Jillian

Jillian and Chad's house was located in a small subdivision just off the tiny main street in downtown Carlton, which had a handful of restaurants and wine tasting rooms overseen by a large silo. Their house was painted light green and the dogs barked whenever someone walked up the front path. As they waited for their home visit to begin one late February afternoon, Jillian had reruns of *Friends* playing on the TV while she tidied up; the channel was airing the season when Rachel was pregnant, which felt appropriate. Chad was in the garage eating ribs that he had smoked himself, exiled because the smell made Jillian sick.

Jen, an apprentice at Andaluz, arrived first. She and Jillian were good friends, and Jillian had been a student midwife at Jen's birth, which she thought created a lovely symmetry. Marilyn arrived next in her usual bohemian-chic attire, a long gray sweater over a black dress and black boots. Jillian showed them both into the kitchen, where donuts were laid out in sticky, colorful glory on the counter, next to a fresh pot of coffee. Everyone sat around the kitchen table chatting until Carrie arrived, sporting a flowing brown linen dress and matching sneakers. She pulled up a chair at the kitchen table and jumped right into the conversation, which ranged from the light pink dress Jillian recently bought to how expensive housing in Portland was getting.

Every so often, Marilyn caught Jillian's eye and slipped in a prenatal-y question—"How are you feeling, sweetie?"—the response to which Jen subtly recorded on her laptop, parsing the relevant clinical information from the small talk. Before long, Marilyn got down to business. How was Jillian's collection of birth supplies? Jillian listed her inventory: she had a stash of old towels she didn't mind getting dirty and she and Chad had picked up a stack of new towels at Target the day before (she knew from experience that there was no such thing as too many towels at a birth). She also noted her new receiving blankets, cookie sheet (in the event a baby needed resuscitation during a home birth, a cookie sheet could serve as a flat surface to lay them on), and the pink inflatable birth tub she'd bought from Birthingway when it closed, planning to use it for Blooming Dahlia. After Target, they'd gone to Home Depot, where she and Chad bought a converter that would enable them to run a hose from the bathroom faucet into the inflatable birth tub in the bedroom, and a pump to dispose of soiled water. At the mention of the pump, Carrie signaled her approval. She recalled how once she had been present at a birth without a pump, forcing her to toss bloody tub water out of a window onto the snow. It had looked like a crime scene.

Then, attention turned to the forms and documents Jillian had laid out on the table. The first was a hospital transfer plan, in which she selected the hospital closest to her house, about a twenty-five-minute drive away. They also reviewed the newborn consent forms that Jillian and Chad had filled out. Immediately after a baby is born, there is a raft of tests and medicines that newborns typically get in the US, like shots of vitamin K, which help with blood clotting, and antibiotic eye drops or ointment that protect babies from bacterial eye infections that can occur during birth. Jillian was intimately familiar with all the procedures and forms and had her own opinions, but she wanted Chad to approach all the questions with a blank slate so they could discuss and decide together. They had done so prior to the meeting, so everything was figured out.

The next form was a copy of the birth plan. For people giving birth in hospitals, birth plans can be a way to convey preferences regarding pain relief or medical interventions to staff. Since there are fewer interventions available in birth centers and homes, Andaluz's birth plan form prompted clients to answer more philosophical and personal questions in addition to practical ones, which not only gave clients the chance to evaluate and express their thoughts, but also offered the midwives more detailed insight into their clients' minds, so they could provide the right kind of help at different stages. These questions included "What's your greatest fear for the birth?" (Jillian had written, "Not being able to turn off my midwife brain") and what type of support would be most helpful and wanted when things got hard (Jillian answered "verbal encouragement").

After they reviewed the paperwork, it was time for the tour of the house. Midwives like to be familiar with clients' homes before the actual birth so there's less of a learning curve. When the day comes, they already know where to set up their equipment, have sketched out where they will sit or stand during labor, and understand which bathroom they should use.

Jillian and Chad's front door opened directly into the living room, which hosted the squishy couch pregnant Jillian had come to revile, a chair with a blanket covered in dog hair where Paisley liked to nap, a TV, and a wood-burning stove in the far corner. To the left of the front door was a small alcove with deer antlers mounted on the wall, a gift from Chad's grandfather, who had hunted the deer himself in 1953. At the back of the living room, the airy kitchen opened to the left, lined with windows on two sides and sliding doors that led to the back deck.

Past the kitchen and living room, the hallway narrowed. There was a bathroom on the left and the small nursery on the right, with a crib and a mobile already set up, and a table covered in baby gifts. The stuffed fox that Jillian had clutched crying on the plane home from St. Louis was nestled cheerfully in the crib. Across the hall from the nursery, there was a small guest room with a futon and a floor-to-ceiling bookcase lined with

Jillian's midwifery books and an anatomical model of the female reproductive system, which Jillian had also salvaged from Birthingway.

Jillian and Chad's bedroom was at the back of the house, with windows that looked out onto rolling fields. They had a king-size bed with a light blue comforter and a dresser under the window, along the back wall, lined with bonsai trees. When Marilyn inquired about the bonsais, Jillian explained that they were Chad's and she was not allowed to touch them, kind of joking, but kind of not. Years before, just after they moved in together, Jillian had moved bonsais that Chad had lovingly tended for fifteen years onto the porch while she cleaned—in the summer, in 110-degree heat, for hours—and caused their untimely demise. Chad had since replaced the plants, but Jillian still steered clear. Carrie and Marilyn pledged to set up their midwifery supplies on the other dresser, lest the bonsais be placed in the line of peril once again.

Once the tour was complete, Jillian laid on her bed so Carrie could take her blood pressure and listen to the baby's heartbeat. Chad stood nearby. As she pulled up her shirt, her belly moved as the baby did, and the Doppler began to pick up little hiccupping sounds. Marilyn stood in the doorway, leaning against the frame and running through the rest of her routine prenatal questions.

"Are you staying hydrated?"

"Yes," Jillian assured her.

"Do you have a baby carrier?"

"Yes."

"Are you planning to breastfeed?"

"Yes."

"Are you planning to get a third-trimester ultrasound?" Carrie chimed in. "It's optional, but it can confirm the baby's position."

"No. The baby's head-down and the head is low. Breech isn't likely."

Then Marilyn switched to more emotional questions.

"Is there anything you're particularly nervous about, honey?"

Jillian repeated the answer she'd put on her birth plan. "The thing I'm most nervous about is if I will be able to turn off my midwife brain and not midwife myself or analyze what's going on," she said.

"It can be a challenge, letting other people be the midwife and knowing when to ask for help," Carrie agreed. "But you will get to a place of survival and desperation where you will have to turn it off."

"I've wondered that," Chad added. "If because Jillian is a midwife, she will be more stubborn or reluctant to say when something is hard or she needs help."

"That's why we will be there," Carrie reassured him.

Jillian asked Chad if he had any other questions and he asked about postpartum depression—how to notice it and if there were specific things he should look out for. Carrie was impressed. For many first-time parents, and particularly dads, postpartum depression wasn't really on their radar.

"There's a normal, expected amount of emotion," she began, "and then there are some signs, like an almost manic anxiety or not wanting to hold the baby." It could be confusing, she explained, because there was a lot of change happening at once on many levels for a new mother, and some degree of travail was to be expected—the so-called baby blues. But it wasn't always easy to parse what was normal and what wasn't until things became more serious. Luckily, conversations had been shifting and people were talking more openly about the issue.

Despite how much medical attention pregnant people receive during their pregnancies, most of that attention pivots to the baby after birth. That transition can be jarring, like having a blanket ripped off. It can also create the sense that the physical, emotional, and mental health needs of the mother are a lower priority during a time characterized by extreme hormone swings, milk coming in, lack of sleep, and all sorts of other factors that can leave new parents feeling sad, anxious, exhausted, isolated, alienated, overwhelmed, and discombobulated. Perineums and surgical scars and nipples and pelvises hurt. It might not be easy to walk, to go up stairs, to pee, or to shower. And amid all that, there's suddenly a squalling, fragile little creature that needs constant attention. For all these reasons, and many others, postpartum depression and anxiety are common, affecting an estimated one in seven mothers in the US, but these conditions are largely ignored and undiagnosed.

The general consensus is that postpartum care in the US is woefully inadequate. Certainly, there are physiological and hormonal factors underlying postpartum depression, but there are also social ones that make the situation worse. The US is the only high-income country that does not guarantee paid leave to mothers after childbirth. One study found that one in four employed women returns to work within two weeks of giving birth and one in ten go back after four weeks. The lack of paid leave exacerbates financial stress and prevents people from taking the time they need to heal, to process, and to regain some semblance of equilibrium. It can also cause new mothers to feel swamped with feelings of shame, stress, fear, and guilt.

Carrie continued on, explaining that the hardest part of dealing with a perinatal mood disorder could be acknowledging the truth of the feelings and asking for help. Depending on the case, midwives (and other care providers) should be able to help connect clients with more specialized resources, such as talk therapy or psychiatry. For more minor cases, getting rest, carving out time for self-care, spending time with friends and other new parents, and accepting practical support, like dropped-off meals, could go a long way, but those measures were rarely simple or even remotely feasible when caring for a newborn. She also mentioned that physical and emotional health were tightly linked—it was hard to be in a good mood when feeling like an old cut of roast beef—and suggested a slew of items Jillian should have around for physical postpartum care, a flurry of words that sounded like a foreign language: Dermoplast, Frida, flange, HaaKaa, sitz bath. Jillian was familiar with all those terms but appreciated being guided through it all as if she wasn't. It made her feel like all the bases were being covered.

After that conversation, the group filed out of the bedroom and back into the living room, where everyone perched on chairs and couches. Chad crouched down to stoke the fire he'd built in the stove, while Carrie asked Jillian a few remaining questions, including what music she had on her birth playlist. Jillian said the baby seemed to really love the Police, Santana, and rap from the 2000s; she wanted to add some Talking Heads into the mix too. Jen remembered aloud how, at one birth, the family had blasted opera music the whole time. Carrie laughed and recalled how at the birth center in Tualatin, in the days before iPods and iPhones, the only music available was Jennifer's CD collection, which was entirely comprised of worship music with a few Loreena McKennitt ("eclectic Celtic") and Enya albums sprinkled in.

"I haven't been to an Enya birth since 1998," Marilyn said. "They always take so long." One birth story begat another and another. Before wrapping up, Marilyn asked what Jillian planned to do with the placenta. Although there is no hard scientific evidence to support it, many cultures and midwives believe that consuming placenta (often by dehydrating it and putting it into pill form) has benefits that include raising energy levels, boosting breast milk, leveling hormones, and lowering the chance of postpartum depression. Jillian said she would like to encapsulate it, and Jen offered to do it for her. Then Jillian inquired about everyone's dietary restrictions. She wanted to have meals and snacks prepared for the midwives to eat during the birth. When she envisioned her birth, she liked the idea of everyone hanging out in her home, chatting and snacking, like they were now. *There's a birth story for everything,* she thought. *And soon, I'll have one too.*

CHAPTER 21
T'Nika

Throughout her pregnancy, T'Nika spent a fair amount of time on the *What to Expect* app. It was fun to see what type of fruit or vegetable her baby was in terms of size, and she had joined a couple of message boards, both for people in the Portland area and for people who were due in the same month from around the country. She didn't post much herself—she was more of a lurker who occasionally hit the like button—but she enjoyed feeling linked to a larger community of people who were also pregnant and could validate any number of experiences, feelings, or random side effects she was facing. It was nice to know that she wasn't the only person dealing with round ligament pain or weird discharge. She also found it interesting to learn what others were experiencing during their prenatal care—how many ultrasounds they'd had, for instance, or how many times their cervix was checked—and use that to keep her own nerves in check. Whenever T'Nika started wishing she was getting more tests and checks and scans, because it felt like reassurance that she and the baby were healthy, a post would appear in her feed from someone who had their cervix checked and was told they had to be induced. That wasn't what she wanted, she reminded herself, as she kept scrolling.

More than anything, though, T'Nika found herself enthralled by the cultural trends that circulated on the forums. It was almost like watching an anthropological study happen in real time. One in particular that she noticed was the rise of 4D ultrasounds. No longer was a professional maternity photo shoot—looking ripe and fecund in a belly-hugging dress in front of a flowering tree—sufficient. Now, people were scheduling private sessions to take detailed images of babies in utero and then posting them on social media. The funny part was that the images were objectively weird-looking, almost like smushed little mummies or encapsulated aliens, but still people liked and commented, gushing over how "cute" the babies were. T'Nika might chuckle at the antics, but she understood the impulse that drove expectant mothers to try to visualize and document as much as they could. Sure, a 4D ultrasound might be a lot, but it reflected the desire for the baby on the inside—an odd combination of physical reality and abstract concept—to be manifested externally. To see it, rather than just feel it, and to share that experience with the world.

And then there was the forum drama. It was better than reality TV.

As with all things on the internet, the forums were a blend of kindness and chaos, nonsense and real information, judgment and support. They could show how factionalized people could be, how defensive, combative, or uninterested in posts that didn't align with their belief system. Sometimes people would lay out a fact, or an alleged fact, and someone else would say they were wrong. There were rousing debates with data points and opinions flying about, and plenty of misinformation. One poster asked if it was okay to drink a glass of wine and the hordes chimed in, some cheering, "Yes, girl, go for it, you do you," and others, aghast, fuming, responded, "Absolutely not, how could you even consider doing that to your baby?"

On occasion, though, people shared experiences or information that were beneficial. One woman who went into labor early posted a photo of her baby and said, "This is what a thirty-four-week baby looks like," a post that T'Nika found comforting. T'Nika knew that Black women were more likely to experience preterm labor, so seeing that photo reassured her that if she went into labor at thirty-four-weeks (when the baby "is as big as a pineapple"), everything could still turn out okay.

On the forums, T'Nika saw how many women felt lost, confused, and uncertain during pregnancy, buffeted by tailwinds of conflicting and contradictory information coming from all sides and not sure how to sort out what was legitimate from what wasn't. The app didn't make it easier to weather those winds, per se, but it was a place where they didn't have to be weathered alone. The forums were a reminder—a helpful one, as she made her way through her final trimester—that so many people had done this before her, and would continue to do so for long after.

When she was thirty-five-weeks pregnant, T'Nika opted to do a third-trimester ultrasound. She was confident the baby's head was down but eager for any opportunity to see her daughter and get more information. Once she knew which direction the baby was facing, it was fun to poke her belly and tickle where she thought the head was. It became a game between the two of them; sometimes the baby moved in response, as if indignant that T'Nika put her thumb in her face. T'Nika liked that the baby had spunk and that her personality was coming through. The ultrasound also showed that the baby already had hair. *Oh good,* T'Nika thought. *She won't be a baldy.*

During the ultrasound, the doctor provided an estimate for the baby's weight and the length of her femur (femur measurements can be used as a marker for growth and health), which T'Nika used later that week for a Target trip, strolling around the baby section with a ruler, measuring tiny onesies and pants to see what sizes would fit. Even though T'Nika knew that estimates about the baby's weight were just that—estimates—she clung to the number. *Six pounds, nine ounces.*

Two weeks later, the couple was back at Andaluz for an appointment with Marilyn. T'Nika's hair was in two braids, and her sage green sweatshirt matched the color of the walls. Her hot pink compression socks were pulled up over black leggings. While they waited in the lobby, T'Nika noticed Jillian standing behind the desk, wearing jeans and a long-sleeve striped shirt that stretched over her belly, teaching her maternity leave replacement how to use the computer system. T'Nika didn't know Jillian well, but it was amazing to see how they were having this experience at the same time. How they each looked and felt at this stage of their pregnancy. It was a cool thing to be connected by, and reminded her of the way she'd felt tethered to the people in the birth center where she and her siblings had been born.

Before long, one of the midwifery students, Harper, walked in, wearing a long, flowy paisley skirt and a band T-shirt with a cardigan over it. She waved at T'Nika and Daniel and called them into the Tierra room. When they entered, T'Nika placed her wallet, keys, and phone on the bedside table and sat on the bed while Daniel, in a gray hoodie and sneakers, perched with a cup of tea at the foot of the bed. Harper sat in an armchair with a laptop on her knees, ready to take notes. As everyone got settled, Marilyn swept into the room.

"I'm happy to see you," she told T'Nika, leaning against the tub with crossed arms as she took a longer look. "You look well!"

To start, T'Nika caught Marilyn up on everything that had gone on since she'd last seen her—the progress on the nursery, the death of their cat Kimet, starting the new job.

"Did you end up getting all the paperwork you needed to get more breaks at work?" Marilyn asked. "Are they going to give it to you?"

"Yes," T'Nika said. "And I'm starting some night shifts soon, which should be a little more low-key."

"How are you sleeping?"

"Last night, I had some Braxton-Hicks. They started at two thirty a.m. and were seven to eight minutes apart. They were keeping me up, so I showered and braided my hair because I didn't want it to be a mess if I was actually in labor."

"Sometimes Braxton-Hicks means the baby is getting lower and the cervix is ripening," Marilyn replied, "but it sounds like some part of you knew it might not be labor and you didn't need to call. That's good."

"I figured if it was labor, I was coming in anyway." T'Nika shrugged. Marilyn smiled before giving T'Nika a serious look.

"Now, honey," she continued with gravity. "I want to talk to you about your nipples."

T'Nika nodded. That was the main issue she wanted to discuss that day. Lately, she'd noticed her nipples were inverted (reminding her of the Pokémon character Dugtrio), which she knew could make it more difficult to breastfeed. At first, she'd thought that some internet research might help her figure things out, but when she looked at photos of other people's bodies, there seemed to be such a range, so she'd showed her own to Marilyn.

"Have you looked into nipple shells?" Marilyn asked. "Or is it nipple shields? Breast shells? Breast shields? Whatever they are called—"

"Breast shell," Harper chimed in.

Marilyn nodded in thanks, explaining that a breast shell went under the bra, to put constant pressure on nipples and release the inversion.

"Any idea how long you want to breastfeed?" she asked T'Nika.

"Not really," T'Nika replied. "As long as it works out, I guess."

"Well, the gold standard is six months exclusively," Marilyn said. "But sometimes babies have their other ideas. My daughter was just a few months old and pulling food off my fork. We want to build flexibility into all our plans, just like with labor." T'Nika agreed and said she hadn't set specific goals for breastfeeding because she didn't know what to expect. She planned to breastfeed but didn't want to have unrealistic expectations if, as Marilyn said, her body or the baby had other ideas. She would give it her best shot.

Breastfeeding, she knew, was yet another aspect of new motherhood that could be stressful and where opinions ran hot. A majority of new mothers—84 percent—start out breastfeeding, but by six months, the rate is under 60 percent. While there are salient benefits to breastfeeding, it is also a tremendously time-consuming, emotionally draining, and physically grueling practice that does not work out for everyone. Sometimes breasts don't produce enough milk or people develop mastitis. Some people have no way to pump in their workplace. For others, orienting their life around breastfeeding makes them miserable. Families must figure out, often on the fly, what works for them and their baby, weighing their particular circumstances and priorities. While Marilyn encouraged her clients to breastfeed, she was always careful to emphasize that other options existed and there was nothing wrong with using them, as long as everyone was healthy.

Over the course of the twentieth century, infant formula ascended as the superior, more scientific option. Breastfeeding hit a low in the early 1970s and then rates began to steadily climb. Today, breastfeeding is generally encouraged inside and outside of hospitals and promoted by organizations like the American Academy of Pediatrics, but resources like formula and donor milk are a lifeline for many families.*

"We'll just have all the tools, honey, and see what we need," Marilyn reassured her.

As the appointment continued, Marilyn asked T'Nika whether both her mother and Daniel's were planning to be present for the birth. T'Nika hoped so—they just had to figure out when to call them up from Eugene. Daniel's mom was retired, so her schedule was flexible, but T'Nika's mom was still an endoscopy technician and might not be able to come right away if, as T'Nika put it, "her scope was in someone." They talked more about T'Nika's swelling feet and compression socks, and then they ran through her vitals—blood pressure was at 112/70, and her pulse was 84 (both in healthy range).

"Are you taking iron?" Marilyn asked.

"Yes, Hema-Plex," T'Nika said. "Also I've been wanting to eat toothpaste because of the baking soda or, like, laundry detergent because it smells fresh."†

---

* In 2021, investigators identified multiple strains of the dangerous *cronobacter sakazakii* bacteria in a Michigan plant that produces 20 percent of the nation's baby formula supply, leading to a severe shortage.

† Pica, unusual cravings for nonfood items, can be a symptom of pregnancy.

Marilyn paused, seemingly surprised by the cravings. "That's weird, dear."

Everyone laughed.

"Have you had heartburn?"

"Oh yes," T'Nika said. "It was real bad two weeks ago."

"What did you do about it?"

"Suffered and drank water," T'Nika replied.

T'Nika then lay down on the bed and pulled up her shirt so Marilyn could examine her belly.

"Oh my gosh, look how this belly has changed," Marilyn marveled.

"I have all the fun coloring," T'Nika said, not sounding enthused as she peered at the shades of brown and beige striating over her baby bump. The baby visibly moved under Marilyn's hands as she palpated and measured. Thirty-eight inches, one inch for every week of gestation.

"Are you eating well?" Harper asked.

"Uh, yes?" T'Nika said. "I mean, I've been eating."

Daniel nodded. "Oh, she is," he said.

And was she drinking enough water? Having normal bowel movements? Were there any visual disturbances?

"Yes, I see stars a lot," T'Nika replied. "On Saturday, I saw stars after we ran some errands and Daniel asked if I remembered to eat my breakfast sandwich and I hadn't. He's my patroller."

"I'm glad he's keeping an eye on you," Marilyn said with a wink.

The remaining two orders of business were to review T'Nika's first- and second-choice birth suites: Solana, Marilyn read from the paperwork, followed by Clara. They also talked through her plans for the placenta. T'Nika had seen a way to make a print with it on Instagram and was interested in doing the same. She wasn't sure what type of paper to use, but because Daniel's mother was an artist, she had a generous stock of art supplies to choose from. Andaluz would handle the disposal; she didn't feel the need to eat, bury, or encapsulate it.

Before it was time to go, Marilyn and Harper asked if T'Nika would take a group B strep test, which would detect the presence of bacteria in the gastrointestinal tract that could cause complications during pregnancy and serious infections in newborns, if not treated with antibiotics. Harper handed T'Nika a swab and instructed her to swipe from her vagina to her anus and then put the swab into the sterile tube. T'Nika went into the bathroom and reemerged a minute later, handing the tube back to Harper. Then she stepped on the scale one last time so Marilyn could record her weight. She'd gained thirty-five pounds so far during pregnancy.

"You could beat me in wrestling," Daniel said with an impish grin.

T'Nika nudged him with her elbow as they walked out.

CHAPTER 22
Alison

In January, when she was thirty-four weeks along, Alison and Steve took part in a hallowed rite of pregnancy—the baby shower. Their friends Susan and Wes helped organize the event for a Saturday at noon, bringing over bunches of balloons, and biscuits and gravy for brunch. All the other guests participated on Zoom, and one upside of holding the event virtually was that Steve's family members were able to join from Michigan. Susan tried to position Alison on the couch so she faced the camera with the balloons arrayed behind her, but she balked. *Oh no,* she thought. *This is not good for my flashlight.*

At a recent prenatal appointment, Gina had shared the "flashlight trick," telling Alison to imagine her belly button was a flashlight and to be mindful of where it was aiming. Pointing the "flashlight" straight out or downward created space in the pelvis and encouraged the baby to get into the optimal position. It could also help reduce the chance of back labor, which is when the back of the baby's head presses against the spine and tailbone during labor, creating a seismic amount of pain. Since then, Alison had been mindful of where her flashlight was pointing anytime she sat down, but she didn't want to derail or complicate

Susan and Wes's vision for the shower. She decided not to worry about it, touched that so many people had pitched in to orchestrate and attend the event.

Alison and Steve kicked things off by giving the guests a tour of Theo's nursery and played games like decoding children's book titles by emoji sequences (for *The Very Hungry Caterpillar,* a caterpillar followed by all the things he ate; for *Where the Wild Things Are,* a cat, a crown, a sailboat, an island, and two devils) and "Who's more likely to" (Be nervous? Everyone said Steve). They played a few rounds of pregnancy trivia and there was a slide show with baby pictures of Alison and Steve. Alison's favorite was a photo from her own birth. Her mother's hair was perfectly coiffed at 1980s amplitude, and she had on a full face of makeup. She looked polished and beautiful. Alison's dad, meanwhile, looked worse for the wear, prompting a laugh from the attendees. She'd had the baby, but he looked like the mess.

Then, Alison and Steve opened gifts. They had created a registry on Amazon and received a laundry hamper meant for cloth diapers, a stroller, an adapter for the stroller to go in the car, a Mickey Mouse toy, baby hats, a basket for stuffed animals, a changing pad, more cloth diapers, a mobile to hang over the crib, a baby carrier, blocks to record the baby's age, swaddles, and more. Susan knit them a baby blanket with a sailboat pattern, and Alison's brother bought them a book called *You Are New,* which Alison adored and read twice that night.

The following weekend, the festivities continued. Alison and Steve ventured with Susan and Wes and a few other friends on a trip to Leavenworth, Washington, a quaint old-world Bavarian-style village in the Cascade Mountains, a five-hour drive away. Alison liked the idea of taking a trip before the baby came and had always wanted to go to Leavenworth, which was snowy and charming in the winter. She wasn't sure if it was okay or advisable to travel so close to her due date (most airlines have rules that prevent pregnant women from flying after thirty-six weeks), but she checked with the birth center and friends who had kids, and everyone said it was fine, especially since they were driving. Leavenworth was only two hours from Seattle in the unlikely event Alison needed to get to a hospital.

On the trip, Alison had no trouble keeping up with the group during a hike or staying up late chatting around the fireplace. She felt exhilarated and powerful—she was thirty-five weeks pregnant, and here she was, in the home stretch, hiking up a mountain. She almost couldn't believe how strong she felt. She could do this, and she was almost there.

A couple of weeks later, with the fun of the baby shower and trip to Leavenworth behind her, Alison turned her focus to getting organized for the baby's arrival. Her biggest and most pressing task was to finalize plans for her maternity leave. She had been granted up to twelve weeks of parental leave after the baby was born, and that would take her through the end of the school year, after which she had the summer off. Then, in January, the school district announced that it was moving from fully remote school to a hybrid model that blended in-person and online teaching. When she read the notice, her heart sunk. Teachers would be expected to return to the classroom, which Alison—nearing her due date during a pandemic in which schools were transmission points—was unwilling to do. The data on how Covid affected pregnant women and babies was still inconclusive, and if she tested positive for Covid when she went into labor, she would not be able to give birth at the birth center.

Upon closer reading, she learned that high-risk workers, including pregnant people, could apply to the state for a special accommodation. If she applied, it would enable her to start her maternity leave early, rather than returning to school, but she had to file additional paperwork to get approved. She had already prepared the letter for her standard maternity leave request, but now she needed a revised version that included specific language for the high-risk accommodation. She called the WHA network's general line and was connected to an advice nurse who worked as a generalist (meaning not specifically with the birth center), who told her somewhat brusquely that they wouldn't be able to help.

Alison was taken aback. What? How was that possible? She couldn't be the only patient with this kind of a request. If she couldn't get the letter, she would either have to go back to in-person school, which made her fear for her health, or take unpaid leave, which would be a financial hit. Both of those options were nerve-wracking. And even if the answer to her request was "No," for whatever reason, was it necessary for the nurse to be so abrupt and dismissive? Alison wasn't sure what to say or do and felt rejected and lost. She started to cry, which startled the nurse enough that she asked if there was anything else she needed. Alison, indignant and shook up, said yes. She was upset, and it would be nice if one of the midwives could call and check on her.

The nurse replied that it was unlikely anyone would call her that same night (it was 4:45 p.m.) and asked again if there was anything else Alison needed. Yes, she replied. She hadn't felt the baby move very much that day. What should she do? Alison was already agitated, so everything else—all the benthal concerns lurking deep below the surface—seemed amplified, rising inexorably toward the top. The nurse suggested that Alison lie down and do a kick count, looking for ten kicks in two hours. Once she tallied ten kicks, she should call back and let the birth center know.

Alison walked down the hall to the bedroom and heaved herself on top of the fluffy gray comforter. The late-afternoon light filtered through the windows, and she took deep breaths, going over and over the exchange in her mind. Alison knew her request hadn't been unreasonable or unfulfillable, and while she might be inordinately upset, she felt her frustrations were justified. Yet again, she felt resistance anytime she asked for something that deviated from protocol. She just wanted to be able to get a midwife on the phone directly, not call a central line and have a receptionist patch her through to a random advice nurse who told her midwives were unavailable. As she reflected, she continued to count kicks. Slowly, the feelings of frustration and fear seeped away in the quiet. Theo's movements were consistent and robust. Everything was fine.

When the two hours were up, Alison called WHA back. This time, she was connected to a midwife named Catherine, one of the higher-ups at the birth center. Alison explained the situation with the kick count and with the letter. Catherine immediately understood and told Alison to email her the letter with the required wording. She would get it taken care of.

At her prenatal appointment the next day, Gina handed Alison the letter, updated and revised as promised. Alison appreciated the quick turnaround, but this time, she decided to speak up and be honest with Gina that she was entertaining the possibility of moving her care elsewhere. Alison knew the midwives were busy with full schedules of other patients, but she needed to trust that her care team would be present when she needed them. She hadn't liked the care she received from the OB clinic in Vancouver during her miscarriage, but at least when she'd called them, she was able to get ahold of her doctor. She sometimes felt like she was on her own, and that troubled her.

Gina took everything in, listening closely to each of Alison's grievances before responding. She was sorry that Alison had encountered those barriers, she began. And, in fact, it wasn't the first time the issue had come up. The midwives knew patients wanted a direct line and had discussed getting their own answering service before; maybe this feedback would push them to do so. If Alison felt like moving care was the right choice for her, then Gina said she supported that decision, but she hoped she would stay.

Alison knew Gina's sympathy and concern were genuine, and she admitted that she couldn't imagine starting over with a new care provider with only four weeks to go until her due date. The chance that she'd find one she liked more than the midwives at the birth center, who she really did like, seemed highly unlikely. Leaving would be more stressful than staying, and Alison didn't want to introduce more anxiety into the situation. She was already overwhelmed by the shift to weekly prenatal appointments. Making time for them every week on top of her full-time job and graduate school *and* getting ready for the baby was stretching her thin. Gina reassured her that a lot of moms felt that way toward the end of pregnancy and offered to forgo next week's appointment, to Alison's relief, unless something came up in the meantime.

Later that night, Alison told Steve how her day had gone. When she was done, he gently suggested that maybe part of why she had been so upset had been due to unrealistic expectations. Yes, having a baby was probably the biggest thing that Alison had ever been through, but for the staff at the birth center, it was their everyday work. She was only seeing things from her own point of view, where her experience was at the center of her universe. That rationale made sense, Alison agreed, but *he* had to understand that she had put so much effort into finding a birth center practice where her needs were respected; to still feel sidelined and to question her choices after all that work was demoralizing. Steve got that, but he teased her for having a flair for the dramatic. Alison laughed. Maybe he was right. She had never thought of herself as being particularly dramatic or needy or anxious, but pregnancy seemed to bring out those traits in her, in varying degrees in different situations. Her emotions felt as though they were climbing over one another with no rhyme or reason, like puppies scrambling for the top of a pile. She hoped that once her maternity leave started, she would have time to relax and decompress, and maybe every little thing wouldn't feel so charged.

With the letter situation sorted, Alison started maternity leave in February, and one of her first tasks was to pack her suitcase for the birth center. The black suitcase, which she placed in the hall, had a bag of toiletries, including mascara (the more pregnant Alison got, the frumpier she felt, and mascara helped her feel less frumpy), and a bag of comfort items, including string lights with a battery pack and a framed photo of Alison and Steve. Then, there was a bag labeled "For Theo." In it was the baby blanket from Susan and two baby outfits—one from Alison's brother and his girlfriend and another from Alison's friend Elaine.

She also spent time working on graduate school assignments, writing essays, and finishing a grant proposal for her internship. She wanted to get as much work done as possible so she didn't fall too far behind, and as she wrapped up her projects, she thought a lot about how much, or in what ways, having a baby would affect her ambition. She recalled a conversation with a friend who said that once she had kids, her professional goals stopped feeling as important. Alison did not want that to happen to her. She knew her priorities would shift, and that was expected and okay. But she also knew that a perceived lack of ambition and commitment was part of what stigmatized working mothers in the first place. After reaching her goal of becoming a school principal, Alison envisioned earning her PhD someday. She had her eye on a program at the University of Michigan, where they would be close to Steve's family. Or maybe they could move to Mexico or Thailand or Berlin. She knew traveling with a child presented logistical hurdles, but it wasn't impossible. She wanted to be a good mother, but she didn't want her child to be her entire world to the exclusion of all else, or to make it smaller.

Although she had plenty of work to do, Alison made sure to savor leisure time on her maternity leave as well. She and Steve were enjoying the final moments with it just being the two of them. It felt like a romantic time in their marriage. They cooked dinner together and watched movies and sometimes hung out in the nursery, imagining what it would be like to have a baby. One night, Alison pulled on a pair of sweatpants and a small T-shirt that Steve had made her a few years before. Now, it didn't even reach below her belly button. She had become the "burrito mom," but it wasn't as bad as she'd anticipated all those months before. It meant they were close to the end.

With this realization, Alison felt like she'd emerged on the other side, into a place of equilibrium. Certainly there had been frustrations and emotional ups and downs along the way, but considering how wrecked she had been after her miscarriage experience, Alison thought she'd weathered the fluctuations rather well. She had gotten bolder in speaking up when something bothered her and, in some ways, she'd learned to let go a little. In nine months, she had evolved from someone who meticulously weighed out coffee beans and worried about every potential mistake to someone who strolled to her favorite coffee shop on sunny afternoons and ordered whatever she felt like. She no longer felt compelled to follow every single pregnancy rule and dicta to the letter, putting more trust in her own discretion and judgment. That felt like meaningful, personal growth, and she hoped it would stick with her once the baby was born.

CHAPTER 23
Jillian

By late February, Jillian still hadn't put her NARM paperwork in the mail. All the signatures were complete, but the further along she progressed in pregnancy, the more she felt shrouded in a mental fog. She'd once prided herself on her organizational skills, but now she kept forgetting tasks on her to-do list. Before she knew it, weeks had passed. It was exasperating, even more so because it was unlike her. Her mind had a million thoughts running through it, and while she had lots to do, she couldn't seem to get things done because of how tired she was. Her sleep had been fragmented because her body was so uncomfortable, and she spent half the night struggling to find a position that didn't ache.

At thirty-six weeks, she finally conceded it was unlikely she would get her application processed and take the test before the baby came. She was disappointed with herself and with the situation. If only she'd gotten it together, if only she'd pushed harder or moved faster, maybe she could have earned her certification. When she shared her disappointment with Jennifer, her boss told her not to worry—she had no doubts about Jillian's professional future. Juggling a baby and a midwifery career would be tough, but Jennifer had done it, as had most of the other Andaluz midwives. She even offered to cover the cost of the exam if Jillian couldn't afford it when the time came. Beyond wanting Jillian to succeed, Jennifer had her own stake in Jillian's certification—she was looking to hire a midwife or two to work full-time at the birth cottage in Dundee. A few members of her staff were retiring or moving away, and having the midwives circulate between the two Andaluz locations wasn't always convenient, especially for those who didn't live in the Willamette Valley. Jillian, who lived nearby, was an ideal candidate. And although it was technically a birth center, the cottage offered a kind of home-birth-away-from-home option that appealed to Jillian.

Others offered to pitch in as well. Jen, Jillian's friend and fellow Andaluz apprentice, said she could babysit when Jillian needed to study, and Chad pledged to take the day off work so he could watch the baby during the exam. Jillian had been feeling defeated, but the outpouring of support reassured her that she wasn't alone in trying to achieve her goals, and people believed in her. Once she let go of the compulsion to submit her application, it was like a burden had been lifted and she realized that all the emotional turbulence and pressure and self-doubt and anxiety she'd been channeling toward the NARM exam was about something deeper: a fundamental reckoning with all the ways in which her life was about to change.

Soon, how Jillian spent her time and where she focused her energy would be on someone other than herself, and that was daunting. The couple didn't have family who lived close by, childcare was outrageously expensive, and there were not many childcare options in their tiny town. Chad got only a few weeks off from his job and he earned a higher income than Jillian did, so it didn't make financial sense for him to stay home. Plus, Jillian planned to breastfeed, which required proximity to the baby.

All those factors meant that Jillian was going to be the primary caregiver, at least in the beginning. Jennifer had told her to take as long as she needed for maternity leave, and not to set a hard timeline for returning because she didn't know how she would feel. Jillian was grateful that she had the ability to stay home, as so many people had no choice but to go back to work right away, but she also anticipated the shift of being home, alone, with the baby, all day, every day, without going to work, would be a difficult one. Isolating, probably, and wearisome.

Jillian had started working out of the house as a teenager and, since then, had never been home without a job to go to. She wondered with trepidation how she would handle it. What would it be like? Would it change how others viewed her? She had friends and family members who were full-time caregivers for their kids and had heard stories about snide remarks they received, from "What do you do all day?" to "It must be nice to stay home and not work." Through her years of nannying, Jillian had also seen how working mothers faced the flipside of that stigma. In one family, the mom had had a career in international aid and traveled all around the world on business trips. She was successful and adventurous and had close relationships with her partner and kids, and yet she sometimes received snide comments from other parents at school or on the playground for spending so much time away, as if it meant she wasn't truly committed to her family.

Really, there was no way to win. Between nannying and midwifery, Jillian had seen how every choice would elicit disapproval or judgment from somewhere and perfection was an illusion. Best intentions aside, parenting required winging it, adapting in the moment, and responding to the individuality of the kids. As long as they were cared for and loved and their needs were met, Jillian thought, that was all that mattered. And that, she knew she could do.

The first week of March was Jillian's last week of work at Andaluz, two weeks before her due date. Due dates are really due months—the majority of babies are born between thirty-eight and forty-two weeks and the babies born within that range have better outcomes, so due dates are estimated at forty weeks. First-time moms generally go a week past their due date, and Jillian was expecting to do the same. She told members of her extended family that her due date was two weeks later than it was because she didn't want people peppering her with questions about whether she'd gone into labor.

On Thursday, March 4, Jillian spent the morning driving around Portland to visit families she'd nannied for who wanted to see her, wish her good luck, and give her their hand-me-down baby gear, including an expensive ergonomic high chair that Jillian could never have afforded on her own. She arrived at Andaluz midday, and after helping with a newborn hearing screen appointment, she settled in to wait for Marilyn to call her into her own prenatal appointment. Marilyn had attended a birth that morning, so she'd been at Andaluz since 1:00 a.m. and was running behind schedule, but Jillian didn't mind. While she waited, she drank a murky dark green liquid out of her water bottle and chatted with the other midwives and students circulating through the kitchen to grab snacks or fill out paperwork, regaling them with a story about the time Chad tried to take her bow hunting at night and how scared she'd been of the dark.

"You're looking better today, honey," Marilyn told her once they were seated in the Solana suite. "I've been fretting about you."

"I wasn't feeling good on Tuesday, so I decided to splurge on thirty-dollar chlorophyll powder," Jillian replied, looking between Marilyn and the student assistant, Samantha. "It was expensive and I wasn't sure if I wanted to spend the money, but I'm glad I did because it's definitely making me feel better. Also, this is my last day, so now I can relax and prepare for the baby—and, Marilyn, you're almost done too!"

"We tried to calculate last week how many babies Marilyn has delivered," Samantha said with a hint of pride. "We estimated forty-five babies a year for forty years. That's, like, eighteen hundred babies."

"Oh no, it can't be that many," Marilyn protested.

"Your hands have helped so many people into this world," Jillian said.

Marilyn held her hands out in front of her. "I guess they have."

Jillian took another big swig of the green drink.

Samantha asked Jillian if she'd been feeling the baby move (yes) and if she was eating well (yes, craving lots of sweets). She asked her about bowel movements and headaches and swelling, and Jillian said her hands were a bit swollen, but she assumed it was from organizing the Andaluz basement earlier in the week.

Once the questions were done, Jillian lay on the bed and pulled her shirt up and her waistband down. Marilyn walked over to take her pulse and blood pressure. Then, she palpated the belly, noting that the baby was either ROT (right occiput transverse) or ROA (right occiput anterior). ROT means the back of the baby's head (the occiput) is toward the mother's right and it faces and kicks toward the left side; ROA means the back of the baby's head is toward the mother's front and slightly rotated to the right. Babies can also face the other way, for LOT (left occiput transverse) or LOA (left occiput anterior); or they can be in the occiput posterior position, in which the back of the baby's head is in the pelvis, also referred to as "face-up" or "sunny-side up."*

"I feel like my belly just went *poof*!" Jillian said, her hands expanding outward as Marilyn's hands moved around her. "And I finally know what 'lightning crotch' feels like," referring to the sharp shooting pain in the vagina that people often feel late in pregnancy.

"Carrie told me that people in the UK call them 'fanny daggers,'" Samantha said with a giggle.

After the standard questions, Jillian said she had one incident she wanted to bring up. While grocery shopping on Saturday, she had been in the produce section, reaching to grab a box of dates. There had been water on the floor near the shelf, and no caution sign, so Jillian hadn't seen it. She'd slipped but caught herself on the shelf right before she hit the floor. The only victim had been a jar of minced garlic, but the sound and the sight of a heavily pregnant woman falling attracted a fair amount of attention.

"I was more embarrassed than anything," Jillian explained. "It made such a mess." She was sure everything was fine but felt it was important to tell them nonetheless.

---

* Occiput posterior position can lead to increased risk of complications and interventions.

Marilyn made sympathetic sounds and agreed that it was good to know as she moved to grab more equipment. Then, she said it was time to listen to the baby.

The heartbeat came through loud and clear on the Doppler.

"It feels like I was just upstairs with you looking for a heartbeat for the first time," Marilyn said with a kind smile, looking Jillian in the eyes. "Aren't you just so excited to know when labor will start?"

"It's here all of a sudden," Jillian murmured. "With clients, it always feels so long."

She looked toward the monitor, listening to the rhythm. She was about to give birth not just to a baby, but to a new family, and to a new self. She'd seen it at just about every birth she'd ever been to—how something alchemical happened to new parents, how they melted into puddles of love. Anthropologists refer to the transition as "matrescence," the psychological passage into parenthood, and as with adolescence, her mind and body would never be the same again. *I'll still be Jillian,* she thought, listening to the beats from the Doppler. *But part of my old self will probably die in the fire of birth.* Maybe it was cheesy, but she kept thinking of the metaphor of the phoenix, a new being rising from ashes. What would that new version of her be like? What parts of herself would stay, and which would be discarded?

In a couple of weeks, she would find out.

CHAPTER 24
T'Nika

By late February, T'Nika was ready to go on leave. She had only two night shifts left to complete, and they were proving to be physically and emotionally grueling. There had been one patient who had made T'Nika feel particularly vulnerable and unsafe, a large middle-aged man who had been violent upon entry to the hospital for complications from a drug addiction, and even after he was discharged, she felt tense and rattled. She wanted to be at home, relaxing and resting, not worrying about navigating patients and workplace dynamics. At full term, she felt stretched in every way, like the only thing preventing her from bursting was a piece of tissue paper. Her maternity scrub pants, which had been too big when she'd first bought them, were now too tight and left marks across her belly. She wore her tightest pair of compression socks to prevent swelling and showed coworkers how her "squishy" ankles still bubbled over her shoes. Someone joked about requisitioning a wheelchair for her to use for the night. Luckily, there weren't many patients and she felt free to rest as needed, propping her feet up on a trash can at the nurses' station as she chatted with her fellow nurses.

During the final stretch of her last shift, T'Nika had one patient on the floor who was her primary responsibility, a young Black woman in her mid-twenties named Jada. Jada had been a nursing student but dropped out of school when her daughter was born, though, as she explained to T'Nika, she hoped to go back someday. Jada took an immediate shine to T'Nika, asking questions about her pregnancy and her nursery setup. She also asked clinical questions, following each step T'Nika took and asking her to explain what she was doing and why as she switched IVs or changed dressings. T'Nika answered each one, indulging her curiosity because she hoped the encouragement might play a small part in inspiring Jada to return to nursing school someday, just as the school nurse in Boston had done with her.

In the morning, before her shift ended, T'Nika received a page from the nurses' station. Jada had called asking if T'Nika could come to her room. When T'Nika walked in, Jada looked at her with a smile.

"This is for you," she said, holding out a small bundle. "You were so nice last night, thank you so much."

T'Nika looked more closely. It was a cream-colored macramé hanging in a half-moon shape. T'Nika had mentioned that most of the furniture in the baby's room was white with a celestial theme, so Jada had spent the night making an accessory to match. T'Nika was moved. *This is why I do what I do,* she thought as she gathered her things to go home for the next few months. *And this is what I want to come back to.*

Maternity leave gave T'Nika time to run errands and finish up things around the house to get ready for the baby, but it also gave her time for some much-needed self-care. She got a manicure and pedicure and had her hair done. She lounged around and watched episodes of *The Bachelor,* got back into the rhythm of practicing her viola, and did some light yoga.

She also worked on her birth playlist. Music was important to her and integral to her life, and what she played during her birth would have an impact on the mental state she hoped to achieve. T'Nika was a "bass-head." Music that was too mellow allowed her mind to wander; heavy bass, although a little more intense, calmed her down. It helped her find her center, focus, and get done what she needed to get done. That was the mode she wanted to be in for the birth. She created her playlist with a mix of bass and ambient music from *Lord of the Rings*—she and Daniel had rewatched the series together during her pregnancy—and video games. The music soothed her and provided a background story her mind could sink into.

Labor snacks were also a priority. Andaluz had food on hand that both she and Daniel could eat, but they liked the idea of bringing their own favorites. They were devoted string cheese lovers, so that made the cut, and T'Nika planned to buy cups of yogurt from Trader Joe's in her favorite flavors—mango and peach cream. (The challenge would be not eating all of them before contractions began.) Daniel loved jerky and even though it required some gnawing, which maybe wouldn't be appealing for her during labor, she knew it would be a helpful quick hit of salt and protein. If she had time to make it, she also wanted to bring some of her homemade granola.

As she neared her due date, T'Nika also reconsidered her desire to use nitrous oxide for pain relief. She had watched videos online and observed the process of inhaling nitrous during labor, which required taking the mask on and off, on and off. To her, it looked like relief pretty much ended once you stopped inhaling, which seemed like a hassle. When coping with the pain, and whatever other sensations birth would entail, she did not want to be worrying about where the mask was and how often to put it on or take it off. T'Nika had never had nitrous before and didn't know how her body would react. Plus, it cost $500, regardless of how much she ended up using. She didn't want to spend that money only to discover she didn't want or need it.

As she neared forty weeks, her nerves about the birth itself subsided. Birth, T'Nika knew, wasn't something she could control, and that powerlessness somehow made her feel less anxious. What she was most worried about was the fact that soon she'd have a baby to take care of, which was surprising given all the experience she had with babies from her siblings and nieces and nephews, not to mention her years as an infant-toddler teacher. But she knew it would be different with her own child. Pregnancy could be an insane adventure, but really it was only the prelude to the actual adventure. The finish line was the starting point.

Worries aside, she enjoyed contemplating what kind of mother she would be and how she would parent. During her second trimester, she and Daniel had watched a series of documentaries about child brain development. Daniel majored in psychology in college, and T'Nika had loved her developmental psychology classes, so they were both fascinated by the subject. One film talked about how mouse mothers who actively groomed their babies tended to have babies who grew up to groom their babies too. A mouse mother who did the opposite had babies who followed suit. In one experiment, a mouse baby was taken away from the grooming biological mother and put with a different mouse mother who didn't groom as much. Did they inherit the proclivity to groom, or was it a function of their early environment? The mouse babies grew up mimicking the mouse mother who raised them, not their biological mouse mother. T'Nika thought about that a lot. She had never been that physically affectionate with family or friends, but she wanted to be a mouse mother who groomed her baby.

"It looks like the baby has dropped a lot," Marilyn said during their next, and maybe final, prenatal appointment on March 16.

T'Nika adjusted herself on the bed in the Tierra suite, looking down at her belly, which now protruded out in an oblong cone shape.

"Yeah, it's . . . weird-looking," she replied. "We took a picture of me resting a cereal bowl on it the other night."

Daniel pulled out his phone to show Marilyn. In the image, T'Nika was sitting on the couch. He had angled the camera from below, so her belly looked extra huge.

As they continued running through updates, T'Nika told Marilyn that the baby had been in an uncomfortable position for a while, huddled over on one side, but one night while lying in bed, she'd managed to get her to move. Since then, she'd felt much spryer, able even to keep up with Daniel when they went for walks. Earlier that day, she spent hours doing karaoke by herself, singing Rihanna, Michael Jackson, Seal, and *The Wiz*'s soundtrack.

Marilyn asked if they had any questions, and T'Nika said Daniel was curious about dates.

"What do you mean?" Marilyn said, unsure if she meant a calendar or the fruit.

"If labor doesn't start before a certain time," T'Nika clarified.

Marilyn explained that Andaluz's postdate protocols started at forty-one weeks and three days. If labor hadn't started by then, there were steps the midwives could take to "push the river," including herbs, castor oil, and "midwives brew," a formula of almond butter, apricot nectar, lemon verbena tea, and castor oil. Foley blubs, which were inserted into the cervix, were another option. Marilyn said that she didn't conduct vaginal exams at every appointment (a more standard practice in regular OB) but offered to send T'Nika home with nitrazine papers, so she could test herself for amniotic fluid.

T'Nika also asked Marilyn if they could peek into other rooms in the birth center for a refresher on what they looked like. There was a family who had given birth that morning still in the Solana room, but Marilyn said they could go look at the Clara, which had also interested T'Nika because of its privacy and the common space for family. That common room was nice to have, Marilyn said, because at the birth that morning, six people—not including the woman giving birth or the midwives—had all crowded into the Solana suite. The imminently expecting mother ended up going into the bathroom to find peace and quiet and gave birth in there. T'Nika shook her head. She wanted her and Daniel's families to be present, but she didn't want people milling around or getting in her way.

Then Marilyn told T'Nika to lie back on the bed and lift up her shirt. She palpated and pulled out a measuring tape.

"I just love your belly so much. It kind of looks like Mount St. Helens—it's up and down, with no peak. It's measuring at forty-three. You look grand."

As she walked out of the birth center, T'Nika thought how strange it was that that might have been her last prenatal appointment. She hoped it was, anyway. At the beginning of her third trimester, she had worried about what would happen if the baby came early. Now, she was worried about what would happen if the baby was late. *Great, here goes another night,* she thought at the end of each day, another without a sign of actual labor. She had started waking up every one to two hours with Braxton-Hicks contractions; sometimes it was hard to get back to sleep afterward, or just as she fell back asleep, another contraction rolled through. She was already pretty tired and really hoped she didn't have to keep going for another week or two.

CHAPTER 25
Alison

Alison's due date, March 3, came and went. It began at 3:30 a.m., with contraction pains that felt stronger and more frequent than Braxton-Hicks. She had lain in bed for two hours, unable to fall back asleep and not feeling great. Finally, at 5:30 a.m., she got up to make French toast and work on a grad school paper that was due in a few days. Her professor had said it wasn't a big deal if she couldn't submit before the baby came, but she wanted to get it done if she could.

As she moved around the house, she ate a few dates. She had been trying to force herself to eat six every day, but she hated the taste and texture and usually only managed to choke down three. She hoped the frequent Braxton-Hicks contractions were a sign the baby was coming soon. On a recent afternoon, she'd watched a forty-five-minute YouTube video of a woman in Tennessee who was in labor for five days and ended up having a surgical birth. It was hard to wrap her mind around being in labor for five days, but overall, the video made her feel weirdly at peace about the prospect of a cesarean. After five days of labor, the option to go into the operating room might feel welcome. Like an escape hatch.

As the intermittent contractions continued, Alison felt a weird mix of wanting them to stop, because they were annoying, and wanting them to ramp up, because that would mean she was in labor.

She had asked Gina to check her cervix at her most recent appointment, and it was soft, open about the size of a fingertip. The baby, too, had been low. Alison didn't find the cervical check painful, which Gina said meant she had a high pain tolerance—all good signs—but Alison's apprehension about the realities of labor remained. She wondered if she'd bitten off more than she could chew. How could she know if she'd be able to make it through a birth without anesthesia? Had she been overly confident about her ability to manage whatever pain might occur? Was she being naive? What if she'd made a mistake? Most of the people in her world seemed to think of her choice to go to a birth center and forgo an epidural as akin to fire walking or polar plunging—a trial of mettle and fortitude, an unfathomable invitation to unnecessary suffering. Alison didn't think of it as any of those things. She had mainly wanted to avoid interventions that might lead to a C-section, which, from the outset, she had thought of in terms of her experience with the D&C. She assumed that going into an operating room would be the result of something going wrong during labor, which was terrifying, or the result of a doctor or hospital system trying to pressure her into a surgery that was unnecessary, which was also terrifying.

Whenever Alison verbalized these fears to her mother, she had been reminded that both Alison's mother and grandmother had had healthy hospital births and delivered their children by C-section. Alison didn't find that reassuring—what she feared wasn't the surgery itself, so much as the circumstances that might ultimately lead to it. Alison had always interpreted her mother's reminders as a form of disapproval of her decision not to give birth in a hospital, but now, as she reflected on just how personal birth decisions were, she wondered if perhaps the reverse was true. Maybe her mom felt that Alison's decision to go to a birth center was a rejection of *her* choices, a critique and judgment about *her* beliefs and experiences. Maybe, Alison considered, she had been too quick to dismiss what her mom was trying to tell her. Maybe she hadn't given her mother enough credit, or the space to explain to her how her C-section births had been just as compassionate, moving, or beautiful as Alison's ideal.

Continuing that line of thought, Alison realized that there was a universe in which she could have a cesarean and look back on the experience in a positive light. That hadn't really occurred to her before, until her mom's words sunk in. It was fair to be disappointed if things didn't work out as planned, but Alison would only make that disappointment worse by being too rigid. If she needed to transfer to the hospital, she would have to roll with the punches, recognize the expertise of the people around her, and make the best of the situation. And depending on the reason for the transfer, Alison would still be in a nurse-midwifery program in a progressive hospital that had cordless monitoring and big birth tubs, just like the birth center. She had to keep an open mind.

These internal debates—and the Braxton-Hicks—stayed with her for another week. Even though Alison knew that due dates were estimates, it was still an odd feeling to have passed the forty-week mark by a wide margin and still not seem any closer to giving birth. Obviously, the baby would come out at some point, but when? How?

To monitor the situation, she was scheduled for an ultrasound appointment at the birth center, followed by a prenatal. The ultrasound was quick, fifteen minutes or so, and during the second appointment, she and a midwife she was meeting for the first time discussed induction protocols. The risk of perinatal mortality and stillbirth increases after forty-two weeks, the midwife explained, so patients who went past forty-two weeks were transferred to the Providence hospital to be induced. She advised Alison to schedule an induction because the following Tuesday, March 16, was the last day that she could give birth at the birth center.

Alison walked out of the birth center in tears and called her doula from the parking lot. It was hearing the word "stillbirth" that shook her. It felt like an invocation or omen, as if someone had uttered "Macbeth" in a theater.

Katherine explained to Alison that the midwife didn't mean that the risk of stillbirth was increasing now, at that very moment, with each passing hour—which was how Alison had interpreted the warning—but that it would after forty-two weeks, which was why it made sense to schedule an induction in advance. It was a just-in-case, not a surrender.

"It seems like you're waiting for them to say that everything will be fine and turn out great," Katherine told her smoothly. "They won't say that, but that doesn't mean it won't work out. I will be there with you, Steve will be with you, and we will do everything to give you a natural birth."

The next day, Alison called to schedule the induction for Wednesday, March 17, at Providence. The nurse who helped her make the arrangements was peppy and positive on the phone—"Oh my gosh, how exciting, you are going to have a leprechaun baby!" she'd exclaimed—and her enthusiasm reminded Alison that hospitals weren't necessarily the dens of terror she sometimes made them out to be in her head.

Later that afternoon, Alison walked to the coffee shop and sat at a wrought iron table on the patio, soaking up the early-spring sun. It was unseasonably warm enough that she ordered an iced coffee and didn't need a jacket over her white long-sleeve T-shirt and black jeans. She sipped her coffee and then walked home to get her car and drive to acupuncture. During the appointment, Alison felt a pulsating sensation in her abdomen. She also felt wetness in her underwear. It wasn't discharge or urine, but it was . . . something.

After the session, Alison had planned to go see some friends, but given the various physical sensations—the contracting, the moistness—she thought it wiser to go straight home. She didn't want to be separated from Steve if something was about to happen, especially not during rush hour. When Alison walked into the house, Steve was surprised to see her back so soon.

"I think my water broke," she said.

CHAPTER 26
Jillian

On Saturday, March 20, Jillian woke up on her due date feeling like crud. She hadn't slept well, and though Chad was usually the first one to wake up and take the dogs for a walk, she had been up first with cramping.

"I can't lay down," she told him as they both started to get out of bed. "I feel things."

"Maybe it's the beginning of labor?" he replied.

Jillian wasn't so sure. She was exhausted, irritable, and achy, but she knew that first-time moms often think labor is starting when it isn't. She texted Jen to ask what early labor felt like, and Jen replied it could be hard to tell. There was a range of symptoms, but Jillian would know if she was in labor.

Jillian didn't want to jump to conclusions. That was a rookie error. She and Chad took Diesel and Paisley for a ten-minute walk up to a small, family-owned cemetery near their house. The month before, a big ice storm felled a huge tree, and the owners said they could take the firewood for free if they chopped it up. While Chad chopped, Diesel and Paisley ran around, and Jillian thought about all the things they had to do that day.

When he was done, Jillian suggested they drive to the grocery store. What she was feeling now definitely felt like something, and she wanted to buy Prosecco and snacks for the midwives and oat milk for coffee, in case it was labor. As she walked around Fred Meyer, the contractions became more pronounced.

When they arrived back at home, Jillian got into the bathtub, still not sure if it was prodromal or "real" labor. She got out around 7:00 p.m. to eat dinner and realized the contractions were closer together, increasing in intensity and frequency so much that Jillian had to lean over and focus through them. There wasn't a dramatic moment of her water breaking or a contraction hitting hard out of nowhere. Instead, the subtle pressure and cramping she'd felt that morning mounted until it was undeniable.

She was in labor. The baby was coming. This was it.

CHAPTER 27
T'Nika

T'Nika could sense that labor was about to start before it did. Years as an athlete, along with her deep understanding of her body from years of health issues and her nursing training, made her intimately and acutely attuned to even the subtlest twinges and pangs. When something changed, she noticed.

It began on the morning of Wednesday, March 17. T'Nika and her mom were running errands when she experienced a strong wave of cramps. She had also been leaking what looked like a combination of watery discharge and mucus, going through sanitary pads at a rapid rate. T'Nika and her mother had swung by Andaluz to pick up the pH strips that tested for amniotic fluid, but the test was negative.

The next afternoon, when she went to the bathroom, she felt something strange and looked in the toilet. There was a big glob of goo there, and in her panty liner. She touched the substance, and it was thick and sticky, almost like a jellyfish. T'Nika realized that it must be her mucus plug.

She texted Marilyn that she was having contractions about six to ten minutes apart, which had the intensity of strong period cramps. Marilyn replied that what she was describing sounded like early, irregular labor. All she could do was relax for the time being, and Tracy, the current midwife on call, would check in with her throughout the evening.

Throughout the rest of Wednesday and Thursday, T'Nika continued to have irregular contractions between six and ten minutes apart. Tracy had advised her not to count them too closely, and instead try to rest because early labor could last for a while. T'Nika puttered around the house, doing small tasks and chores and hanging out with Daniel and her mom. Occasionally, she had to stop what she was doing when a contraction hit, but overall, the pain wasn't incapacitating. She managed to sleep that night, waking up only a few times to change positions.

On Friday morning, T'Nika texted Tracy and asked if she was still on duty. Tracy said that she was, and Marilyn would be back on duty that evening. T'Nika's contractions continued to build in intensity and frequency. What had been mild cramping tightened into a viselike clench that seized and released her. At 9:00 p.m., Marilyn checked in, and T'Nika said she was still contracting and uncomfortable. She was also seeing brownish-pinkish stains on her sanitary pads, which she knew was likely from blood vessels popping as her cervix dilated.

Marilyn told T'Nika to hydrate and get some sleep, but T'Nika could no longer sleep through the pain. She called Marilyn twice more that night, unsure of what to do. Her contractions hurt so much, and now the pain was everywhere, unavoidable, and all-consuming. Relentless. Remorseless. Marilyn suggested that T'Nika hop in the bathtub, so between 2:00 and 3:00 a.m., T'Nika took a bath. It helped, but every time T'Nika tried to get out, the contractions knocked her with fresh agony all over again, pulling her back like Sisyphus to the bottom of the mountain. The pain was so acute, she wondered if she was having back labor, or if this was just how labor felt. She only got out of the tub to use the toilet, but it was difficult to make herself sit down. She waited for dawn to come, even though it brought no promise of relief.

On Saturday morning at 10:00 a.m., Marilyn told T'Nika to come to Andaluz. The center usually advised clients to come in once their contractions were three to four minutes apart, each lasting for a minute, and holding to that pattern for an hour (the 3-1-1 or 4-1-1 rule). T'Nika's contractions hadn't yet hit that benchmark, but she'd been in early labor at home for days and it seemed like an appropriate time to check on her progress.

The prospect of driving across town was unappealing, but T'Nika wanted to see Marilyn and, hopefully, get validation that things were moving. She and Daniel clambered into the car and drove over the river to Andaluz. When they arrived, Marilyn checked T'Nika's cervix in the Solana suite. She was three centimeters dilated. *After all that time and struggle, and just three measly centimeters?* T'Nika exhaled a sigh of exhaustion. It was going to be a long day.

Marilyn offered a choice: T'Nika was welcome to go back home and continue to labor there, or she could stay at the birth center. After discussing it with Daniel, she decided to stay. They were already there, and home had become a site of stagnation. Maybe a change of scenery would help.

After a few hours, Marilyn suggested T'Nika go for a walk. T'Nika, Daniel, and her mother ventured out to the Condor stairs, a steep, heavily forested stairway that leads up the hill to OHSU. T'Nika was skeptical that she was capable of the climb, as her contractions were frequent and strong. She had stopped counting, but had to pause whatever she was doing to breathe through them. The prospect of moving things along, though, was powerful motivation. Her mom took one of her arms, and Daniel took the other. Slowly, ever-so-slowly, they went step-by-step up the stairs. When a contraction rolled through, T'Nika stopped and leaned on them for support, gripping and squeezing their arms until the wrenching passed and she could climb up one more stair. They listened to music as they went, and despite the pain, T'Nika started to appreciate the walk. It felt almost ceremonial. She enjoyed breathing the fresh air and seeing the dewy green leaves, sandwiched by the people she loved most.

To distract her, T'Nika's mother told her that she and T'Nika's dad had ventured out on a walk for the same reason, hoping to encourage labor along when she was pregnant with T'Nika. They had intended to do a short loop, but after about three miles, when she was ready for the walk to be over, they realized they had walked three miles in one direction and had no choice but to walk those same three miles back.

T'Nika told herself that if her mom could walk six miles, she could at least make it to the top of the stairs. And they did, but when they reached the top, T'Nika looked at the length and pitch of the stairway with dread. She had no faith she could make it all the way back down.

"You are going to have to bring the car around," T'Nika said. "I don't know how to get the car up here, but I don't know how I will get down those stairs."

"We will make it down," her mother said. And they did.

CHAPTER 28
Alison

Alison and Steve cooked dinner, and as they went about their usual nightly routine, Alison could feel the flow of liquid getting heavier. She and Steve decided to call the birth center to let them know, and the midwife who answered told them to come in. They arrived around 9:00 p.m. It was after hours and the building was dark, the parking lot empty. An assistant let them into the front waiting room, and from the couch, Alison could hear a woman laboring down the hall, screaming and making sounds reminiscent of a jungle-cat fight. The dark and empty building, combined with the ambient shrieks, made her feel like she was in a horror movie, or at the very least intruding on someone else's personal experience. She wondered if they should leave—stand up, walk out, and return in the morning. She assumed her water broke, but nothing else had happened in the time since. Maybe she was wrong. Steve thought they should stay, at least until they checked in with a midwife. After forty-five minutes, the hollering stopped. A hush fell over the building. Then Kori, the on-call midwife, emerged.

"Welp, we just had a baby," she said. "Sorry to keep you waiting."

"Oh, it's okay," Alison replied sheepishly. "I feel really silly that I'm even here. I don't think my water broke."

"We're going to check it out," Kori said with a smile. "The woman who just had her baby was the same deal. She came in, wasn't sure, and now she has a baby."

Kori brought Alison back to an exam room and explained that the first step was to test for amniotic fluid using a swab and a pH test. It barely even touched Alison's vagina before it started to change colors.

"It's dark blue," Kori said. "That's a good sign."

Next, she did a fern test, another way to check for amniotic fluid. It took about twenty minutes to analyze, but Kori confirmed that Alison's water had broken. She took Alison into one of the exam rooms and hooked her up to a monitor to perform a nonstress test to check the baby's heart rate and well-being before the onset of labor.

Alison lay on the bed, atop a white quilt and coral pillow in the same clothes she'd worn earlier that day, trying to stay calm. As she worked, Kori told Alison that they were officially on the clock; she needed to start active labor within twenty-four hours, or, per WHA's protocol, they would admit her to the hospital due to a heightened risk of infection. They used the first sign of fluid, around 4:00 p.m. after Alison's acupuncture appointment, as their start time. That meant Alison had until 4:00 p.m. on Friday, March 12, and in the meantime, they were going to send her home until things progressed further.

When Alison asked what she could do to bring on labor, Kori gave her a few suggestions, including consuming a concoction of verbena tea, castor oil, almond butter, and apricot juice. If Alison wanted to be more aggressive, Kori added, she could blend castor oil with ice cream and milk. Alison could also sit on her birth ball and use her breast pump, alternating fifteen minutes per breast for sixty to ninety minutes, and was advised to "ambulate." Kori encouraged Alison to go to acupuncture the next day as well, as her body clearly responded to it, and throughout the day she should be monitoring her temperature, to make sure it didn't go over 100.4 degrees, which could be a sign of infection.

When they left the birth center, it was 11:30 p.m. Alison texted Katherine to fill her in and ask where they might find castor oil, especially at that late hour. Katherine responded quickly that there was a twenty-four-hour Walgreens nearby. At the pharmacy, Steve teasingly reminded Alison about how she had wanted to slink out of the birth center unseen. And now look where they were. When they got home, Alison called Katherine again, who advised her to be careful with the castor oil. It could cause diarrhea and vomiting, so she should take it only if she really needed it. Alison decided to take one ounce that night and see what happened. She used her breast pump and was excited to see colostrum, a rich milky fluid that emerges before breast milk comes in. With those tasks complete, Alison went to sleep.

At 3:00 a.m., she woke up with her stomach bucking and ran to the bathroom to throw up, just barely making it to the toilet. Then, for the next half hour, strong contractions barreled through like a storm front. They were painful but bearable. Alison welcomed them as a sign of labor, though she could have done without the puking. Once the surge passed, she was able to go back to bed and fall back asleep.

At 5:00 a.m., she woke up again, this time with the worst diarrhea of her life. Through the battery of vomiting and bowel movements, Alison searched frantically on her phone for an acupuncture place that opened early and could squeeze her in that morning. At 8:30 a.m., she got ahold of a practice in Southeast Portland that offered a 9:00 a.m. appointment. She grabbed her coat and dashed out the door as fast as she could.

Thirty minutes later, as she sat quietly in a room with needles sticking out of her, she realized the contractions had stopped. The surge from the night before seemed to be a fluke, a tease caused by the castor oil. She could feel the time ticking by, each minute moving her closer to the 4:00 p.m. deadline.

When Alison got home from acupuncture, she and Steve walked for a mile and a half on a trail near their house. Nothing happened. They went to the grocery store and then cooked macaroni and cheese. Nothing happened. She bounced on the birth ball and took a shower. Nothing happened. She used the breast pump again, hoping nipple stimulation would help kick labor into gear. Still nothing. It was 2:00 p.m., and she was starting to stress out.

Alison called Katherine, who pointed out that while Alison had first felt wetness around 4:00 p.m., it wasn't until 7:00 p.m. that the fluid had become conspicuous enough to prompt Alison to call the birth center. Alison wondered if that was the better way to look at it. She didn't want to fudge the facts, especially if safety was a concern, but she ultimately felt that Katherine was probably right. The wet feeling at 4:00 p.m. was minor and constituted the earliest, most conservative estimate. Nervously, she called the birth center to ask about moving her 4:00 p.m. deadline back to 7:00. They said that as long as she didn't have a fever, that was fine. Alison sighed in relief. There was still time to kick things into gear.

She swallowed another concoction with two ounces of castor oil and sat on her birth ball, using the breast pump, for two hours. She felt like an absurd burlesque circus act, balancing and juggling and bouncing on a ball with her breasts out, but the routine worked. By 5:00 p.m., she was having consistent contractions, which Steve tracked in an app. They paraded through her body every three minutes and lasted for one minute, and they were intense. It was definitely labor. Alison told Steve to call the birth center. She didn't think she could talk on the phone at that point—the pain was acute, and all she could do in response was yell—but she wanted Gina, who was on duty, to hear about her progress. Now that labor was in motion, Alison felt like everything was spiraling out of control. She wanted to make sure someone had a hold of the reins.

As soon as Steve got Gina on the phone, he passed along a suggestion to moan through the contractions, as higher-pitched yelling could aggravate stress. It seemed like such a small suggestion—to lower the tone of her voice—but it made a dramatic difference. Gina continued, through Steve, to coach Alison through contractions, which she responded well to. It made her feel like there was a method to the madness, a path through the wilderness that she didn't have to traverse alone.

Gina suggested Steve and Alison come into the birth center soon, ideally before 7:00 p.m. At 5:48 p.m., Steve texted Katherine to say she should make her way over to their house so they could all proceed together. Katherine said she was on her way, but with Friday-afternoon rush-hour traffic, it might take a while.

Meanwhile, Alison holed up in the bathroom, contracting on the toilet while diarrhea and projectile vomiting from the castor oil returned. Steve placed a trash can at her side for her to throw up into, but it was hard for Alison to stay still, so he followed her around instead. Her aim wasn't great and she threw up all over the bathroom and all over Steve, who tried to clean up as best he could in between rounds. It was a mess, like getting too drunk in college. She felt like she was unraveling, at the complete mercy of her body.

At 7:15 p.m., Katherine arrived, shocked at the scene before her. Many moms threw up at some point during labor, but this was on another level. This was a scene from *The Exorcist*. Alison had returned to the bathroom to sit on the toilet with her head in her hands, while Steve was cleaning both the house and himself. Katherine was also surprised by how deep in labor Alison seemed to be. Things had started only a couple of hours earlier, but every time a contraction struck, Alison had to get down on the ground on her hands and knees and rock back and forth, breathing deeply. She was really in it. They needed to get to the birth center, but the doula suggested they take a beat to catch their breath. She guided Alison out into the living room, where she leaned over on the birth ball and slow-danced with her husband, before rushing back to the bathroom.

Fifteen minutes later, Katherine helped Alison put on fresh undergarments and clothes—a long-sleeve knit shirt and a soft cotton skirt—and drink some water before guiding her to the bathroom one last time. When the surge passed, Alison reentered the living room, put on her shoes, and took a step toward the open door.

"Aren't you forgetting something?" Katherine said with a slight raise of her eyebrows.

Alison looked at Steve in his hoodie and black baseball hat, who was grabbing her suitcase, and around the living room. Then, she looked down and saw that she'd forgotten to pull her skirt down. She'd been about to walk outside with her butt exposed to the world. Had she not been in labor, that probably would have felt embarrassing, but she found she didn't care at all. Embarrassment was no longer an emotion she related to. She was having a baby. It was time to go.

BIRTH

I am the centre
Of a circle of pain
Exceeding its boundaries in every direction.
—Mina Loy, "Parturition"

CHAPTER 29
Alison

When they arrived at the birth center, Gina checked Alison's cervix and found she was one centimeter dilated. Just one.

"I think you need to go to the hospital," she said. "Your waters have been broken for a long time and it's still early labor. It's safer."

Alison agreed. She wanted to do whatever was safest and was too exhausted to argue. She had managed to avoid throwing up in the car on the way to the birth center, but now it was hard for her to walk more than five paces. When contractions hit, she curled up in the fetal position on the floor of the birth suite. Katherine asked if she wanted a pillow under her knees, but Alison said no. She didn't want anything soft underneath her; she needed to be one with the cool ground. She was existing second to second. Gina notified the hospital that they were heading in and told Alison that a midwife named Lauren was on staff and expecting her. She was amazing, Gina said, and knew Alison's birth plan. She would be in good hands.

The drive was surprisingly relaxed. After months of anxiety about ending up in the hospital, Alison found that when the moment came, she didn't care at all. The version of herself that had been so resistant no longer existed. It was only a matter of time before she and Steve would meet their son.

They pulled up to the hospital's ER entrance around 9:00 p.m. Steve needed to park the car, but Alison knew she wouldn't be able to walk very far, so Katherine walked her inside while Steve disappeared into the parking garage. A hospital staff member standing at the entrance asked if Alison wanted a wheelchair, barely getting the full question out before she said yes.

It was Friday night, and the ER was packed. The check-in staff offered Alison a blanket to cover herself up—her skirt had once again migrated up to her armpits and her underwear was showing—but decency was the last thing on her mind. She and Katherine were sent up to Labor & Delivery, and as soon as she pulled up to the main desk in L&D, Alison said, "I think I'm going to be sick," and vomited everywhere. The excretion was complete liquid because, after hours of vomiting, she didn't have anything left in her system except for water. The nurse at the check-in desk handed Alison vomit bags, and she promptly dispatched two of them.

The staff decided to put Alison in a room immediately, before they could get her name or other relevant intake information, in case she vomited all over their desk (or the floor) again. From there, things moved fast. She was ushered into a room, and the hospital staff started to go through the admittance procedures and run tests. Alison puked as she climbed into the bed and again when she was on it. A nurse asked if she could move Alison to put fresh sheets on the bed, but she refused.

"But, sweetie, then you will be sitting in your own vomit," she said.

"I'd rather do that than move," Alison groaned. She had been throwing up and having diarrhea for so many hours that she was severely dehydrated. Her body felt like a wrung-out, desiccated sponge. The nurse hooked her up to an IV so she could receive fluids, but she still felt terrible. She chugged down three Gatorades but threw them all back up. Pain clamored and clawed at every cell. At one point, she started sobbing. She'd never been so miserable in her life.

"I need some sort of drug or something," she told Katherine and Steve.

"I am not okay. This is not okay." The midwife mentioned that the two main pain relief options were an epidural or fentanyl, and Katherine suggested they take a moment to think about it. In the meantime, she floated the idea that Alison get into the tub in the bathroom. At first, Alison resisted. She didn't want to move and really just wanted pain medication at that point, but she was swayed by the promise that the water would lessen the torment. Katherine ran the bath and turned on the shower while Alison sat on the toilet attached to her IV. Then Alison lay down on the floor. Katherine asked if she wanted towels or a pillow, and Alison said no. The midwife brought in a cushion with a sheet over it anyway, just in case. Finally, Katherine coaxed Alison into the tub.

"Oh my God," Alison said as she descended into the water. "This feels *so* good. Yes."

The tub helped Alison rebound. It soothed her. She had gone through three IV bags of fluids, and the rehydration was helping too. She knelt in the tub so the stream of water from the shower could flow onto her back, and though she moved around to find a comfortable position, she kept returning to her hands and knees.

When Steve came in to check on her, she told him she wanted the fentanyl.

Katherine and the midwife helped Alison get out of the tub to guide her toward the bed, but she sunk onto her hands and knees on the bathroom floor and crawled over to the sheet with the cushion. After allowing her a few more moments, Katherine and the midwife resumed their efforts to get Alison up. She threw up again, and when she got her breath back, there was only one question.

"Where is my fentanyl?" she said. "When is the fentanyl coming?"

At 11:30 p.m., the anesthesiologist came in to administer the drug, which knocked Alison out for thirty minutes. She even snored lightly. When she woke up again, the effects of the dose had already started to fade.

"I'm in so much pain," she moaned. "I think I want to do the epidural."

All signs pointed to a long road ahead. For all anyone knew, labor could last for another ten hours. To Alison, the prospect of feeling that wretched for an indefinable period of time was intolerable and the anesthesiology team was summoned to queue her up for an epidural.

The midwife explained to Alison what the epidural process entailed—she'd have to sit up in the middle of the bed and be still for twenty minutes or so. That didn't sound appealing to Alison, and she asked about getting another dose of fentanyl instead. Before they made the order, the midwife tried to get Alison to change positions, with her butt up in the air to take pressure off her back and rectum. Then, suddenly, Alison let out a bloodcurdling scream. It was loud, raw, and primordial. It sounded like late labor. The midwife asked if she could check Alison's cervix. When she did, she gasped. Somehow, Alison had gone from barely dilated at all to fully dilated and ready to push in just a few hours.

"Alison, you're ready to have this baby," she said. "If you can dig deep, you could be done in five minutes. You are ready to have your baby."

Alison rallied. The realization that she was almost done, that the end was in sight, changed everything. She wasn't going to die. She was still in pain, but it felt different, purposeful. She even managed to crack a joke to Steve about how he'd had his water-giving privileges revoked after he'd spilled water on her earlier. It was a total reversal.

"All right!" she said, sitting up. "We're going to do this." She put her hand up for high-fives and then turned back over onto her hands and knees, where pushing felt more instinctive.

"Do you think we can get him out on the next push? The next push?" she asked.

"It's just like reaching van #5 on the Hood to Coast race," Steve encouraged. Alison nodded her head in agreement. It was a milestone marker she understood. She rocked back and forth, moving her hips and chanting.

"All right, come on, baby."

She continued the low moaning, sometimes whispering a soft "Ohhh" to herself as a contraction passed. Steve, who had been sitting on the windowsill, walked over to the bed, rubbed Alison's back, and held her hands as she pushed. She tried several different positions, on her side and at the squat bar, then on her back. What could she do? she asked. Was there something that could make things go faster? The midwife replied that she was doing exactly what she needed to do. It was happening exactly as it should.

Alison pushed for the next hour and a half. Even though labor had progressed smoothly until that point, the midwife was starting to get nervous because of the difficulty of finding a steady heartbeat. If the baby wasn't born soon, they might need to do an episiotomy. At one point, the NICU team came in, standing quietly in the back of the room in case they were needed. Alison didn't know they were there until someone mentioned it later.

"I just want this baby to come *out*," Alison whimpered.

The midwife told her to pull her knees way back and push as hard as she could, that she was so close and just needed to push even longer and harder than she already was. Then, she told Alison to reach down. She'd be able to feel Theo's head. He was right there. With just a little more effort, he would be born.

Alison moved onto her side and held on to the backs of her legs, with one hip higher up than the other so she wasn't directly on her tailbone. She pulled her legs back and pulled herself up in a funhouse version of a sideways abdominal crunch. The midwife eased some of Alison's tissue back over the baby's head as she pushed.

Finally, the head came through. Alison pushed again, and the rest of Theo slipped out at 1:40 a.m. on Saturday, March 13, weighing seven pounds and eleven ounces.

The nurse-midwife immediately put Theo, who was a vibrant shade of pink, on Alison's chest.

"Hi, sweetie," she said, smiling down at him, enraptured. She couldn't take her eyes off him. This was *her* baby she was holding. She almost couldn't believe it. She never wanted to let him go.

CHAPTER 30
T'Nika

When they returned to the birth center, T'Nika got into the tub. Her mother-in-law arrived, and the four of them listened to the playlist T'Nika made. The tub had handlebars, and when a contraction wracked her, T'Nika pulled on them while bracing her feet on the tub. Daniel sat on the other side of the tub, pretending to pull, as if they were playing tug-of-war. In between contractions, T'Nika tuned into the music and the conversation and was occasionally able to venture a comment or crack a joke. She drank water and ate bites of snacks as the contractions built in intensity.

Earlier in labor, she couldn't imagine how the pain could get worse, but then it did, and then it did again and again. It was like being pursued by a massive thundering horde. She didn't think she could handle more, and then more came and she handled it. She had no choice. T'Nika reached the point where she couldn't snack anymore and talking became unthinkable. She tried to find a position that relieved the anguish: she sat in the tub, she bounced on the birth ball, she lay on the bed, she let warm water run over her back in the shower, and she squatted on a birth stool. She grabbed a scarf and hung it over the door so she could hang off it. Then she draped the scarf around Daniel's neck and hung off him. Sitting on the toilet felt excruciating, so any time she needed to pee, she went into the shower where she could stand.

Around 4:00 p.m., Marilyn suggested T'Nika try the peanut ball. She lay on her side on the bed with the peanut between her legs for a few contractions before her water finally broke, making a loud *bop* sound. Liquid gushed everywhere. Suddenly, T'Nika felt a surge of energy and sense of success. Marilyn checked the fluid and there was no meconium, which was a good sign. Then she checked T'Nika's cervix. Six centimeters. Progress, albeit incremental progress.

T'Nika was elated. She got back into the tub, but the excitement quickly vanished as she realized that, with her water broken, the contractions had become more intense. The next four hours were a torturous haze, during which she spun around in the tub like a lost torpedo, trying to find a comfortable position. She shook, but not because she was cold. She made all kinds of crazy sounds. (Her mom said she sounded like a caribou from *The Polar Express*.) She also started vomiting everywhere. Daniel assumed the responsibility of holding the vomit bucket and held it under T'Nika's face when she asked, but the smell made T'Nika feel even sicker. She told Daniel to get away, and he obliged.

"Not *that* far, come back!" she groaned. As Daniel walked back toward her, T'Nika vomited, half in the bucket and half on him. That happened twice.

Throughout all the moaning and mess, the midwives came in to check on T'Nika and the baby. They were both doing fine from a clinical perspective—the baby's heartbeat was strong every single time, and by 9:00 p.m., Marilyn thought she was close to transition. She checked T'Nika but found she was still at six centimeters. She had endured an unfathomable pain for the last four hours, and nothing had changed.

"This is impossible," T'Nika said, on the verge of tears. "This is not legit. I can't go anymore."

"Yes, you can," the midwives and her family encouraged her. "You got this." But T'Nika didn't believe them. Marilyn proposed a plan—T'Nika could do a circuit where she tried one position, then another, then another, including the torturous peanut.

"For how long?" T'Nika asked.

"Two hours," Marilyn said.

"Nope," T'Nika said. "What are the other options? I'm not doing a circuit for two hours."

The other option, Marilyn replied, was to go to the hospital for pain management. T'Nika said that was what they were going to have to do. It had been almost four days since those early labor pangs, and she was done.

Marilyn contacted OHSU, T'Nika's backup hospital, to let them know they were coming and sent along T'Nika's files to smooth the transfer of care. The group packed up their things and pulled on their coats. Marilyn, T'Nika's mother, and Daniel would go with her to the hospital while the others waited at home, as Covid restrictions on the number of guests were still in place.

T'Nika tried to pull herself together for the trip. She was wearing a dress her mom gave her that was designed for labor. It had buttons at the top on the shoulder and all down the back and could be folded to let her belly out. It was similar to a hospital gown, in that all the requisite body parts were accessible, but cute, with a leaf pattern in mint green. T'Nika pulled the dress around her as she made halting steps toward the birth center's back door. It took everything she had to get to the car. Standing in the parking lot, her father-in-law asked what he could do. T'Nika told him to open the car door. He obliged and wished her good luck.

T'Nika hadn't known it was possible to feel worse, but the journey to the hospital felt like a medieval form of torture. The car ride took them to the same destination as their walk up the stairs had earlier, but the road was steep, windy, and curvy. They bumped and wound up around the incline, stopping at stop signs and lights and arcing around hairpin turns. When they arrived at the emergency room, T'Nika immediately extracted herself from the car, yelling and hooting and moaning as she made her way inside. She hadn't put on underwear under her labor dress and tried to maintain a semblance of modesty and composure (she didn't want her private parts "flapping in the wind"), but it wasn't easy. An ER technician brought over a wheelchair, and T'Nika collapsed into it. Somewhere through the pain, in the recesses of her brain, she chuckled to herself about being that stereotypical pregnant woman making a scene in the hospital.

The staff in the ER told T'Nika she was doing great and then launched into a slew of intake questions, including her birthday. That pissed T'Nika off—they had known she was on her way and her medical records clearly stated her birth date. She had been in active labor for nearly forty-eight hours, and they were expecting her to answer "June 24" as if she had nothing better to do?

At last, a staff member came to wheel T'Nika to the Labor & Delivery unit. On the ride to the elevators, a series of bumps sent jolts of pain through her body. She tried to keep her hollering to a minimum, not wanting to disturb other patients or staff, but inside she was fuming about the kind of sadist who would design hospital floors that way. Even the tech pushing her wheelchair apologized and warned her when another bump was imminent. When they arrived at the elevator, the door didn't open, so they had to try a different elevator bank, which involved navigating over a few more bumps. Finally, they arrived at the maternity ward. The nurses welcomed her, but all T'Nika could manage was a request to get her to a bed. She still had the shakes.

Once in her room, T'Nika was hooked up to a fetal heart rate monitor that was attached to her belly with a band. It made the contractions feel exponentially worse, but when T'Nika asked if they could take it off in favor of intermittent monitoring, the care team said that wasn't possible. She had to stay in bed, and soon they would place the IV to prepare her for the epidural. (Because she was six centimeters dilated, she would get the lighter option, called a "walking" epidural.) T'Nika was still shaking and dehydrated, so the nurse had a hard time finding a vein.

As a nurse herself, T'Nika had sympathy for the IV-placement troubles, but as a woman in the throes of labor, her tolerance for being repeatedly poked with a needle waned fast. She suggested she change positions and get on her knees, bracing her arms on the top of the bed in an attempt to curb the shaking. That seemed to work, and the nurse placed an IV in T'Nika's left arm. She was given fentanyl for pain relief, which she hated. The drug made her eyes roll around in her head. She felt strange. Wrong. She was still shaking and could feel pain, but now because of the fentanyl, she was even more out of it. She was high and in pain. *This is so stupid,* she thought. *How do people do this?*

Soon, the anesthesiology team arrived to administer the epidural. Again, T'Nika was called upon to sit still, to arch her back, to do this and that, but she couldn't. After a while the anesthesiologist got the epidural in, and things started to calm down. *Oh, thank Jesus Christ,* she thought, lying back on the bed for a moment of repose, before a spurt of fluid squirted all over her face. While the nurse had been fiddling with the IV, it fell out and started to gush. The nurse apologized, and at that point, all T'Nika could do was laugh.

The nurse placed a new IV in her elbow and T'Nika was started on Pitocin around midnight. Thanks to the epidural, she wasn't in excruciating pain anymore and was able to sleep on and off throughout the rest of the night, waking up when staff members came in to check on her. The whole labor experience up until that point had been anxiety-inducing, especially since it had not gone according to plan, but she was making peace with the change. In the face of the struggle and disappointments, she had decided to seek out the comedy and absurdity in the situation, and to treat it as a learning opportunity. When the staff members on her care team found out T'Nika was a nurse, they were happy to share the nitty-gritty details of their actions and answer her questions. When a nurse placed a catheter, T'Nika paid close attention because she'd never had a catheter before. She asked Daniel to hoist her up so she could see her pee bag. She also liked to monitor the Pitocin dosage level, as it increased over time in increments.

At 10:00 a.m. on Sunday, March 21, a doctor came in to check her [illegible] T’Nika was eight centimeters dilated, only two more than when she’d arrived, and the baby was at station 0, which meant she had not yet descended down T’Nika’s pelvis. (As Marilyn had explained to T’Nika during prenatals, the first part of dilation is up to the mother’s body doing the contractions and dilating on its own, but the second part happens because the baby puts pressure on the cervix.) Because T’Nika’s baby’s head was nowhere near her cervix, the doctor ordered a bedside ultrasound, which showed that the baby’s head was skewed to the right and crooked. With every contraction, the baby’s head had been shoving itself into T’Nika’s hip, instead of down into the birth canal.

Well, she thought, *that explains the clobbering agony.*

Because of that positioning, the length of her labor, and the fact that T’Nika’s contractions weren’t moving the baby down, the doctor recommended a C-section.

T’Nika’s first instinct was to feel sadness. She cried for a few minutes, but then the practical part of her brain took over. She had been committed to the idea of an unmedicated, out-of-hospital birth, like her mother had with her. This wasn’t what she envisioned, but when the doctor said the word “C-section,” she wasn’t surprised. She had always known that surgery was a possibility, and the reasons seemed valid. She had been in labor for days and endured an unimaginable amount of pain and didn’t seem to be getting anywhere. T’Nika was ready to be done with labor. She was ready to focus on all the joy that she expected to come, when she could hold her brand-new baby in her arms and begin the next chapter of her life as a mother. And she trusted the judgment of the midwives, doctors, nurses, and care team around her to make it happen.

“Okay.” She nodded. “Let’s do it.”

In near-perfect rhythm, the staff stopped the Pitocin, unhooked T’Nika from the monitors, and transported her to the OR, while Daniel went to get suited up so he could join her. (T’Nika’s mother and Marilyn had left the night before to sleep; T’Nika’s mother returned to the hospital in the morning and Marilyn went back to Andaluz and checked in throughout the day.) T’Nika, ever resilient, made the best of the situation.

While they prepped for surgery, she chatted with the team in the OR, telling them how she didn't get to do her L&D rotation because of Covid and was excited to be this close to the action. She also joked that she'd had a book about what to expect when birthing in a hospital but hadn't read it because she'd planned for the birth center.

"I guess I should have read it," she said with a laugh.

The anesthesiologist numbed T'Nika's lower half, which felt weird—it was like her legs had disappeared, and all she had was a floating torso. The doctor said T'Nika could try to move her legs, but she couldn't figure out how. It seemed like the top half and the bottom half of her body weren't connected, which confused her brain. She thought of Uma Thurman's character in *Kill Bill*, trying to will herself to wiggle her big toe. The surgical team hung a curtain so that T'Nika wouldn't be able to see what they were doing as they operated. They swabbed her with iodine, which she couldn't feel, and then invited Daniel in.

Even though she couldn't feel her legs, T'Nika was still shaking on her top half. Shaking while she was immobile and her arms were outstretched in a T-shape, an IV in her right arm and a blood pressure cuff on her left, was unpleasant, to say the least. She could feel the doctor digging around and tugging behind the curtain, which was a strange sensation but not painful. It seemed to T'Nika like they were having a tough time getting the baby out. She wondered if something was wrong.

Then, at 11:47 a.m. on March 21, a baby was lifted above the curtain like Simba in *The Lion King*, jutting her bottom lip out in a momentous pout, looking grumpy and startled, an expression T'Nika recognized from her own baby pictures. T'Nika gazed at her with wonder.

This was her baby. Her *daughter*. This was Aaliyah Ruth. T'Nika felt an immediate sense of recognition, like of course this was her baby. *She's so cute,* T'Nika thought.

For some reason, T'Nika had prepared herself for an ugly baby, musing that most looked purple, slimy, and gross when they emerged from the womb, but Aaliyah was perfectly adorable. She was brand-new and yet familiar, foreign, and completely hers. She was seeing her for the first time, but she'd known her forever. It was an incredible feeling. For a moment, everything else faded away.

Then reality seeped back in. The doctor continued to hold Aaliyah up for T'Nika to look at, and though she appreciated the gesture, she was still splayed out, cold, and immobile on the operating table. She was eager to get sewn up and leave the OR but wasn't sure how to say "You can take my baby away now, I'm done looking" without making it awkward.

Finally, the neonatal team took Aaliyah over to a table, where they cleaned and measured her and checked her Apgar scores. She was eight pounds, eleven ounces, twenty and a quarter inches long, and healthy. With those measurements complete, a nurse placed Aaliyah on T'Nika's chest. She was still shaking and lying flat on her back. She couldn't hold the baby with her right arm because of the IV, so she held the baby with the arm that was still wrapped in a blood pressure cuff. It was hard to relax and focus on the baby in that position, so she handed Aaliyah to Daniel, who took her to the recovery room.

Then it was time to stitch T'Nika back up. Someone on the surgical team asked what music she wanted to listen to, and T'Nika requested the video game ambiance music from her birth playlist. She thought about how, soon, she would be tucked into a hospital bed, together with Daniel, holding their baby. She couldn't wait.

CHAPTER 31
Jillian

When Jillian had a contraction that was so strong it made her throw up, she knew it was time to call the midwives. She texted both Marilyn and Carrie to let them know she was in early labor; she still hadn't decided whom she wanted her primary midwife to be because she secretly hoped they could both be at her birth.

Marilyn responded to say she was at another birth—T'Nika's, it turned out—and Carrie, who lived an hour away, said she would drive down soon, so she would be there when things started to speed up. She preferred resting in Jillian's spare room to wresting herself from sleep before dawn or risking hitting morning rush-hour traffic. Jessica, Jillian's friend and an Andaluz apprentice, drove over at 11:00 p.m. to check Jillian's cervix. She was at a "stretchy four or five." It was active labor, but they had time.

Carrie arrived around midnight. She chatted briefly with Jillian to see how she was doing and then went into the spare room to take a nap on the futon next to the bookshelf. Chad and the dogs slept in the bedroom. Meanwhile, Jillian didn't sleep at all. She stayed out in the living room with the TV, then moved to the tub, then back out to the living room, and then into the tub again. The baby was squirming around between contractions, making it impossible to rest or relax.

As the night wore on, labor began to hurt, pulsing and constricting, shattering, raging, and walloping as Jillian desperately tried to claw her way to something—if not comfort, then at least endurance. She was on the inside now, sucked into the chomping vortex, and she couldn't escape or see her way out.

As the gray light of Sunday morning dawned, any cheer or curiosity she'd felt about labor was gone. Had she not been so tired, she could have done a better job handling the pain, but the pain on top of the fatigue from two nights of no sleep was too much. Anything she did to feel better seemed so pointless. She made a smoothie, knowing she needed sustenance, but promptly threw it back up. *I don't know if my body can handle this,* she thought as she tried to steady herself. *I don't know if I can fucking do this.*

Carrie woke up and checked Jillian's cervix again. She was around seven centimeters dilated. That was solid, promising progress, but Carrie could see in Jillian's eyes that she looked defeated.

Jillian spent some time in the inflatable birth tub in the bedroom, but the water didn't help as much as she hoped it would. She started to cry. She still had so long and so far to go. She wasn't sure how much stamina she had left. She was unraveling, feeling weak and vulnerable, like she couldn't control her emotions or keep up her strength. All that was left was a crumpling heap of radiating, battering pain.

Carrie offered to break her water, which Jillian eagerly agreed to, but once it happened she realized the intensity she felt before was nothing compared to what she felt now that there was no cushion. She got into the tub and could feel the baby getting lower, which was bizarre and alarming and should have been motivating, but somehow wasn't. She was encouraged to get up and walk around, but she was just too tired. Around midday, Carrie checked her cervix again. Nine centimeters. She was so close to transition—the last part of active labor before pushing—but Jillian had hung on for as long as she could. She couldn't cope anymore.

"I'm done," Jillian said. "I don't want to do this." She just wanted to rest—and she could have kicked herself for not doing so on Friday when she had the chance. She'd heard the midwives tell mothers-to-be over and over again throughout the years to rest when they felt like labor was starting, and yet when the time had come for her, she had been unable to lie or calm down. Thoughts of going to the hospital for pain relief flickered at the edges of her mind. The mood in the house had turned bleak, tension hovering heavy like a cloud in the air.

Carrie could see how demoralized Jillian was and knew she had to do something.

"Honey, you *are* doing this," she said, reaching for her phone. They needed a change of scenery, a change of mood. She sent a quick text to Jennifer, asking if the cottage was available, and it was. "Jillian, I know you really wanted to have a home birth, but what would you think about transferring to the cottage?" she suggested. It had a much bigger birth tub with powerful jets and a nitrous tank. Maybe with a measure of pain relief, Jillian would be able to rest in between contractions and regain some vigor.

Jillian was skeptical at first that moving locations would help. She didn't want to leave home or deal with a car ride. It was hard to see her way out of her negative mental space, but at this point she felt things couldn't get any worse. Finally, she agreed. It was time to try something new. She needed the baby out of her body.

As soon as the entourage arrived at the cottage, the energy changed for the better. Jillian discarded her clothing and climbed straight into the capacious tub. Chad set up a phone and a Bluetooth speaker with her labor playlist on the bathroom counter next to the sink. Carrie, wearing a black maxi dress, pulled out the nitrous tank from the closet and sat on a low stool next to the tub, coaching Jillian on how to use it. Whenever she felt a contraction coming on, all she had to do was grab the mask, put it over her face, and inhale. Chad, wearing brown board shorts, eased into the tub with Jillian. After a few contractions with the nitrous, Jillian's scowl relaxed, her brows unfurrowed, and a smile crept back onto her face. The nitrous made the pain feel manageable, and knowing she had the ability to provide herself relief gave Jillian a sense of agency. Labor didn't feel so hopeless anymore. Ensconced in warm water with her husband, in the terra-cotta-toned bathroom, with music playing and friends milling around, she was almost able to enjoy herself.

Jessica posted up at the small dining room table with her laptop open. She was working as the primary student midwife, periodically walking into the bathroom to listen to the baby with the Doppler and relaying the numbers to Jen, who sat on the couch with her socked feet propped up on the ottoman, inputting the information. Jillian's friend Taylor, who she'd hired to do birth photography, arrived and settled silently into the armchair. They ordered food, and when the black Styrofoam boxes from Black Bear Diner arrived, everyone (except Jillian) sat around the table to eat.

As the hours of the afternoon ticked by, the team settled into the cottage for the long haul. Other than the sounds of music and the nitrous tank emanating from the bathroom, and occasional peripatetic chitchat out in the main room, the cottage was quiet and calm. In the bathroom, Jillian lay back in the tub, reclining with the nitrous tank in reach, while Chad rubbed her feet. Carrie left her post on the stool to take a brief nap in the bedroom. The small building seemed to possess its own sense of time, as if it was a self-contained island floating separately from the rest of the world. Takeout containers, bags, laptop cords, and jackets were strewn everywhere. It was strange to think of people going about their normal weekends on the outside.

Suddenly, Chad yelled across the cottage.

"Hey, Carrie!"

Carrie dragged herself up from the bed and went back to the bathroom to see what was going on. Chad's holler had made it sound like Jillian needed help.

"Do you know who the fifth member of the Traveling Wilburys is?" Chad asked when Carrie appeared in the doorway. "It's not George Orwell. Not Orson Welles."

"Roy Orbison," Carrie said, amused at the question.

"Roy Orbison!" Chad said, turning to Jillian with a smile.

Carrie sat back on the stool, deciding against a nap for the time being. She settled in with Jillian and Chad, who began to tell a story about the eccentric ninety-five-year-old rodeo financier whom he used to do landscaping work for in central Oregon.

Suddenly, Jillian's face clenched in concentration. Chad peered down into the water and nervously told Carrie that he could see Jillian's vagina starting to bulge.

"Yes, that's what we want," Carrie said. "It's so nice to be in the tub and not hooked up to a bunch of shit, isn't it?"

Around 7:00 p.m., as darkness descended, the vibe in the cottage shifted again, charging up like a low current of electricity. The assembled team got more animated and chattier. Jillian said she was feeling a pushing sensation and was ready to get out of the tub. Carrie walked into the bathroom, and she and Chad helped Jillian step out, wrapping her in fluffy towels.

Jillian leaned on the edge of the tub, and Carrie checked her cervix. "Oh yeah, let's do some pushes and see how it feels. Let's go right into it." She asked Jess to walk to Jennifer's main house and grab the birth stool. Carrie pulled on a pair of purple latex gloves.

Jillian asked Carrie if she should change positions or do anything differently as she pushed.

"You can just play with it," Carrie said. "Remember, the most progress is when you curl around the baby and do one to two pushes for longer than you think."

Before long, Jess returned with the stool and pulled a pair of red scissors out of a drawer to cut a purple foam pool noodle in half. Then she wrapped the noodle around the birth stool to serve as a cushion and placed the stool next to the tub, laying a Chux pad beneath it. Jillian sat on the stool, naked, her friends and midwives arrayed around her like a Rembrandt painting. Chad sat to her side, holding her hand, and Carrie sat on the floor between Jillian's legs.

"Try to relax into it," Carrie said. "Try to push past it because you have a whole baby who needs to come out. Push right into your butt, hard. Push my fingers out. Yes, you're doing it! Do you want me to move your lip?" she asked.

"Yes, do it," Jillian said. "I don't want to be here all night. Chad, do you want to come over here so you can catch? I know you want to be a part of this."

"Can I come closer so I can see?" Chad said.

"There's nothing to see yet," Carrie said. "But it does feel like there's lots of change since we sat down here."

Every time Jillian was hit with a contraction and pushed, she got very quiet and smushed her face up with the effort, squeezing Chad's hand. It was almost as if with each push, Jillian was figuring out how to push, how to work with the contractions to move the baby down the birth canal. Another contraction stampeded through.

"That time you found it right away," Carrie said. "Do you want to feel?"

Jillian nodded and reached her fingers down. "I feel a scrunchy little scalp," she said. Then she sighed, almost in a whisper: "Get out, baby, I am *done* with this."

She blew out her lips and made a whale sound as she did a big push.

"Oh my gosh, that's the ticket," Carrie said. "Feel that baby moving? Oh yeah, that moved your baby down a bunch. You really found your way with that one. That's what it takes each time. You have to get red in the face. Okay, let's get back to that power. Do it more, extra power, yes! Yes. That was a big movement. I'm going to stretch that fascia. It's going to take over."

Jillian closed her eyes and leaned her head back, absorbing every word Carrie was saying.

"There's not much more," Carrie said. "You just have to fingertip it on both sides and can feel the head. You have to release everything that's there. If you pee, that's fine. If you poop, that's fine. Everything must go. You have enough energy. You have everything you need to finish this process.

"That's it, there you go, more, more, more. That's it. Yup, yup, yup," Carrie said, sounding excited. She gestured to Chad, and he scooted toward her. "We can share this space," she said.

Jillian was starting to get louder. Not screams or yells, but aggressive, effortful panting. Chad rubbed her back, and Jillian put her fingers over her eyes and rocked back and forth.

"The head is firmly lodged in your bones right now," Carrie said, turning to Chad. "Put your finger toward her butt, feel that?"

"Oh yeah," Chad said.

"That's your baby's head," Carrie said, and Chad let out a gleeful giggle.

"That's our baby, oh my God, you're getting it, Jillian," he said, his voice resonant and deep in the bathroom and sounding a bit stunned. "You are so close."

Chad seemed galvanized by Carrie's encouragement and got more vocal with his support. He sat with one leg splayed out to the side and the other tucked in, holding Jillian's hand and using his other hand to hold out two fingers below her so he could feel the baby as Jillian pushed.

"Bear down, bear down!" he said with all the fervency of a high school sports coach.

"I can't do it," Jillian whispered, like she was sharing a secret. She grabbed her water bottle from the side of the tub and took a big sip.

"You are bringing it right to the opening, you just have to keep going," Chad said.

"I have to wait for the contraction," she responded gently.

"Hey, I'm learning on the job here," he said, and everyone in the room laughed.

Jillian closed her eyes and rolled her neck. "Okay," she sighed out heavily. She waved her hand at Chad, signaling for him to take it. She took a deep breath in and opened her eyes. Once the contraction passed, her body slumped, gathering her resources.

"You can take a break," Carrie said. "Walk around if you want."

Jillian moved her hips up to stretch and arched and then flattened her back. She braced her hands on the birth stool. A contraction started, and Jillian's shoulders hunched up by her ears.

"Now you're starting to get pissed," Carrie said. "That's good. Get pissed."

"Ooooh," Jillian moaned. "It's intense."

"Let it be there," Carrie said. "Let it burn."

"Every ounce of strength you've got," Chad said.

Jillian exhaled.

After ten minutes, Jillian decided to get back in the tub. She was done with the birth stool. Chad helped ease her into the water, and she sighed with relief, but also excitement.

"Are you ready to be done?" Carrie said, smiling at Jillian.

"I need you to reassure me that that was the hard part," she replied. "I can do this with my body and shove this baby out."

Carrie met her at eye level. "You can do this with your body," she said. "And shove this baby out."

Jessica walked in to take Jillian's vitals, her temperature, blood pressure, and pulse, and to listen to the baby. A contraction rolled through, and Chad cheered.

"I can see dark hair!!!"

By now, it was 10:00 p.m. Outside, the temperature dropped. The stars were out and the frogs croaked, but inside it was warm and bright. Jillian's contractions were closer and closer together.

They say the universe can't give you more than you can handle, Jillian said to herself. *And you can handle this. You aren't alone.* She looked around for a moment, grateful for Chad and the women who surrounded her.

"I love you," she told them. "You're all getting the best thank-you presents ever." She turned to Chad. "Thanks for being a cheerleader, honey," she said to him. "I feel like every time, I get close." She braced for an intense push.

"You're going to get your present today," Carrie said. "It's happening. You are about to meet your baby. Wait for another contraction."

The air in the room felt saturated and heavy like a sponge. It was quiet again, with reverence, with tension, with the effort to create a space into which the baby could emerge. All the attention was directed toward Jillian as she hunched her tired shoulders forward.

Chad started to tear up. "Come on, I can't wait to meet him," he said.

"Let's go slow," Carrie said. "We've got to see if the cord is there. One last push and your baby will come out."

At 11:35 p.m., the baby slipped out into the water into Chad's hands. Carrie delicately took over and with discretion and efficiency unwrapped the cord from around its neck. One. Two. Three. Four. Five wraps. Once unwrapped, she placed the baby on Jillian's chest. It moved its mouth and squirmed. Its head was cone shaped, molded by the journey through Jillian's pelvis.

"I'm done," Jillian said with excitement. She looked down, her eyes wide with disbelief. The baby gave a small cry.

"Five wraps," Carrie said, standing up. "I've never seen anything like it."

Then the baby's tentative cry erupted into a wail.

Jillian looked at Chad.

"What is it?" she asked. "Boy or girl?"

Chad peered down. He hadn't thought to look or ask.

"It's a boy," he said. "We have a son. With the biggest set of balls I've ever seen."

All the midwives burst into laughter.

"What do you think, honey?" Jillian said, looking at Chad. "Is he Sydney?"

Chad nodded his head. "Yes, Sydney."

After some more time in the tub, Chad went to the kitchen to grab the bottle of Prosecco from the mini-fridge, which was otherwise filled with bags of breast milk. He poured Prosecco into coffee mugs and handed them out to the team and then walked into the bathroom to hand Jillian her mug. Everyone followed, standing around the tub, sipping the wine and waiting for the placenta. After a few coughs, it slid out.

"Do you want to cut the cord, honey?" Jillian asked.

"I would love to cut the cord," he said.

Jen grabbed surgical supplies from the cart, and Carrie guided Chad through how to cut. She held the cord, clamped and taut, and Chad snipped.

"I feel like a whole new person," Jillian said.

"You *are* a whole new person," Carrie said.

POSTPARTUM

I can hear the sizzle of newborn stars,
and know anything of meaning,
of the fierce magic emerging here.
—Joy Harjo, *Secrets from the Center of the World*

CHAPTER 32
Jillian and Sydney

After Chad cut the umbilical cord, Jillian stood up in the tub, moving slowly so she wouldn't slip. She attempted to move her breasts and belly out of the way so she could see if she was bleeding, but nothing gushed out. Carrie and Jess helped her step out of the tub and gave her a hand towel to press against her vagina to stem any minor leaking. Chad carried Sydney back to the bedroom, and Jillian stepped into the shower. There were so many things to think about, but the thought foremost in her mind was about her dogs. She'd have to give their neighbor a massive thank-you for checking on them on such short notice.

While Jillian showered, Jen filled out the requisite forms and Carrie took the rest of the baby's vital stats. Chad sat with Sydney on the bed, mesmerized by his every wiggle and movement. From the shower, Jillian continued chatting with Jess—about how unusually long the cord was, her worry about the dogs, and how she was hungry. Her voice, echoing around the bathroom, was buoyant.

After her shower, the new parents lounged in the bed, marveling at the human they'd created, while Carrie, Jen, and Jess tidied up until the postpartum midwife arrived to relieve them. Sydney took to breastfeeding easily and, other than feeling tired, Jillian felt good—great, even. She wasn't bleeding much and didn't have any tearing. She was eager to go home and get into her own bed. Jillian and Chad made smoothies, got their stuff together, strapped Sydney into the car seat, and headed out around dawn.

During the drive to the cottage, Jillian had felt dispirited and defeated. Now, she felt triumphant. She'd had a baby. Birth had tested her in ways she hadn't expected. She was filled with gratitude for the support she'd received and even more committed to guiding other people through the journey, just as her midwives had guided her.

When they arrived home, it was disorienting to walk back into a house they'd so suddenly abandoned the day before. The cottage had seemed like a time capsule, a boat bobbing in the ocean far away from shore, untethered from the rest of the world. But their house was stuck in the pre-Sydney world. Finding that the vestigial clutter—the cups and coffee mugs and towels and blankets and phone chargers—remained after their momentous experience was strange. Jillian's immediate impulse was to tidy, but all she could manage was to climb into bed and sleep. Chad made a motion to drain the inflatable birth tub, which was still in the corner of their bedroom with leftover water in it, but Jillian told him to leave it until the morning. They could clean the next day. Holding Sydney, she sat and then pivoted to lie down in the bed while Chad got in from the other side. Paisley and Diesel lay on their dog beds in the corner.

The next phase of their lives as parents had begun.

As a midwifery student, Jillian was used to sleep deprivation, but after long stretches of wakefulness, she'd always been able to go home and sleep for eight, ten, twelve hours. That, she quickly learned, was not how it worked with a brand-new baby. She was lucky to get a few uninterrupted hours, at most.

The first few weeks with Sydney were a blur, during which Jillian and

Chad's entire world narrowed down to a few basic impulses—feeding and sleeping and changing diapers. They practiced co-sleeping, meaning the baby slept with them in their bed, but he only slept if he was propped up on a chest, so whoever held him had to sleep sitting up. Jillian's body was sore from the birth, and her breasts were heavy, like carrying around boulders. The reality of going from days of being in labor straight into parenting a newborn was grueling. There was no respite, and somehow, in a heavy sleep-deprived haze, she had to tap into deep emotional and physical reserves and figure out how to meet the needs of a tiny, crying creature. Every time Sydney cried and woke her up, it felt a little like being hit when she was down, even though every time she looked at him, she vibrated with love.

After two weeks, Chad went back to work, while Jillian stayed at home with Sydney. Friends stopped by when they could, but people were busy with their jobs and lives and kids of their own. Plus, most of them lived or worked in Portland, so they couldn't casually drop by her house in Carlton, leaving Jillian, who didn't know many people in her neighborhood, for the most part on her own. Time moved slowly and fast. The hours dragged, and she'd count them down until Chad came home and he could hold Sydney while she completed tasks that required two hands. Other times, she looked at the clock and was stunned to see that, all of a sudden, it was 4:00 p.m.

She couldn't imagine spending full days away from Sydney when he was so young, but it was hard to go full days without speaking to another adult human. She missed the hustle and bustle of the birth center, which had been replaced in her life by the persistent routine of meeting Sydney's needs. She fed him and then cleaned up the poop that emerged after the feeding. And repeat. And repeat. And repeat. Every night, she went to bed exhausted, but also astonished—not just that she had made it through another day, but that she'd have to wake up and do it all over again. *Does this feeling ever end?* she thought to herself as she drifted off to sleep.

Beyond direct baby care, even the most minor tasks could sometimes feel like too much to handle. Jillian had envisioned that she, Sydney, and the dogs would go for strolls around the neighborhood when the weather was good, but she tried it once and vowed never to do so again: venturing out with two dogs that had different walking paces, plus a baby, quickly turned to chaos. The leashes got tangled, one dog pulled while another dragged, and Jillian worried she'd trip or fall with Sydney strapped to her chest. Within minutes, she was flustered and retreated to the house, covered in a sheen of sweat. Something as straightforward as going to the grocery store to buy rice for dinner or stopping by the bank, too, came to feel like towering hurdles. A trip to the ATM required driving to the next town, where her credit union had a branch, so if Jillian needed cash, she had to get dressed, or at least take off her light blue bathrobe with pink flowers, dress Sydney, and strap him into the car seat. Once at the ATM, she had to extricate Sydney from the car seat and then navigate through the ATM door, which required swiping her card, with the baby in her arms, and then pulling out her wallet, entering her PIN, and getting the cash. And then she had to do that whole sequence in reverse. It was frustrating to feel like she had nothing but time and yet could accomplish nothing. Anything—even just sitting down and drinking a hot cup of coffee and having some breakfast—felt like a victory.

It was during those early, chaotic days that driving to Jennifer's property became one of Jillian's favorite things. It helped her find balance and connect to the wider world and back to herself. There, she could visit with the midwives on duty at the cottage and stay up-to-date on what was going on at Andaluz. It wasn't a long drive and it was easy to bring Sydney along because if he cried or needed to be fed during the visit, it was no big deal—she could whip out a boob and hang out for a while. Jillian also brought Sydney to Andaluz in Portland for her postpartum appointments and to visit with the staff in the kitchen. Tales of his lengthy umbilical cord and five neck wraps had circulated through the birth center and become the stuff of legend.

By four weeks old, Sydney was sleeping in uninterrupted stretches of four to five hours, which meant Jillian could, too, but a new challenge emerged: even though he was sleeping more, he would start crying hysterically anytime Jillian tried to put him down. The bouncy chair was a no-go, and he wailed with particular and immediate intensity whenever she put him in the car. A few times, he started screaming so loudly as she buckled him into the car seat that she called off the trip.

Jillian had heard countless babies crying over the years, but there was something so different about hearing her own baby cry. Her body reacted to the sound in a way that felt primal, like they were connected by an invisible energy field she was powerless to resist. She would do anything to fix the problem and give her baby what he needed. It was a compulsion, the intensity of which surprised her.

Sydney's need to be held all the time made it even more difficult than it already was to do things around the house or visit friends or run errands, much less eat and shower. Jillian spent most of her time in her robe and PJ pants, with him in her arms and the TV on in the background. (Her go-to was to put on a channel that replayed young adult movies from the '90s and 2000s, like *17 Again.*) At times, she felt trapped and alone. It was so hard to do this without much help. She had a wide community of family and coworkers and friends, but that was not the same thing as having people immediately present to spend time with, commiserate with, rely on, and ask for advice or assistance. She didn't have anyone to call when she needed someone to watch Sydney for thirty minutes while she went to Target. Or whom she could make a date with to meet at a coffee shop in town with their babies. She had tried to search for a new mom group in her area, but the town was tiny and there weren't any close enough to be workable.

Jillian loved Sydney with her entire being and could not imagine her life without him. She couldn't stop kissing his cheeks or tickling his belly or smelling his head. But new motherhood was hard. It wasn't pink-tinted, milk-scented days of bliss. Beyond the physical toll, Jillian felt plagued by anxiety that something bad would still happen. She had been pretty relaxed about her pregnancy, but now that Sydney had arrived, danger seemed to lurk everywhere. A friend suggested that when Jillian wanted to shower, she could bring Sydney into the shower with her, but Jillian was too scared that she'd slip and drop him.

She trusted that at some point, everything would get easier. Sydney would get older and she would get more used to being a parent. She yearned to be connected to the world again, and so when Sydney was six months old, she resumed her part-time administrative work for Andaluz, working from home. She was glad to have something else to think about and a new external purpose, even if it was just for a few hours a week. She loved communicating with her coworkers and knowing that the tasks she completed helped the birth center run smoothly. It wasn't always easy though. It was too hard to work when Sydney was awake because he could only handle five, maybe ten minutes in the bouncy chair before he'd want to be picked up again. She tried to do bursts of work while he napped, but there were often other things to do around the house, and she couldn't resist the impulse to check on him.

Uninterrupted time didn't really exist anymore, but she relished the time they had together. Jillian loved to dress the baby in cute little outfits—itty-bitty Carhartt hats and patterned onesies and teeny-tiny rainboots—and watch him puzzle out new things, like an herb garden or string lights. Watching Sydney figure out the world prompted Jillian to do the same, looking at everything with fresh eyes and embarking, together, on a process of daily discovery. When over the summer, Jillian and Chad flew to Hawaii for a family wedding, Sydney spent the whole plane ride snoozing peacefully in his DockATot. Jillian was relieved that he didn't cry and cause a commotion, and was excited about the possibilities that flight seemed to open up—it seemed like a milestone, a signal that she could reengage with the wider world.

Over time, through trial and error, the couple honed strategies that enabled some semblance of Jillian's life before to resume. In September, Chad planned to switch to a four-day workweek, with longer days Monday through Thursday, so he could be home on Fridays. Jillian was excited because she'd be able to drive to the Portland birth center for midwife meetings or go to a café for a few hours with her laptop—maybe she could even start to pursue her midwifery credential again. She'd thought she had plenty of time to submit her application, but an unexpected deadline had emerged. NARM typically gives midwifery students seven years from when they graduate to submit all their application materials and take the exam, but the state of Oregon, Jillian learned, had a different timeline: to get licensed in the state, midwives must have attended ten births as an apprentice within two years of applying. Since she had completed her apprenticeship in October 2019, her window was rapidly closing. If she didn't apply for her license and pass the exam before then, she would have to "redo" those births.

It was exactly the fire she needed lit under her. She finally sent off the application and scheduled her exam for September 16. Jen came over a couple times to watch Sydney while she studied, and on the day of the test, Chad stayed home from work. Jillian, who was prone to test anxiety, was glad she could take the test from home, with a proctor observing her on camera.

The exam was challenging, as anticipated. It was eight hours in total—four hours in the morning, a break for lunch, and then another four hours, with three hundred questions in total. Jillian had some technical issues getting set up, and at one point, the test-taking platform froze and wiped some of her answers, which absorbed forty minutes of her time. She also had to stop a few times throughout the day to feed Sydney.

After she finished the test that evening, Jillian thought she had done well. There were a few questions she wasn't sure about, with confusing multiple choice options, but overall, she felt good about her grasp of the material.

The next morning, at 7:30 a.m., she saw an email with the results. She opened it. "We regret to inform you that you did not pass," it read. *Well, fuck.* She had failed by one point. It felt like a punch to the gut. *One point?* To be so close, and yet fall short, was something she hadn't expected. She had tried her best, pushed herself, and did what she could to set herself up for success under the circumstances, but it hadn't been enough. Mostly, she felt let down and regretful. She wished she'd hustled to take the test before she had the baby, because maybe then she would have passed. Now she would have to redo a bunch of births as an apprentice. Where would she find the time to do that with an infant?

Dejected, and a little embarrassed, Jillian told Jennifer what happened.

"Plenty of people don't pass the test on their first try," Jennifer reassured her. She also reminded Jillian that she had taken the test six months after having a baby, months in which she had not gotten enough sleep and barely had time to study. The test was hard, even under the best circumstances. It was impressive she hadn't failed by more. There was still time. And she would help Jillian with whatever she needed to take the test again, whether that meant helping her find childcare, or subsidizing the testing fee, or both.

Jillian was touched by the offer. She had so much admiration for Jennifer and for the birth center and midwifery community she'd built. After she had been out of the game for so long, and doubting her own abilities, Jennifer's belief in her was a major boost to Jillian's confidence. If Jennifer didn't doubt that she was capable, she wouldn't doubt it either. She just needed to be patient and understand that it might not happen as quickly or as easily as she wanted it to.

Eventually, Jillian came to see her test score as a blessing in disguise. Had she passed the exam and received her license, she would have wanted to start practicing as a midwife right away, but there was absolutely no way that would have been feasible. If taking a shower or running an errand was too much with a baby, how could Jillian possibly spend hours away at births? And if finding childcare was already difficult, how would she find any that could accommodate such an unpredictable schedule? Some of the options she'd considered required a full-time commitment, which Jillian wasn't looking for. She needed someone she could call if or when she got summoned to a birth in the middle of the workweek, who could watch Sydney part-time. That didn't appear to exist. Without that, there was no way she could pursue her career until Sydney was older. But what if she and Chad wanted to have another baby? Then the clock would start all over again.

Those were problems for down the road. In the near term, Jillian needed childcare a few hours a week so she could handle her administrative responsibilities at Andaluz. Once again, Jennifer offered a solution: the Gallardo family's accountant was a longtime family friend whose wife had recently retired and babysat for their infant niece. She offered to watch Sydney, too, at a very reasonable rate. They worked out an arrangement for childcare four to five hours, twice a week. The woman lived close by, and she and Sydney immediately took a liking to each other.

Suddenly, Jillian had ten hours a week all to herself. At first, she luxuriated in the time to simply take a shower, be alone, and get her Andaluz work done. Once she acclimated to the new routine, she set her sights back on her midwifery exam.

In June 2022, Jillian retook the NARM exam and passed. She also started going to births again to satisfy the state's licensing requirement. Jillian was determined. She was a mother now, but she could be a midwife too.

CHAPTER 33

T'Nika and Aaliyah

After a few hours in the recovery room, T'Nika, Daniel, and Aaliyah moved to the postpartum floor, where, despite her exhaustion, T'Nika struggled to sleep. She was proud of how she'd handled the tumult of her birth experience, but now her emotions seemed to be bubbling up through her subconscious. Every time she dozed off, anxiety dreams rolled through in rapid succession. She had one in which the baby dislocated her shoulder, and another where someone tried to put a bag over Aaliyah's head. They were intense and terrifying. Over the course of the three days and three nights that she and Aaliyah stayed in the postpartum recovery unit, they started to subside, but then, a new set of challenges emerged.

As she anticipated, breastfeeding proved difficult at first: T'Nika's nipples had been inverted during pregnancy, but using her breast pump caused them to come out too far. All the skin that had been on the inside was exposed and super sensitive, which doctors refer to as "frayed ends." After her second attempt at pumping, they started bleeding and T'Nika wasn't producing any milk. The hospital offered donor breast milk, which Daniel fed to Aaliyah in a bottle.

Then, one morning, T'Nika woke up from a nap shaking uncontrollably, wracked with discomfort and pain. She was taking oxycodone, and the medication was causing constipation, which was causing everything to push on everything. A nurse gave T'Nika a heating pad and warm blankets, which helped quell the shaking, but it was hard not to feel scared. T'Nika's edema, or swelling, continued to alarm her. It was like she had a balloon on top of her foot, and when she pressed the skin, it stayed indented. The fact that she had never seen "pitting" like this, to this degree, on any of her own patients, scared her more.

Finally, she and Aaliyah were discharged to return home and she hoped being in her own bed would make her feel better, but she was still in so much pain that comfort was hard to come by. Every movement, every reach of her arm or twist of her body, seemed to irritate the wound from her C-section. The area around her surgery scar was a pulsing, searing kind of sore. She couldn't stand for long or easily sit up, but sometimes lying down hurt too. She had left the hospital with a prescription for oxycodone but tried not to rely on the opioid too much, preferring to take ibuprofen and Tylenol instead.

Of all forms of movement, going up and down stairs hurt the most. The physical maneuvering necessary to lift one foot up after the other or to step down tore at her scar in a specific and unbearable way. Before long, T'Nika was orienting her life around minimizing trips between floors; in the early days, she mostly stayed upstairs with Aaliyah while Daniel and her mother ferried up tuna fish sandwiches and water and medicine and whatever else T'Nika needed.

It wasn't just the stairs though. Even getting out of bed was tough. If she wasn't gentle enough, she would pull on the scar, which caused it to bleed and sent pain careening around the incision point. T'Nika had heard of the "C-section shuffle," and that was what she did on every trip to the bathroom. She wished she'd known to buy a stepstool to make getting in and out of bed easier. Sometimes, thinking about how to work around the pain took as much out of her as actually doing so. She didn't have energy to do much other than pick up Aaliyah and feed her, so they spent most of their time snoozing and cuddling in bed, watching endless hours of *Property Brothers*.

After an initial rocky start with breastfeeding, T'Nika's nipples got their act together, but Aaliyah had a tough time latching on and sucking. Marilyn noticed that Aaliyah had a tongue tie during a postpartum checkup, which could make it difficult for babies to breastfeed, so they made an appointment at OHSU to fix it with a simple procedure. T'Nika knew it was necessary, but seeing her baby looking like a bloody vampire, screaming her head off, with nothing she could do to help, was distressing in the moment. T'Nika cried too. On top of all that, Aaliyah developed infant torticollis, meaning that during breastfeeding, her head favored one side, and she seemed to suck without moving her jaw, so the milk didn't transfer. The lactation consultant at OHSU had a scale to measure precisely how much milk the baby transferred, which confirmed T'Nika's suspicions that it wasn't enough. As they worked to resolve the issue, T'Nika continued using a combination of formula, donor milk, and her own breast milk to feed her.

During her second week at home, T'Nika felt like she was coming apart at the seams. Literally. Her cesarean incision opened in what's known in medical parlance as a "dehiscence," causing a small infection. The doctors treated the wound and prescribed T'Nika antibiotics, but it refused to heal. A second hole opened next to the first one, so there were two holes as big as T'Nika's pinky right next to each other. Then the second hole closed, but meanwhile a third hole opened on the left side. Between the incision issues and her visits with the lactation consultant and their pediatric appointments, T'Nika was going to the hospital two to three times a week. It was the only time she left the house, the only time she moved in any significant way. Daniel tried to make the journeys as easy as he could by carrying the baby and opening doors, but there was only so much he could do.

In early May, about six weeks after the surgery, the incision had still not healed completely, but T'Nika was bored and frustrated with sequestering herself to one floor of her house for the entire day. It was spring and she could see the sun shining and flowers blooming out her window. Like a woman in a Victorian novel, all she could do was stare out forlornly at the world beyond. T'Nika hated to be confined. She hated that she had to rely on someone to bring her basic items. She hated trekking all the way downstairs, only to realize she forgot something upstairs. If Daniel was out running errands and T'Nika wanted something to eat, she had to decide whether to wait, hungry, for him to come back, or put herself through the slog of making her way to the kitchen. That wasn't going to be sustainable for much longer. Once Daniel went back to work (even though he would be working from home), he wouldn't be as available as before.

One day, not long before he started work again, T'Nika attempted a trip downstairs by herself. She picked up Aaliyah and packed a small purse with ibuprofen and her phone. Slowly, carefully, she took the stairs one step at a time. When she made it to the bottom, she stopped and sat down, in an abnormal amount of pain. This wasn't a standard ache, but something sharper. She lifted her shirt to look at the incision. It was bleeding again, angry and red and oozing. She went to the doctor, who found the incision site was reinfected and put T'Nika on a second round of antibiotics. Daniel pushed back his return-to-work date by another week.

All T'Nika wanted was to heal and be active and self-sufficient. Her pregnancy had seemed like ailment after ailment, the birth hadn't gone like she'd hoped, and now her recovery felt interminable. As she lay in bed, T'Nika thought about the things she wished she'd done differently, in retrospect. She wished she'd been more assertive and honest about her pain scale when the midwives asked—she'd said a "7" when it felt like a "9" or "10," thinking she should reserve the higher number for later. She wished she'd done more research about OHSU when she'd selected the hospital as a transfer site, and maybe even taken a tour. And she hadn't thought to check whether her insurance covered care at OHSU, since she hadn't expected to end up there. Her insurance did cover it, but had it not, that simple oversight could have cost her and Daniel tens of thousands of dollars.

T'Nika also dreaded the prospect that in the future, she might have to have another C-section if she and Daniel had another baby. (After getting the surgery, she'd learned that, because she was a Black woman, she had a higher likelihood of having a repeat C-section.*) T'Nika knew that she couldn't have avoided a C-section in her situation. It was what needed to happen, but that didn't make it any easier to reckon with the consequences. Postpartum was complication after complication from the surgery, just as she'd feared. The toil of trying to heal for six full weeks, to seemingly no avail, wore her down to a nub. She felt low, crying off and on all the time. It might be one thing if her injury was something she could manage or work around, but it got in the way of her ability to be independent. She couldn't just go and sit outside by herself or take a walk or run errands. She couldn't live her life or do the things that usually cheered her up. And she couldn't go back to work as soon as she planned, so her doctor wrote a note to extend her maternity leave by a few more weeks.

And then, she would look at Aaliyah. Throughout it all, the main joy and solace she found was in her delightful, jolly, cheeky baby. Taking care of Aaliyah felt fun, and—dare she say it—easy. She cried like any baby, but as soon as she got what she wanted, she stopped (unless it was the "baby witching hour" of the late afternoon/early evening, when nothing seemed to soothe her), and T'Nika and Daniel quickly became experts at anticipating her needs. At night, when Aaliyah stirred ever so slightly in her bassinet, one of them would swing into action to get the bottle ready, change her diaper and feed her before she started to wail, and she'd slip seamlessly back into sleep.

The love T'Nika felt for Aaliyah was all-consuming, and almost painful sometimes. She loved her so much that it caused her intense anxiety around her baby's survival. T'Nika had felt connected to Aaliyah when she was pregnant, but she'd been more of an abstract idea then, rather

---

* Doctors use what's known as a "VBAC calculator" to determine how likely a patient with a previous C-section is to have a subsequent vaginal delivery. The calculator factors in things like a patient's age, height, and weight—and race. In 2019, a group of researchers at Harvard Medical School and Brigham and Women's Hospital found that all else being equal, the algorithm gave patients of color a significantly lower chance of having a VBAC.

than a unique and special human with her own personality who was alive in the world. Now that she was born, now that T'Nika had met her and knew her, the worst thing she could imagine was a world without her in it. Her mind ran through scenarios of all the bad things that could happen, at times drowning her in dark thoughts. The nightmares that had begun in the hospital continued—in one, she put Aaliyah down for a nap and heard a noise on the baby monitor. When she went upstairs to check, the baby had turned into Sméagol from *The Lord of the Rings* and was choking on her own spit, with blankets wrapped around her head. It was terrifying, and even though it had just been a dream, T'Nika had stopped laying Aaliyah in that direction in the crib. When Aaliyah got sick with a minor, common baby ailment, T'Nika checked her temperature constantly, unable to relax until all the symptoms subsided.

T'Nika knew other mothers felt that way sometimes, too, and she did her best to push the scary thoughts out of her mind, to remind herself the fears were in her head and Aaliyah was okay, and to focus on the good. And there was so much good to focus on.

T'Nika loved to watch her figure out her own body and the world around her. She was a curious baby and liked to lift her head up and look around. She cooed, smiled, and did a baby version of a laugh, which made T'Nika giggle because it sounded so strange. She liked to move her hands and arms through the air and chew on her fingers and swat at the shapes hanging from her mobile. A small mirror hung from her playmat, and if Aaliyah turned herself around and could no longer see the mirror, she'd whine until she got turned back around. T'Nika liked to tease her for being vain. Aaliyah continued to grow like a champ. She was in the ninety-sixth percentile for her weight and height and had a big head (just like her dad). She was strong too. If T'Nika held her by the waist, she could hold her body up and stand tall. After putting on a bunch of weight, Aaliyah got too chubby to roll around and she'd get stuck on her back, kicking her arms and legs around like a capsized turtle. She was also very vocal. Sometimes, she'd trill her lips and let out a shriek, which T'Nika thought sounded like a pterodactyl. She made a lot of "gah" sounds too. When she woke up from a nap, T'Nika and Daniel could hear her in the crib, gabbing to herself on the baby monitor. Eventually, after twenty minutes or so, Aaliyah would start to get sad, as if she realized she'd just been talking to herself and no one was listening. T'Nika and Daniel started calling her "Chunky Gabby."

As she got bigger and stronger, the baby started to move on her own, albeit very slowly. One night, Daniel and T'Nika sat at their table eating dinner and Aaliyah was a few feet away on her playmat. She had been facing the mirror, but the next time T'Nika looked over, she had rotated about fifteen degrees. The next time T'Nika looked, Aaliyah was facing the window. She reminded T'Nika of a starfish—she never saw her moving, but every time she was in a different position.

T'Nika loved to hang out at home with her baby, whom she found endlessly entertaining. And even as new parents, she and Daniel had been able to stick to their favorite habits and routines. They still played video games and watched TV and played with their cat, but now Aaliyah was there with them. T'Nika joked about photoshopping Aaliyah's face into old family photos to pretend like she had been there all along.

Medical problems aside, T'Nika had savored her maternity leave because it gave her time to recover and for the three of them to bond as a family. They felt like such a precious, intimate little unit. She wasn't thrilled with the prospect of returning to work but knew it was important to keep investing in her career. Still, it was difficult to separate from Aaliyah. T'Nika cried the first time she left for a shift, but once she was back in the busy routine of her nursing rotation, there wasn't much time to focus on those feelings. Her colleagues were helpful and supportive and made sure she didn't have to lift anything heavy. She pumped during her breaks, often looking at pictures of Aaliyah on her phone while she did so. (At that point, she was producing so much milk that she began to donate the surplus to a friend's sister who needed it.) She didn't love her surgery scar, which looked like a thin knotted rope, but it wasn't having too much of an impact on her mobility. It still hurt sometimes, but lidocaine injections helped. T'Nika was nowhere near back to her old self, but she could finally move through the world on her own.

As with her pregnancy, though, old problems receded only for new ones to take their place. She developed bacterial vaginosis and diastasis recti, or abdominal separation, at her belly button—four fingers apart and two knuckles deep, for which she was "prescribed" a workout program targeting her core and pelvic muscles. There were also incontinence issues, a very common aftereffect of childbirth, which required her to wear special, super-absorbent pads at work. During one shift, T'Nika was in the room of an elderly patient and had an inkling that she might need to use the bathroom soon, but she had already started the process of passing the patient's medication. It wasn't like T'Nika could pop the pills into her pocket, go to the bathroom, and come back. Since she'd already started, she had to finish administering the pills before she could leave the room, which involved listening to the patient's heart and lungs, examining her feet, logging in to the computer, scanning the patient's wristband, and then giving her the medication—all while clenching with every fiber of her being and trying not to pee.

It had been about ten minutes since T'Nika first felt the pressure in her bladder, and the situation was getting more urgent. At last, she was ready to open the pill packet and grappled with the packaging, trying frantically to open it and get the pills into the cup for the patient, when the floodgates opened. *I just straight-up peed my pants in someone's room,* T'Nika thought to herself, as she hustled down the hallway to the bathroom. Fortunately, the twelve-hour protection pad she was wearing saved the day, her scrubs were dry, and the patient hadn't noticed anything was amiss. T'Nika changed the pad and went on with her day. There were so many indignities to new motherhood—all she could do was laugh.

As the fall began, T'Nika started to think about how she could turn some of the challenging, hard experiences she'd encountered over the past year into a positive. How she could use them to help people. She had always focused her ambitions on working in an L&D ward, and she was still drawn to that idea, but other possibilities had dawned on her as well.

She had never considered nursing in a postpartum unit before and now realized just how important that was. To T'Nika, it seemed like a real opportunity to help new mothers figure out the brave new world they were in. To help them navigate a situation it was impossible to be prepared for. To let them know that after the baby was born, whatever they had been through, and whatever they were still going through, mattered. And she could be the one to do it.

CHAPTER 34
Alison and Theo

Almost as soon as Theo emerged from her body, Alison felt strong, powerful, and thrumming with energy. Completely transformed. She couldn't believe what she'd just been through, what she'd just accomplished. It had been the most intense experience of her life. She kept reliving the birth in her head, returning to the story, and asking questions to fill in gaps she couldn't remember to etch the memory in place. She sat in bed holding Theo, propped up by a throne of pillows, feeling like a queen holding court as various hospital staff came through to check on them. He was doing great. A bit jaundiced, it turned out, but after a pediatric consultation, Alison wasn't too worried.

On Sunday, March 14, the family was discharged from the hospital around 7:00 p.m. When Alison and Steve got home, they found their neighbor had kindly prepared a meal, baked gingersnap cookies, and left a pack of two hundred paper plates. They ate dinner and collapsed into bed, with Theo in his bassinet next to them. They woke up throughout the night to tend to Theo, still in a state of suspended disbelief about being home with a baby. *Their* baby. Before they had time to get their bearings, it was time to leave again and drive back to the hospital for an 8:30 a.m.

appointment at the Mother & Baby clinic, where Theo's bilirubin levels were tested to monitor the jaundice, and Alison had to meet with a nurse and lactation consultant about breastfeeding. During the session, the nurse expressed concern that Theo was losing weight and therefore "failing to thrive." Alison's optimism evaporated. *Failure to thrive?* He'd been alive for only two days! The nurse explained that some of the weight loss could be because Alison received so many bags of IV fluid during labor—eight bags in total. Some of Theo's birth weight was probably water weight, she continued, in which case the weight loss might be less dramatic than the numbers indicated. It was important to build up her milk supply by pumping, breastfeeding, and feeding with formula, and repeating that sequence every two hours. She also recommended a particular type of formula and emphasized the importance of keeping it sterile. Alison nodded, but she was already feeling overwhelmed. That was three approaches of feeding to manage and keep track of.

While pregnant, Alison had almost taken it for granted that she would breastfeed. She'd read and heard plenty about its benefits, and she wasn't keen to spend money on formula if she didn't have to. She figured that she would breastfeed Theo for a year, at minimum. Now, facing down the visceral specifics of what it would entail, she wasn't so sure. It was a tremendous commitment of her time and her body, and she was the only one who could do it. It was important to Alison and Steve that they were equal partners in caring for Theo, but breastfeeding was a task that fell solely on Alison's shoulders (or breasts, as it were). If they used formula, Steve could participate more actively in feedings. Plus, she found she loathed the breast pump. Sitting plugged into that contraption made her feel like a cow being milked. Alison disliked breastfeeding, but with all the pressure and opinions, she couldn't help but feel that she was falling short by not giving it her all, that she was somehow deficient as a mother because she found she preferred to feed with formula. The lactation consultant encouraged her to keep trying, despite her frustrations.

Later that week, at one of Theo's pediatrician appointments, she broke down. The stress of going to so many appointments with a brand-new baby and to breastfeed was too much. To her surprise, the pediatrician said that was fine—Alison didn't have to breastfeed if she didn't want to. Formula was a great option, he said, and the prescription to feed Theo in a rigid cycle of every two hours, as the lactation consultant had advised, wasn't very "child-centered." They could just feed him when he cried. Alison had assumed the pediatrician would push breastfeeding, just like everyone else, but he emphasized that whatever worked for her and her family was fine. That was a relief, and the validation Alison needed in a blizzard of conflicting advice.

The next day, Alison had another visit with the Mother & Baby clinic's lactation program and told the consultant that she was leaning toward formula feeding. She wasn't closed off to their advice about what was best, but somewhere between pregnancy and motherhood, her confidence had grown. She had resolved to be assertive about setting boundaries and say no to things if she hoped to keep her sanity.

During that same appointment, the nurse took Alison's blood pressure. It was high, and she said if the level didn't go down, Alison might have to be readmitted to the hospital. Alison had monitored her blood pressure during pregnancy, but it hadn't occurred to her that the risk continued postpartum. She called WHA, and Gina booked her in for an appointment the next day. When she told Gina about all the stress she was under from the postpartum and lactation and pediatric check-ups and their barrage of instructions, Gina said that the stress probably had something to do with why her blood pressure was high. It was a lot to handle for someone with a new baby, and it sounded like what Alison needed was to stay home, drink water, rest, and recuperate.

After talking it through, Alison decided to drop out of the Mother & Baby program. She had wanted to try breastfeeding, but wasn't deeply committed to it. She had the support of the midwives at the birth center and her pediatrician. She just needed time to chill—and that was exactly what she did. For the next few days, she lounged around in a black maxi skirt, a gray T-shirt, and a fluffy white robe, carrying around a jumbo cup with a straw she'd taken home from the hospital, and she and Steve spent that weekend watching March Madness on the couch with Theo and eating takeout off paper plates.

The respite was desperately needed. In all the running back and forth to appointments, Steve and Alison hadn't had the chance to take a moment and figure out how to exist as parents. When they'd first returned home, they decided that whoever was more awake would be "on duty" for Theo and they would take turns. After trying that approach for a while, they found they were both completely exhausted all the time, so they switched to shifts. Steve didn't mind getting into bed at 4:00 p.m. and Alison didn't mind staying up late, so they changed the guard around 1:00 a.m. It gave each of them a period of rest and calm, but it meant that they barely had any time together. Sometimes if one of them was in bed, or "off duty," they texted the other for a favor, like a cup of coffee. They had Google Voice set up in the house, and Alison thought it was funny to broadcast messages to Steve when he was out in the living room.

They were managing as best they could, but there was no way around the disrupted sleep. After a couple of weeks, the exhaustion sunk into the marrow of their bones. Alison's energy was tapped out, and she was left feeling like a zombie. There were nights when Theo wouldn't stop screaming for hours, which she'd heard about, of course, but living through it was a whole other experience. She felt besieged. It was sensory overload, until salvation came in the form of a mamaRoo, a bounce-chair-rocker-swing contraption that aims to mimic the swaying motion of a parent holding a baby. Alison, ever skeptical of gear, hadn't been sure if she would use it, but it turned out to be essential. If Theo was fussy, or if Alison or Steve needed to do a task that involved both hands, they could put him in the mamaRoo and he'd calm down and smile, as if by magic.

While pregnant, Alison had heard the term "kangaroo baby" and grasped on to it, as she had with breastfeeding. She had read about attachment parenting and the purported benefits of continuous closeness and assumed she'd be a kangaroo mom who had her baby strapped to her all the time. But once she had become a mother, she realized that carrying a ten-pound baby around all the time wasn't feasible. To her, it made much more sense to put Theo into the swing while she did tasks like cook dinner, rather than carrying him while standing over a hot stove. As with breastfeeding, there were ideas that sounded nice and then there was reality, and as a new mother, Alison found herself increasingly emboldened to discard suggestions or ideas that weren't serving her or her family. If she hoped to make it through the maelstrom of new motherhood, she had to trust her own judgment about what was best for her and Theo instead of what was considered "best" by others.

Once the novelty of life with a baby settled down a bit, life started to feel somewhat normal again. Alison and Steve had the closest to a date night they could muster. They ordered sushi and talked about how Theo was born almost a year exactly after the miscarriage. Now that they had him, it felt like he was meant to be their baby. And not only had she had a healthy baby, but her husband was thriving as a father and partner. Seeing Steve take to fatherhood had been a whole other level of joy. He was the same, but different. Sleep deprived though they were, it felt like a time in their lives to cherish. Alison had the sense that motherhood never stopped being hard, but the specific ways in which it was hard would change, and things that had once felt hard would someday feel like no big deal. They might even become fond memories.

Before giving birth, Alison had thought she'd be happy to skip the labor part of having a baby. Now, she felt like it was a critical piece of understanding the universe. Her birth hadn't happened where or how she expected, and the whole castor oil situation had been gruesome, but Alison still surfaced from the experience feeling fulfilled. She had been surrounded by a team of people who respected her wishes, listened to her requests, and cared for her needs. She never felt pressured or judged. In retrospect, she felt a little silly for being so afraid of the hospital, especially given that it had a midwifery program, but all of it was part of how Theo got there.

Alison had once watched a documentary called *Fantastic Fungi* on Netflix, in which Michael Pollan talked about his research into how psilocybin mushrooms can be used for medicinal purposes. Patients take the mushrooms, have a psychedelic experience, and for some, their worldview radically changes. That was what childbirth felt like for Alison—a deeply spiritual, mind-expanding, and life-altering experience. It was an experience she had to surrender to. She did what she could do to manage the circumstances and environment, but once she was on the ride, she was on the ride. All she could do was hold on and press her way forward.

Alison had invested so much into having a physiologic birth with midwives at a birth center because she wanted to have more control. And yet, despite all her preparation, things easily could have gone another way. Alison knew she had the experience she had through a combination of privilege, determination, and luck. She could have made different decisions and had the same outcome or made the same decisions and had a different outcome. It was all random and yet felt ordained. Alison wasn't sure if that justified all her planning or undermined it, but she felt stronger and wiser for having gone through it.

The deep understanding that she could, and should, only try to control so much carried over into how she parented. To her own surprise, she found she was more relaxed than many of the other new moms she knew. During the Doula Love birth classes, a woman named Grace had gathered all the participants' phone numbers and started a group text thread. She and Grace had continued to text, especially after their deliveries (Grace had a cesarean a few days before Theo was born), and soon those conversations became walks and coffee with a few other women from the group, which became a valued source of support, socializing, and perspective. The moms shared tips and information and talked about their birth experiences. Hearing that others had had more difficult paths to bringing their babies into the world, or harder recoveries, made Alison realize, yet again, how fortunate she was.

It was also fascinating for her to observe the relationship between people's pregnancy and birth experiences and their approach to parenting. Some of the moms in the group who seemed to have sailed through their pregnancies with minimal anxiety or angst were tightly wound, nervous, and a tad obsessive as parents. Meanwhile, Alison, who had dedicated countless hours to research before making decisions and grappled with anxiety throughout her pregnancy, was comparatively laid-back. Some of the concerns the other moms had were things that hadn't even occurred to her to worry about, and she liked it that way.

Some of the women in the group said that they had felt immediately, powerfully, and blissfully bonded to their babies. Others, like Alison, found that an intimate emotional bond took time. She did feel bonded to Theo, but more out of a primal sense of responsibility for him, rather than a deep-seated personal connection. She thought he was the cutest baby in the world, but like any human, he would take time to get to know. A relationship was something they would build together. The feeling of connection became stronger once Theo's personality started to show. He could lift his head and smile. He loved to watch birds and responded to music. When he slept, he moved his fingers in a fan motion like he was counting. One night, while they lay in bed, Steve told Alison that she did the same thing in her sleep. It was such a small thing, but knowing that she and Theo shared that in common made her feel closer to him. They were all learning more about one another.

By the time the school year started, Alison was ready to go back to work and thankful that she had her childcare lined up. A retired teacher from Alison's school district ran a daycare out of her home, specifically for the children of teachers. She was nearby, had availability, and her prices were relatively affordable, which felt like an incredible stroke of luck. Alison looked forward to leaving the house, getting back into a work routine, and having professional goals to direct her energy and mind into. She was slated to teach fourth grade and complete an internship with the school principal as part of her graduate work.

Back at work, Alison was pleased to discover that she felt just as passionate about her career as she had before Theo was born. Instead of feeling like one identity or priority had subsumed the other, her world was expanding to make room for both. She was excited for work and then excited to go home at the end of the day and be with Steve and Theo. For so long, she'd been hung up on "being perfect."

And now she realized all she had to do was "be."

AFTERWORD

Jillian, T'Nika, and Alison are only three, out of over three and a half million, women who give birth in the US each year. Their stories are specific and unique for so many reasons, but there are threads in each for anyone to relate to and learn from. Even for someone who has no interest whatsoever in midwifery or community birth, who lives in a state where it's not available, or who is ineligible due to a risk factor; who comes from a different background than these three characters; or perhaps who has no interest in having children of their own, there are aspects of these narratives that are universal. And I hope that through their stories, idiosyncratic as they may be, one thing has been made clear: everyone has a right to bodily autonomy, safety, and respect in their reproductive lives. In their own distinct ways, that is what Jillian, T'Nika, and Alison were each seeking when they walked through the doors of a birth center.

For too many people in America, their experiences of pregnancy and childbirth are missing at least one of these elements, if not all three. Improving maternal healthcare in the US is not a simple or straightforward goal, but through reporting this book, I've come to hope that we are on the precipice of meaningful and lasting change. So much important and impactful work is being done to improve pregnancy and childbirth from different angles—in hospitals and outside them, within and across communities, from the top down and the bottom up and in all the space in between.

At the vanguard of that change is the reproductive justice movement. Reproductive justice is defined as "the human right to maintain personal bodily autonomy, have children, not have children, and parent the children we have in safe and sustainable communities." The framework, formulated and advanced by women of color, situates pregnancy, childbirth, abortion, and miscarriage as all part of the same life cycles and argues that issues like climate change, police violence, and wage equity—all the various elements that shape people's lives and whether and how they raise children—are directly, intrinsically related to health and equality. "Reproductive safety and dignity depends on having the resources to obtain good medical care and decent housing, to have a job that pays a living wage, to live without police harassment, to live free of racism in a physically healthy environment," wrote Loretta Ross, a founder of the movement, and the historian Rickie Solinger in the book *Reproductive Justice: An Introduction.*

The framework was developed in the 1990s by a coalition of groups who found that the mainstream reproductive rights movement—which was largely led by white, middle-class women—failed to represent their needs, ignoring key issues of race and class. The focus on abortion as the "right to choose," as primarily a legal or political question, sidelined poor women, women of color, and queer folks. For people who didn't have hundreds of dollars to spare on the procedure or reliable transportation to a clinic or the ability to take multiple days off work (a particular issue in states with mandatory waiting periods), access to abortion remained a right only in theory, not practice.

Moreover, 60 percent of people who have abortions already have children. Most of the remaining 40 percent will go on to do so. Access to contraception, abortion, miscarriage, and childbirth are intrinsically linked, and yet they have been treated as separate silos. And though essential, the feminist emphasis on abortion rights has sometimes occluded other important aspects of bodily autonomy. "One of the things we talked about was that, since the Civil War, the African-American community has been subject to strategies of population control, trying to make sure that we don't have children," Ross told *The New York Times Magazine*. "So we have to fight equally hard for the right *to have* the children that we want to have. As we thought about it further, we said, Well, once we had kids, no one seemed to care. So we have to fight for our right to parent our children in safe and healthy environments."

In 1997, sixteen organizations representing women of color came together to form SisterSong, a national organization dedicated to reproductive justice. One part of applying the reproductive justice framework to maternal healthcare is advocating for greater access to midwifery care—which evidence shows can improve outcomes, lower costs, mitigate racial inequities, and reduce the prevalence of mistreatment and bias—and for greater access to birth workers who reflect the communities they serve, including midwives and doulas. Some of the most radical, powerful possibilities for midwifery exist for people who have been traditionally marginalized and disadvantaged by the mainstream hospital-based system.

The esteemed midwife Jennie Joseph runs one of the first and longest-running midwifery clinics in the US based on these values. (She also owns the only independent midwifery school run by a Black person in the country.) Joseph was born in England and has practiced as a nurse-midwife in Winter Garden, Florida, for thirty years. Joseph's birth center, Commonsense Childbirth, follows her signature approach, known as the "JJ Way," which includes accepting all patients, regardless of insurance status, and ensuring that all patients are treated with dignity, respect, and compassion in an environment where they feel cared for and safe.

An evaluation of the birth center conducted by a local health department found that Joseph's clients of African descent were almost 40 percent less likely than women of a similar race throughout the nation to have a preterm labor or a child with a low birth weight. "It's a model that somewhat mitigates the impact of any systemic racial bias," Joseph told *ProPublica*. "You listen. You're compassionate. There's such a depth of racism that's intermingled with [medical] systems. If you're practicing in [the midwifery] model you're mitigating this without even realizing it."

The US would benefit from more birth centers like Joseph's, however, it can be prohibitively expensive to open and run a birth center, and extremely difficult to keep one open. The startup costs for a freestanding birth center are estimated around $1 to $2 million. According to the Birth Center Equity Fund, the number of community birth centers led by people of color, like Joseph's, is less than 5 percent. "The majority of birth centers in this country are owned by white women, and the majority of women who have access to them are white women," said Leseliey Welch, a co-founder of the Birth Center Equity Fund, in an interview with *Today*. "And those centers are fed by funds from previous practices, family income, family gifts—all of these things that our racialized history around wealth and the economy has given people of color a disadvantage."

Despite the financial barriers, a growing movement of midwives, doulas, and even a few physicians of color are opening birth centers around the country. Welch is also the co-founder and CEO of Birth Detroit, which offers community-based maternal and infant healthcare and is raising money to open a birth center. In 2011, the Family Health and Birth Center opened in Northeast Washington, DC, to serve low-risk women in the community, led by CNM Ebony Marcelle. That same year, Racha Tahani Lawler—a fourth-generation midwife whose grandmother delivered more than one thousand babies in Los Angeles hospitals—opened the Community Birth Center, the only Black-owned birthing center in LA at the time. In October 2020, midwives Kimberly Durdin and Allegra Hill opened the doors of their birth center, Kindred Space LA. Dr. Nicola Pemberton, a Black OB/GYN, is the founder and owner of the Birth Center in Union, New Jersey, which primarily serves people of color.

There's the Roots Birth Center in Minneapolis, and CHOICES in Memphis, which opened a nurse-midwife run birth center as part of its larger reproductive health practice and has provided abortion care for over forty-five years.* The new sixteen-thousand-square-foot building,

* On August 25, 2022, CHOICES stopped offering abortion services in Memphis due to a new law banning abortions in Tennessee.

which opened in 2020, is a physical manifestation of the fact that people who need abortion care and people who need pregnancy and childbirth care are often the same. (In Buffalo, Buffalo Women's Services also provides birth center and abortion care under one roof.)

In New Mexico, Nicolle Gonzales is a Navajo nurse and midwife and the founder of the Changing Woman Initiative. Many Native American women have few options other than to give birth at Indian Health Service hospitals, which are notoriously underfunded and have a fraught history that includes the forced sterilization of as many as seventy thousand Native women. Gonzales is working to open a birth center that will provide members of New Mexico's northern Pueblos with maternal healthcare that decolonizes, reclaims, and honors Indigenous birth practices. Gonzales has consulted with Indigenous architects and plans to design a space with a roundhouse center, as well as space for a sweat lodge and a garden to grow traditional herbs.

There are also indications that more Black and minority-owned birth centers are on the way. In 2020, Stephanie Mitchell, a CNM and CPM, raised $163,808 on GoFundMe to open Birth Sanctuary Gainesville, which would be a freestanding and Black-owned birth center in Alabama. In Euclid, Ohio, CNM Da'na M. Langford recently opened the Village of Healing Center, a women's healthcare and midwifery clinic. In Ferguson, Missouri, Jamaa Birth Village, a practice that provides "culturally-congruent traditional midwifery care," is raising money to open a birth and postpartum retreat center. In Chicago, CNM Jeanine Valrie Logan is working to open the Chicago South Side Birth Center, which would be the area's first freestanding birth center, where Logan has said she aims to create a "utopia" of Black birth workers.

Along with midwives, doulas and grassroots community collectives are a key part of working toward birth equity and justice. Organizations like Ancient Song in Brooklyn, Oshun Family Center in Philadelphia, and Uzazi Village in Kansas City, Missouri, offer accessible doula services and doula training courses. Ancient Song was founded by Chanel Porchia-Albert in 2008 to provide sliding-scale doula services to women of color and low-income families who otherwise would not be able to afford them, as well as training doulas to address health inequities in their work. Oshun Family Center was founded by Saleemah McNeil, a doula and traumatic birth survivor who created a Maternal Wellness Village program "after watching years of unfair treatment and inhumane conditions, reproductive injustice, systemic racism, and trauma." In Delaware, the Ubuntu Black Family Wellness Collective, led by CNM Michelle Drew, provides full spectrum reproductive health services, prenatal and parenting classes, and community doula services. In 2022, the nurse-midwife and professor Lucinda Canty opened Lucinda's House in Connecticut, which provides advocacy, education, and support for Black women and other women of color as they navigate pregnancy and childbirth. In 2019, a doula named Kelsey Carroll launched Rainbow Doula DC, a local doula service and childbirth community for people who are gay, lesbian, nonbinary, trans, and queer. In addition to hiring queer doulas, Rainbow Doula DC is building out a referral system and database that lists local queer-friendly providers, including midwives, primary care providers, and lactation consultants.

This list is not exhaustive and there's still a long way to go, but organizations like these are all part of reshaping the maternal health landscape in the US. They are not only establishing new paradigms for pregnancy care, but also for reproductive healthcare in general. They are helping to position midwifery and community birth work as a critical part of efforts to reduce inequities and improve the outcomes and experiences of giving birth in America.

Although they would make a difference, more midwives and birth centers are not a one-size-fits-all solution. There is no one-size-fits-all solution. Improving maternal and infant health outcomes is a complicated, multilayered, multifaceted problem that demands change on many levels.

Here are a few other measures that are necessary to build the reproductive health landscape that every pregnant person deserves:

- Universal access to affordable family planning resources, contraception, and abortion care is critical to ensuring people have control over if and when they become parents. Improving maternal healthcare requires enshrining the right to abortion into federal law. It requires removing barriers to abortion access such as state-wide bans, gestational bans, waiting periods and other TRAP laws that target clinics, and the Hyde Amendment. And it requires making medication abortion, a highly safe and effective method, more widely available and decriminalizing self-managed abortion. Organizations like Aid Access and Plan C offer valuable resources for how people in all fifty states can access abortion pills at home, while abortion funds and practical support organizations are a vital network helping people access legal, clinic-based care across the country.

- In 2021, the Black Maternal Health Momnibus Act, which aims to "comprehensively address every dimension of the maternal health crisis in America," was introduced in the House. The bill includes provisions for growing and diversifying the perinatal workforce, improving data collection processes and quality measures, supporting maternal mental health, and investing in social determinants of health that influence outcomes, like housing, transportation, climate-change-related risks, and nutrition.

- Passing a federal mandate to extend postpartum Medicaid coverage to twelve months would have a significant effect on outcomes. The current requirement is sixty days, which is woefully inadequate. Efforts to expand Medicaid eligibility outside the perinatal period are also key, as Medicaid expansion improves access to prenatal care and to preventative and primary care, enabling people to enter pregnancy in better health.

- On the hospital front, the development, dissemination, and promotion of toolkits for managing common obstetrical complications, such as those successfully deployed in California, have shown promising results. The Alliance for Innovation on Maternal Health (AIM)—which is funded by the US Health Resources and Services Administration and supported by medical societies including ACOG, the American College of Nurse-Midwives, and the American Academy of Family Physicians—has created a series of safety bundles for states and interested hospitals. Current safety bundles include obstetric hemorrhage, severe hypertension in pregnancy, safe reduction of primary cesarean birth, cardiac conditions, care for people with substance use disorders, and postpartum discharge, with a bundle for sepsis in development. The goal is for these evidence-based approaches for managing complications to become the widely adopted standard of care.

- Understanding the causes of and reducing the likelihood of preventable maternal death requires more consistent data collection and maternal death reviews, which are standard in countries like the UK. These review boards help provide greater insight into what went wrong and areas for improvement, so the same mistakes don't happen again. They are key to reducing the numbers of preventable deaths.

- The indiscriminate use or overuse of medical interventions during childbirth is one of the reasons why mortality and morbidity rates, not to mention costs, are so high. Reducing the prevalence of interventions and cesarean surgeries will require tort and malpractice liability reform, as well as changes to medical education and training. And by offering tools like birth tubs or cordless/intermittent monitoring to interested patients, and by having midwives on staff, hospitals can promote physiologic birth for the patients who prefer that approach.

- It should go without saying that listening to patients, respecting their wishes, and treating them with dignity and compassion are essential to improving maternal healthcare. Adhering to the principles of informed consent and shared decision-making should be an integral part of maternal healthcare (or any) practice. Obstetric violence and reproductive coercion are unacceptable and should be treated like the violations of human rights that they are.

- Birth choice is reproductive choice. Everyone having a baby should have the ability to give birth in the environment and with the provider that is the right fit for them. To that end, we need community midwives to be legal everywhere, and we need more midwives and more birth centers, which requires improving the access to and affordability of midwifery education and training. And while increasing the number of midwives is important, it's not enough. We also need to increase the diversity of the midwifery workforce and increase the number of midwives of color and community-based midwives who can offer culturally congruent care.

- Midwifery and community birth need to be a more integrated part of the maternal healthcare system. Deeper integration requires more insurance carriers to cover community midwives, payment reform so midwives and birth centers are paid fairly, and malpractice and tort reform so liability insurance isn't prohibitively expensive. Achieving those goals requires a greater standardization in how midwives are trained and certified, in line with international standards. It also requires greater willingness on the part of doctors, hospital administrators, nurses, and midwives to work together, collaborate, and treat one another with respect for the good of the clients. Productive relationships between community birth practices and local hospitals encourage the smooth transfer of care.

- The same principles apply to doulas. There needs to be funding for community-based practices and greater support for those practices so that midwives and doulas can earn a sustainable living. That support needs to include public and private insurance coverage for midwifery and doula services, so they are affordable to all.

- And finally, we as a country need to do a better job of caring for pregnant people and mothers, and supporting families postpartum. The Pregnant Workers Fairness Act, which was introduced in the Senate in 2021, would require employers to provide reasonable accommodations for pregnant women whose healthcare providers say they need them. There needs to be stronger screening and treatment for postpartum depression and anxiety and other perinatal mood disorders. Universal paid leave and childcare are critical to giving new parents the time they need to heal, bond, and get their bearings. It shouldn't be a Herculean feat or require vast troves of money to balance work life and family life.

ACKNOWLEDGMENTS

First and foremost, I would like to thank Jillian, T'Nika, and Alison for your time, your patience, your honesty, and your courage. I will forever be grateful for the ways you let me into your lives and your personal commitment to telling a new kind of birth story.

I'd also like to thank Jennifer, Marilyn, Carrie, and the whole Andaluz crew for opening the birth center and sharing your midwifery practice with me. I know that inviting me in was an act of trust, and I do not take that lightly.

A big thanks to the publishing team who sparked this book and who believed in me and this project before I did. My agent, Sarah Phair, for giving me the confidence to even think about writing a book proposal, and my editor, Julianna Haubner, for seeing the potential to tell these stories in a new way and for helping to shape the malleable mountain of research and reporting into an actual, cohesive book.

Many friends and loved ones encouraged and supported me along the way, and I would have been adrift without them.

To Ashley Tucker, who helped me celebrate my book deal with $80 worth of cheese in my favorite Brooklyn hot spot—your backyard. You never let a milestone go by without making it feel special and momentous. Your friendship is são magical to me and I am eternally grateful for your arguably too-fervent support.

So much love and gratitude to Kelsi George: ever since that fateful day in Lopburi when you were reading *Marley & Me,* I knew we were destined to be best friends. Okay, maybe I didn't know at that exact moment, but we've been through it all together. I wouldn't be the person I am without you. I wrote this book with the memory of Colette in my heart.

And to the rest of the Jazzy Galz—Heather Chadwick and Sarah Brooks—whose regular Polo dispatches, Peace Corps reminiscences, love of books, and thirst for details keep me laughing and motivated every single day.

To Kelsey, Summer, Avery, Cade, Kara, Skylar, and Max—I feel so lucky to be part of the dirty Wilson clan. I'm writing this on your dad's birthday, and can only hope this book has just a sprinkle of Buddy Style throughout its pages. He was one-of-a-kind, and is deeply missed.

To Jake Patoski, Dené White, Rachael Pike, Vicki Brown, and all my Portland pals. Thank you for being my PNW community and for making the city feel like home.

I want to give a shout-out to the Group for making me a better journalist, for inspiring me with your own work, and for creating the space to support one another in this shitshow of a profession: Spenser Mestel, Margot Boyer-Dry, Britta Lokting, Stephanie Russell-Kraft, Alex Kane, and Ted Brown. I might have given up on journalism a long time ago if it wasn't for you all.

Of course, the deepest of thanks to my amazing family, whom I love roof to sky. To my mom, Lauryn Guttenplan, who carried and raised me and modeled what a strong, ambitious, independent, caring, curious woman could be.

To my dad, Chris Grant, who never misses an opportunity to say you're proud of me. You challenge me to think harder and differently about everything and always encouraged me to forge my own dauntless future.

To my sister, Sarah, who makes me look lazy by comparison. I'm still sorry I said you would grow up to be a duck all those years ago, but I'm grateful that we always push each other to be better, go further, and climb higher.

And finally, a huge thank-you to my husband, Cullen Wilson, and our dog, Yoshi. Cull, I told you if you weren't nice to me, I would give Yoshi top billing in the book acknowledgments. His constant companionship and excess of fluff got me through the inevitable struggles of writing my first book, but it was you, all those years ago, who asked me why I was making sandwiches and helped me find my way back to journalism. Your support is unquantifiable and unwavering. I can't imagine my life without you, nor do I want to. I love you. Thank you for everything.

BIBLIOGRAPHY

Block, Jennifer. *Pushed: The Painful Truth About Childbirth and Modern Maternity Care*. Cambridge, MA: Da Capo Press, 2007.

Bovard, Wendy, and Gladys Milton. *Why Not Me? The Story of Gladys Milton, Midwife*. Summertown, TN: Book Publishing Company, 1993.

Bridges, Khiara M. *Reproducing Race: An Ethnography of Pregnancy as a Site of Racialization*. Berkeley: University of California Press, 2011.

Cassidy, Tina. *Birth: The Surprising History of How We Are Born*. New York: Grove/Atlantic, 2006.

Cottom, Tressie McMillan. *Thick*. New York: The New Press, 2018.

Davis, Dána-Ain. *Reproductive Injustice: Racism, Pregnancy, and Premature Birth*. New York: New York University Press, 2019.

Dekker, Rebecca. *Babies Are Not Pizzas: They're Born, Not Delivered!* Lexington, KY: Evidence Based Birth, 2019.

Dusenberry, Maya. *Doing Harm: The Truth About How Bad Medicine and Lazy Science Leave Women Dismissed, Misdiagnosed, and Sick*. New York: HarperOne, 2018.

Ehrenreich, Barbara, and Dierdre English. *Witches, Midwives & Nurses: A*

History of Women Healers. New York: Feminist Press at the City University of New York, 2010.

Epstein, Randi Hutter. *Get Me Out: A History of Childbirth from the Garden of Eden to the Sperm Bank*. New York: W. W. Norton & Company, 2010.

Fett, Sharla M. *Working Cures: Healing, Health, and Power on Southern Slave Plantations*. Chapel Hill: University of North Carolina Press, 2002.

Fraser, Gertrude Jacinta. *African American Midwifery in the South: Dialogues of Birth, Race, and Memory*. Cambridge, MA: Harvard University Press, 1998.

Gaskin, Ina May. *Spiritual Midwifery*. Summertown, TN: Book Publishing Company, 1976.

Goan, Melanie Beals. *Mary Breckinridge: The Frontier Nursing Service and Rural Health in Appalachia*. Chapel Hill: University of North Carolina Press, 2008.

Harjo, Joy, and Stephen Strom. *Secrets from the Center of the World*. Tucson: University of Arizona Press, 1989.

Holmes, Linda Janet. *Into the Light of Day: Reflections on the History of Midwives of Color Within the American College of Nurse-Midwives*. Silver Spring, MD: American College of Nurse-Midwives, 2011.

Karkowsky, Chavi Eve. *High Risk: Stories of Pregnancy, Birth, and the Unexpected*. New York: Liveright, 2020.

Leavitt, Judith Walzer. *Brought to Bed: Childbearing in America 1750–1950*. New York: Oxford University Press, 1986.

Lenz, Lyz. *Belabored: A Vindication of the Rights of Pregnant Women*. New York: Bold Type Books, 2020.

Litoff, Judy Barrett. *American Midwives: 1860 to the Present*. Westport, CT: Preager, 1978.

Logan, Onnie Lee, and Katherine Clark. *Motherwit: An Alabama Midwife's Story*. San Francisco, CA: Untreed Reads, 2014.

Loy, Mina, *The Lost Lunar Baedeker: Poems of Mina Loy*. Edited by Roger L. Conover. New York: Farrar, Straus and Giroux, 1996.

Luke, Jenny M. *Delivered by Midwives: African American Midwifery in the*

Twentieth-Century South. Jackson: University Press of Mississippi, 2018.

Meckel, Richard A. *Save the Babies: American Public Health Reform and the Prevention of Infant Mortality, 1850–1929*. Rochester, NY: University of Rochester Press, 2015.

Morris, Theresa. *Cut It Out: The C-Section Epidemic in America*. New York: New York University Press, 2013.

O'Connell, Meaghan. *And Now We Have Everything: On Motherhood Before I Was Ready*. Boston, MA: Little, Brown and Company, 2018.

Oparah, Julia Chinyere, et al. *Battling Over Birth: Black Women and the Maternal Health Care Crisis*. Amarillo, TX: Praeclarus Press, 2018.

Oster, Emily. *Expecting Better: Why the Conventional Pregnancy Wisdom Is Wrong—and What You Really Need to Know*. New York: Penguin Books, 2013.

Owens, Deirdre Cooper. *Medical Bondage: Race, Gender, and the Origins of American Gynecology*. Athens: University of Georgia Press, 2017.

Reagan, Leslie J. *When Abortion Was a Crime: Women, Medicine, and Law in the United States, 1867–1973*. Berkeley: University of California Press, 1998.

Roberts, Dorothy. *Killing the Black Body: Race, Reproduction, and the Meaning of Liberty*. New York: Vintage Books, 1997.

Ross, Loretta J., and Rickie Solinger. *Reproductive Justice: An Introduction*. Oakland: University of California Press, 2017.

Savitt, Todd L. *Medicine and Slavery: The Diseases and Health Care of Blacks in Antebellum Virginia*. Urbana and Chicago: University of Illinois Press, 2002.

Smith, Margaret Charles, and Linda Janet Holmes. *Listen to Me Good: The Life Story of an Alabama Midwife*. Columbus: Ohio State University Press, 1996.

Smith, Susan L. *Japanese American Midwives: Culture, Community, and Health Politics, 1880–1950*. Urbana and Chicago: University of Illinois Press, 2005.

Tuteur, Amy. *Push Back: Guilt in the Age of Natural Parenting.* New York: Dey Street Books, 2016.

Ulrich, Laurel Thatcher. *A Midwife's Tale: The Life of Martha Ballard, Based on Her Diary, 1785–1812.* New York: Alfred A. Knopf, 1990.

Varney, Helen, and Joyce Beebe Thompson. *A History of Midwifery in the United States: The Midwife Said* Fear Not. New York: Springer Publishing, 2016.

Vincent, Peggy. *Baby Catcher: Chronicles of a Modern Midwife.* New York: Scribner, 2002.

Wagner, Marsden. *Born in the USA: How a Broken Maternity System Must Be Fixed to Put Women and Children First.* Berkeley: University of California Press, 2006.

Wertz, Richard W., and Dorothy C. Wertz. *Lying-In: A History of Childbirth in America.* New Haven, CT: Yale University Press, 1977.

Woo, Victoria G., and Neel T. Shah, "Cost Outcomes and Finances of Freestanding Birth Centers." In *Freestanding Birth Centers: Innovation, Evidence, Optimal Outcomes,* edited by Linda J. Cole and Melissa D. Avery, 147. New York: Springer Publishing, 2017.

Zucker, Jessica. *I Had a Miscarriage: A Memoir, a Movement.* New York: Feminist Press at the City University of New York, 2021.

ENDNOTES

Foreword

xv *23 percent of hospital stays*: Kimberly W. McDermott, Anne Elixhauser, and Ruirui Sun, *Trends in Hospital Inpatient Stays in the United States, 2005–2014*, Healthcare Cost and Utilization Project: Statistical Brief #225 (Rockville, MD: Agency for Healthcare Research and Quality, June 2017), https://www.hcup-us.ahrq.gov/reports/statbriefs/sb225-Inpatient-US-Stays-Trends.pdf.

xv *That's 3.6 million babies*: Bracy E. Hamilton, Joyce A. Martin, and Michelle J. K. Osterman, *Births: Provisional Data for 2020*, National Vital Statistics Rapid Release, no. 012 (Hyattsville, MD: National Center for Health Statistics, May 2021), https://www.cdc.gov/nchs/data/vsrr/vsrr012-508.pdf.

xv *Each year in the US*: Center for Medicare and Medicaid Innovation, *Strong Start for Mothers and Newborns Evaluation: Year 5 Project Synthesis*, Volume 1: Cross-Cutting Findings (Baltimore, MD: Centers for Medicare & Medicaid Services, October 2018), https://downloads.cms.gov/files/cmmi/strongstart-prenatal-finalevalrpt-v1.pdf.

xv *One in three babies*: Joyce A. Martin et al., "Births: Final Data for 2019," *National Vital Statistics Reports* 70, no. 2 (Hyattsville, MD: National Center for Health Statistics, March 2021), https://www.cdc.gov/nchs/data/nvsr/nvsr70/nvsr70-02-508.pdf.

xv *Six of the sixteen most common*: Carol Sakala, *Maternity Care in the United States: We Can—and Must—Do Better* (Washington, DC: National Partnership for Women & Families, February 2020), https://www.nationalpartnership.org/our-work/resources/health-care/maternity-care-in-the-united.pdf.

xv *On average, a vaginal birth costs*: Gene Declercq, "Is There a Problem with U.S. Maternity Care Outcomes?," Birth by the Numbers, Fall 2020, https://www.birthbythenumbers.org/wp-content/uploads/2020/09/BBN-Website-Slides-Fl2020.pdf.

xv *Spontaneous vaginal birth*: Jessica Glenza, "Why Does It Cost $32,093 Just to Give Birth in America?," *The Guardian*, January 16, 2018, https://www.theguardian.com/us-news/2018/jan/16/why-does-it-cost-32093-just-to-give-birth-in-america.

xv *Thousands of families go*: Ibid.

xvi *"The modern medical system was built"*: Karkowsky, *High Risk*, 186.

xvi *According to an exhaustive report published*: National Academies of Sciences, Engineering, and Medicine, *Birth Settings in America: Outcomes, Quality, Access, and Choice* (Washington, DC: National Academies Press, 2020), https://doi.org/10.17226/25636.

xvi *Around 85 percent of women*: Carol Sakala et al., *Listening to Mothers in California: A Population-Based Survey of Women's Childbearing Experiences* (Washington, DC: National Partnership for Women & Families, September 2018, 39).

xvi *Around one in three pregnant people*: Eugene R. Declercq et al., *Listening to Mothers III: Pregnancy and Birth* (Washington, DC: National Partnership for Women & Families, May 2013, XI).

xvi *52.4 percent of women said*: Morris, *Cut It Out*, 7.

xvi *75 percent get an epidural*: Sakala et al., *Listening to Mothers in California*, 11.

xvi *Most patients are restricted*: Declercq et al., *Listening to Mothers III*, 19.

xvii *Between 2004 and 2017*: Marian F. MacDorman and Eugene Declercq, "Trends and State Variations in Out-of-Hospital Births in the United States, 2004–2017," *Birth* 46, no. 2 (June 2019): 279–88, https://doi.org/10.1111/birt.12411.

xvii *Between 2019 and 2020*: Elizabeth C. W. Gregory, Michelle J. K. Osterman, and Claudia P. Valenzuela, "Changes in Home Births by Race and Hispanic Origin and State of Residence of Mother: United States, 2018–2019 and 2019–2020," *National Vital Statistics Reports* 70, no. 15 (Hyattsville, MD: National Center for Health Statistics, December 2021), https://www.cdc.gov/nchs/data/nvsr/nvsr70/NVSR70-15.pdf.

Chapter 2

12 *As a result of gaps in insurance*: National Academies of Sciences, Engineering, and Medicine, *Birth Settings in America*, 81.

12 *People with employer-sponsored health insurance*: Michelle H. Moniz et al., "Out-of-Pocket Spending for Maternity Care Among Women with Employer-Based Insurance, 2008–15," *Health Affairs* 39, no. 1 (January 2020), https://www.healthaffairs.org/doi/abs/10.1377/hlthaff.2019.00296.

Chapter 3

22 *The former carried enslaved*: Varney and Thompson, *A History of Midwifery in the United States*, 10.

22 *During the crossing*: Ibid., 5.

22 *During this era, and for white women*: Wertz and Wertz, *Lying-In*, 4.

23 *"Female slaves were commercially valuable"*: Roberts, *Killing the Black Body*, 24.

23 *Midwives did what they could*: Luke, *Delivered by Midwives*, 17.

23 *They helped to spread culture*: Liese M. Perrin, "Resisting Reproduc-

tion: Reconsidering Slave Contraception in the Old South," *Journal of American Studies* 35, no. 2 (2001): 255–74.

23 *During the twentieth century, more than*: Alexandra Minna Stern, "Forced Sterilization Policies in the US Targeted Minorities and Those with Disabilities—and Lasted into the 21st Century," *The Conversation*, August 26, 2020, https://theconversation.com/forced-sterilization-policies-in-the-us-targeted-minorities-and-those-with-disabilities-and-lasted-into-the-21st-century-143144.

23 *The practice was so common that*: Roberts, *Killing the Black Body*, 90.

24 *Outside of the South, there were*: Varney and Thompson, *A History of Midwifery in the United States*, 10.

24 *German midwives had thriving practices*: Charlotte G. Borst, "Wisconsin's Midwives as Working Women: Immigrant Midwives and the Limits of a Traditional Occupation, 1870–1920," *Journal of American Ethnic History* 8, no. 2 (Spring 1989): 24–59.

24 *In 1908, 86 percent of*: Litoff, *American Midwives*, 27.

24 *In the Pacific Northwest*: Smith, *Japanese American Midwives*, 41.

24 *Doctors, however, were largely unwilling*: Ibid., 42.

25 *In 1905, a Finnish midwife*: Varney and Thompson, *A History of Midwifery in the United States*, 39.

25 *In 1913, 40 percent of births*: E. R. Declercq, "The Trials of Hanna Porn: The Campaign to Abolish Midwifery in Massachusetts," *American Journal of Public Health* 84, no. 6 (June 1994): 1022–28.

25 *In 1921, the US passed the Sheppard-Towner*: Wertz and Wertz, *Lying-In*, 209–15.

25 *Logan was born around 1910*: Logan and Clark, *Motherwit*, 1.

26 *Smith also received a midwifery permit*: Smith and Holmes, *Listen to Me Good*, 67, 2.

26 *One clever technique to gauge*: Luke, *Delivered by Midwives*, 42–50.

26 *They were subject to strict uniform*: Ibid., 49–50.

27 *By 1938, there were thirty-five*: Smith, *Japanese American Midwives*, 41.

27 *Three hundred of his followers*: Gaskin, *Spiritual Midwifery*, 15–30.

27 *In her book,* Spiritual Midwifery: Ibid., 16.

28 *In 1974, the midwife Raven Lang*: Cassidy, *Birth*, 45–47.

29 *The passage of the Civil Rights Act*: Fraser, *African American Midwifery in the South*, 57.

29 *"Nothing in my life has ever made"*: Logan and Clark, *Motherwit*, 187.

29 *As of 2020, 2,572 CPMs*: Ida Darragh et al., *2020 Annual Report* (Summertown, TN: North American Registry of Midwives, 2021), https://narm.org/pdffiles/2020NARMAnnualReport.pdf.

30 *Thirty-seven states had some kind*: "PushStates in Action," The Big Push for Midwives Campaign, accessed December 2, 2021, https://www.pushformidwives.org/pushstates_in_action.

32 *Episiotomies were routine*: David Banta and Stephen B. Thacker, "The Risks and Benefits of Episiotomy: A Review," *Birth* 9, no. 1 (March 1982): 25–30, https://doi.org/10.1111/j.1523-536X.1982.tb01599.x.

Chapter 4

36 *It is extremely common*: James M. Lepkowki et al., "The 2006–2010 National Survey of Family Growth: Sample Design and Analysis of a Continuous Survey," *Vital Health and Statistics* 2, no. 150 (June 2010): 1–36.

36 *12 percent of reproductive-aged*: Anjani Chanda, Casey E. Copen, and Elizabeth Hervey Stephen, "Infertility Service Use in the United States: Data from the National Survey of Family Growth, 1982–2010," *National Health Statistics Report* 73 (January 2014):1–21.

37 *Fertility treatments are exorbitantly*: Amy Klein, "I.V.F. Is Expensive. Here's How to Bring Down the Cost," *The New York Times*, April 18, 2020, https://www.nytimes.com/article/ivf-treatment-costs-guide.html.

37 *More often than not, infertility*: Andre M. Perry, "We Should All Be Able to Have Babies Like White People," *The Nation*, March 9, 2021, https://www.thenation.com/article/society/maternity-fertility-black-women.

42 *It's estimated that 10 to 15* [illegible] Miscarriage," Mayo Clinic, accessed May 13, 2022, https://www.mayoclinic.org/diseases-conditions/pregnancy-loss-miscarriage/symptoms-causes/syc-20354298.

45 *A 2015 study found that*: Lenz, *Belabored*, 43.

45 *"We cannot assume the stage"*: Zucker, *I Had a Miscarriage*, 45.

45 *This, combined with other factors*: Jessica Farren et al., "Posttraumatic Stress, Anxiety and Depression Following Miscarriage and Ectopic Pregnancy: A Multicenter, Prospective, Cohort Study," *American Journal of Obstetrics & Gynecology* 222, no. 4 (April 2020): 367.e1–367.e22, https://doi.org/10.1016/j.ajog.2019.10.102.

Chapter 5

51 *80 to 85 percent of midwives are white*: *2020 Demographic Report* (Columbia, MD: American Midwifery Certification Board, August 19, 2020), https://www.amcbmidwife.org/docs/default-source/reports/demographic-report-2019.pdf.

Chapter 6

61 *Birth, up to that point*: Wertz and Wertz, *Lying-In*, 6.

61 *In 1762, a physician named William Shippen*: Leavitt, *Brought to Bed*, 38–39.

62 *As awareness of forceps spread*: Wertz and Wertz, *Lying-In*, 40.

62 *One forceps proponent, William Smellie*: Ibid., 41.

62 *In 1817, Princess Charlotte Augusta*: Epstein, *Get Me Out*, 30–34.

62 *A new era of unusual birthing gadgets*: Ibid.

63 *In 1828, an English doctor*: Wertz and Wertz, *Lying-In*, 66.

63 *The first maternity clinics*: Cassidy, *Birth*, 54.

64 *Some lying-in hospitals*: Ibid., 55–56.

64 *J. Marion Sims, historically referred to*: Owens, *Medical Bondage*, 35–38.

64 *"Slavery's existence allowed for"*: Ibid.

64 *In 1852, Sims published a paper*: Epstein, *Get Me Out*, 44.

65 *The use of the drug remained the subject*: Cassidy, *Birth*, 89–90.

65 *In 1848, the American Medical Association*: Wertz and Wertz, *Lying-In*, 54–55.

65 *Physicians collaborated and organized*: Ibid., 212–13.

65 *Doctors presented themselves as paternalistic*: Ibid., 93.

66 *Attempts at "scrupulous cleanliness"*: Leavitt, *Brought to Bed*, 160–62.

66 *"The lure of medicine and the progress"*: Ibid., 84.

66 *In an effort to restructure*: Melissa Pandika, "How the Flexner Report Whipped Medical Education into Shape," *OZY*, May 15, 2014, https://www.ozy.com/true-and-stories/how-the-flexner-report-whipped-medical-education-into-shape/31516.

66 *Though the document would ultimately*: Dusenberry, *Doing Harm*, 7.

67 *By 1910, the US had more than*: Goan, *Mary Breckinridge*, 34.

67 *the numbers of women giving birth*: Wertz and Wertz, *Lying-In*, 133.

67 *After World War I*: Ibid., 137.

67 *In the first volume of the*: Leavitt, *Brought to Bed*, 179.

67 *As the journalist Jennifer Block*: Block, *Pushed*, 72.

67 *Pioneered in Freiburg, Germany*: Cassidy, *Birth*, 91–94.

67 *They accused doctors of being*: Epstein, *Get Me Out*, 89.

68 *The doctors who opposed twilight sleep*: Leavitt, *Brought to Bed*, 139.

68 *Doctors would no longer have to*: Ibid., 135.

68 *Popular literature of the 1920s and '30s*: Ibid., 175.

68 *In 1933, the White House published a report*: Wertz and Wertz, *Lying-In*, 161.

69 *That shift, while improving safety*: Leavitt, *Brought to Bed*, 189.

69 *By 1945, the percentage of hospital*: Cassidy, *Birth*, 62.

69 *The Hill-Burton Act of 1946*: Luke, *Delivered by Midwives*, 103.

69 *Moreover, Black doctors*: Ibid., 97.

69 *Black mothers and infants continued*: Davis, *Reproductive Injustice*, 130.

69 *After desegregation, Black women embraced*: Keisha La'Nesha Goode, "Birthing, Blackness, and the Body: Black Midwives and Experiential Continuities of Institutional Racism" (PhD diss., City University of New York, 2014, 61).

Chapter 7

73 *Breckinridge was born to a powerful*: Goan, *Mary Breckinridge*, 15.

73 *by 1910, one out of every four*: Ibid., 34.

73 *In the aftermath of the First World War*: Ibid., 52.

74 *"Her plan to make maternity safer"*: Ibid., 106.

74 *Leslie County, where the FNS*: Ibid., 70.

75 *Over rushing rivers, rickety bridges*: Ibid., 89.

75 *Outposts were opened in neighboring*: Wagner, *Born in the USA*, 102.

75 *In 1937, the FNS registered*: Goan, *Mary Breckinridge*, 171.

75 *The FNS delivered more than*: Ibid., 2.

75 *In 1939, eighteen of the service's*: Ibid., 173–75, 186.

75 *Back then, the only other nurse-midwifery*: Luke, *Delivered by Midwives*, 67–70.

76 *In 1935, as the federal government*: Smith, *Japanese American Midwives*, 112.

76 *That tiered model was intended*: Danielle Thompson, "Midwives and Pregnant Women of Color: Why We Need to Understand Intersectional Changes in Midwifery to Reclaim Home Birth," *Columbia Journal of Race and Law* 6, no. 1 (2016): 35.

76 *To address those divisions*: Holmes, *Into the Light of Day*, 11.

76 *In 1951,* Life *magazine ran a feature*: Luke, *Delivered by Midwives*, 64.

76 *A few years later, in 1955*: Ibid., 70.

76 *That same year, Columbia-Presbyterian-Sloan Hospital*: Cassidy, *Birth*, 44.

77 *The organization had folded in*: Goan, *Mary Breckinridge*, 235.

77 *ACNM did not bar members*: Holmes, *Into the Light of Day*, 12.

77 *In 1971, there were 1,200 certified nurse-midwives*: Cassidy, *Birth*, 44.

77 *In 1933, a British doctor named Grantly*: Ibid., 95, 144–48.

78 *The book was a hit*: Epstein, *Get Me Out*, 111.

78 *By all accounts, he was an arrogant male*: Ibid., 115.

78 *He also endeavored to capitalize*: Ibid.

78 *The Lamaze movement originated*: Cassidy, *Birth*, 148–51.

79 *One reader, named Elisabeth Bing*: Ibid., 153–54.

79 *The film showed a woman*: Ibid.

79 *It was an exam*: Wertz and Wertz, *Lying-In*, 193–94.

79 *As they grew more motivated*: Epstein, *Get Me Out*, 118–21.

79 *One of the first modern birth centers*: Cassidy, *Birth*, 69.

80 *"In Berkeley, in 1977"*: Vincent, *Baby Catcher*, 56.

80 *When Mutual Fire, Marine and Inland Insurance Company*: Kitty Ernst and Kate Bauer, "Birth Centers in the United States," American Association of Birth Centers, 2020, https://cdn.ymaws.com/www.birthcenters.org/resource/collection/028792A7-808D-4BC7-9A0F-FB038B434B91/Birth_Centers_in_the_United_States__2020_.pdf.

80 *"It was as if the gains"*: Vincent, *Baby Catcher*, 313.

80 *Today, there are around 385 freestanding*: Ernst and Bauer, "Birth Centers in the United States."

80 *They may employ only CPMs, only CNMs*: National Academies of Sciences, Engineering, and Medicine, *Birth Settings in America*, 67.

81 *although representing just 0.5 percent*: MacDorman and Declercq, "Trends and State Variations in Out-of-Hospital Births in the United States, 2004–17."

Chapter 8

87 *"It's like an auto mechanic"*: Wagner, *Born in the USA*, 39.

87 *"When the women in our study"*: Oparah et al., *Battling Over Birth*, 105.

87 *In 1989,* The New England Journal of Medicine: J. P. Rooks et al., "Outcomes of Care in Birth Centers: The National Birth Center Study," *New England Journal of Medicine* 321, no. 26 (December 1989): 1804–11, https://pubmed.ncbi.nlm.nih.gov/2687692.

87 *In a study of 16,924 women*: Melissa Cheyney et al., "Outcomes of Care for 16,924 Planned Home Births in the United States: The Midwives Alliance of North America Statistics Project, 2004 to 2009," *Journal of Midwifery & Women's Health* 59, no. 1 (January/February 2014): 17–27, https://doi.org/10.1111/jmwh.12172.

88 *"Increasingly better observational studies"*: Ole Olsen and Jette A. Clausen, "Planned Hospital Birth Versus Planned Home Birth," *Cochrane Database of Systematic Reviews* 9, no. 9 (September 2012), https://doi.org/10.1002/14651858.CD000352.pub2.

88 *However, for every study*: Amos Grünebaum et al., "Neonatal Mortality in the United States Is Related to Location of Birth (Hospital Versus Home) Rather Than the Type of Birth Attendant," *American Journal of Obstetrics & Gynecology* 223, no. 2 (August 2020): 254.e1–254.e8, https://doi.org/10.1016/j.ajog.2020.01.045.

88 *In part, these discrepancies*: Annalisa Merelli, "The Data on How Many New Mothers Die in the US Are in Shambles," *Quartz*, October 29, 2017, https://qz.com/1108268/maternal-mortality-data-in-the-us-is-so-bad-we-dont-actually-know-how-many-new-mothers-die.

88 *"To be frank, it seems very unlikely"*: Oster, *Expecting Better*, 265–270.

88 *The National Academies of Sciences, Engineering, and Medicine reached*: National Academies of Sciences, Engineering, and Medicine, *Birth Settings in America*, 152.

89 *All this fragmentation and variation*: Emily Le Coz, Josh Salman, and Lucille Sherman, "The Injustice: How a Burgeoning Industry Fails to Hold Midwives Accountable," *USA Today*, November 25, 2018, https://stories.usatodaynetwork.com/failuretodeliver/the-injustice.

89 *In 2018, GateHouse Media*: Ibid.

90 *Most pregnancies are uncomplicated*: "4 Common Pregnancy Complications," Johns Hopkins Medicine, accessed July 12, 2021, https://www.hopkinsmedicine.org/health/conditions-and-diseases/staying-healthy-during-pregnancy/4-common-pregnancy-complications.

90 *Even among eligible clients*: Cheyney et al., "Outcomes of Care for 16,924 Planned Home Births in the United States."

90 *This dynamic is harmful*: Saraswathi Vedam et al., "Mapping Integration of Midwives Across the United States: Impact on Access,

Equity, and Outcomes," *PLoS ONE* 13, no. 2 (February 2018): e0192523, https://doi.org/10.1371/journal.pone.0192523.

90 *"In the United States, integration of midwifery"*: National Academies of Sciences, Engineering, and Medicine, *Birth Settings in America*, 251–53.

91 *Eilers was a member of a group within WHA*: Donald M. Berwick, Thomas W. Nolan, and John Whittington, "The Triple Aim: Care, Health, and Cost," *Health Affairs* 27, no. 3 (May/June 2008), https://www.healthaffairs.org/doi/full/10.1377/hlthaff.27.3.759.

91 *Most of the money paid*: Sakala, *Maternity Care in the United States,* 10.

92 *If just an additional 10 percent*: Betty-Anne Daviss, David A. Anderson, and Kenneth C. Johnson, "Pivoting to Childbirth at Home or in Freestanding Birth Centers in the US During COVID-19: Safety, Economics and Logistics," *Frontiers in Sociology* 6 (2021).

92 *In 2021, the Midwifery Birth Center*: "Oregon Birth Data," Oregon Health Authority, updated May 2, 2022, https://www.oregon.gov/oha/PH/BIRTHDEATHCERTIFICATES/VITALSTATISTICS/BIRTH/Documents/2022/facilmonth22.pdf.

Chapter 9

103 *The Portland Andaluz location*: Karina Brown, "Midwives, Moms Say State Harassed and Investigated Them in Bad Faith," *Courthouse News Service,* September 14, 2010, https://www.courthousenews.com/midwives-moms-say-state-harassedand-investigated-them-in-bad-faith.

103 *a malpractice suit filed*: Aimee Green, "Waterbirth Center Didn't Know Baby Was Breech Till Informed by Mom, $7.5 Million Suit Says," *The Oregonian*, July 8, 2016, https://www.oregonlive.com/tualatin/2016/07/waterbirth_center_didnt_know_b.html.

103 *disagreements with the state about*: Andaluz Waterbirth Center, "Today I (Jennifer Sue Gallardo) gave a speech to over 30 law makers, Oregon state employees, and heads of CCOs (Medicaid insurance

care providers)," Facebook, August 7, 2019, https://www.facebook.com/andaluzwaterbirth/posts/today-i-jennifer-sue-gallardo-gave-a-speech-to-over-30-law-makers-oregon-state-e/3015948398476869.

Chapter 10

109 *In 2002, the Institute of Medicine*: B. D. Smedley, A. Y. Stith, and A. R. Nelson, eds., *Unequal Treatment: Confronting Racial and Ethnic Disparities in Health Care* (Washington, DC: National Academies Press, 2003), https://www.ncbi.nlm.nih.gov/books/NBK220355.

109 *For example, cesarean sections are*: Marco Huesch and Jason N. Doctor, "Factors Associated with Increased Cesarean Risk Among African American Women: Evidence from California, 2010," *American Journal of Public Health* 105, no. 5 (May 2015): 956–62, https://www.ncbi.nlm.nih.gov/pmc/articles/PMC4386542.

109 *but Black women are*: Bridges, *Reproducing Race,* 112.

110 *"Like millions of women of color"*: Cottom, *Thick,* 85–86.

Chapter 11

116 *Today, one in three people*: Martin et al., "Births: Final Data for 2019."

116 *a rate that is roughly*: Katherine Ellison and Nina Martin, "Severe Complications for Women During Childbirth Are Skyrocketing—and Could Often Be Prevented," *ProPublica,* December 22, 2017, https://www.propublica.org/article/severe-complications-for-women-during-childbirth-are-skyrocketing-and-could-often-be-prevented.

116 *Entities like the World Health Organization*: World Health Organization, *WHO Statement on Caesarean Section Rates* (Geneva: World Health Organization, Department of Reproductive Health and Research, 2015), https://apps.who.int/iris/bitstream/handle/10665/161442/WHO_RHR_15.02_eng.pdf.

116 *The risk of severe maternal complications*: Elliott Main et al., *Cesar-*

ean Deliveries, Outcomes, and Opportunities for Change in California: Toward a Public Agenda for Maternity Care Safety and Quality (Palo Alto: California Maternal Quality Care Collaborative, December 2011), https://www.cmqcc.org/resource/2070/download.

117 *Babies are impacted as well*: "Overdue: Medicaid and Private Insurance Coverage of Doula Care to Strengthen Maternal and Infant Health," National Partnership for Women & Families, January 2016, https://www.nationalpartnership.org/our-work/resources/health-care/maternity/overdue-medicaid-and-private-insurance-coverage-of-doula-care-to-strengthen-maternal-and-infant-health-issue-brief.pdf.

117 *For too many people giving*: Ellison and Martin, "Severe Complications for Women During Childbirth Are Skyrocketing—and Could Often Be Prevented."

117 *As Emily Oster wrote in* Expecting Better: Oster, *Expecting Better,* 211.

117 *Instead of prioritizing prevention*: National Academies of Sciences, Engineering, and Medicine, *Birth Settings in America,* 101.

117 *The anthropologist Robbie Davis-Floyd*: Robbie E. Davis-Floyd, "The Technocratic Model of Birth," in *Feminist Theory in the Study of Folklore,* eds. Susan Tower Hollis, Linda Pershing, and M. Jane Young (Champaign: University of Illinois Press, 1993), 297–326, http://www.davis-floyd.com/wp-content/uploads/2016/11/TECHMOD.pdf.

117 *"We designed the birth environment"*: Emily Kumler Kaplan, "Reducing Maternal Mortality," *The New York Times,* March 5, 2019, https://www.nytimes.com/2019/03/05/well/family/reducing-maternal-mortality.html.

118 *all stressors that can slow down*: Sarah J. Buckley, *Hormonal Physiology of Childbearing: Evidence and Implications for Women, Babies, and Maternity Care* (Washington, DC: National Partnership for Women & Families, January 2015), https://www.nationalpartnership.org/our-work/resources/health-care/maternity/hormonal-physiology-of-childbearing-exec-summary.pdf.

118 *"Women may find that technologies"*: Morris, *Cut It Out*, 84.

118 *In one* Listening to Mothers *survey*: Sakala et al., *Listening to Mothers in California*, 49.

118 *About one in three women*: Ellison and Martin, "Severe Complications for Women During Childbirth Are Skyrocketing—and Could Often Be Prevented."

118 *Another commonly cited justification*: Ibid.

118 *In the 1950s, during the era*: Dekker, *Babies Are Not Pizzas*, 47.

119 *Research suggests that labor*: Morris, *Cut It Out*, 89.

119 *Despite this marked increase*: Sakala et al., *Listening to Mothers in California*, 36.

119 *In 25 percent of C-sections*: Morris, *Cut It Out*, 8–10.

119 *A pattern of dips*: Ibid.

119 *"Many C-sections done for"*: Tuteur, *Push Back*, 100.

120 *"You have to almost prove"*: Morris, *Cut It Out*, 78.

120 *A suspected macrosomic*: Roni Caryn Rabin, "When a Big Baby Isn't So Big," *The New York Times*, January 11, 2016, https://well.blogs.nytimes.com/2016/01/11/high-birth-weight-predictions-are-often-inaccurate.

120 *One study found that only*: Ibid.

120 *A small percentage of women*: ACOG Committee on Obstetric Practice, "Cesarean Delivery on Maternal Request," Committee Opinion 761, American College of Obstetricians and Gynecologists, January 2019, https://www.acog.org/clinical/clinical-guidance/committee-opinion/articles/2019/01/cesarean-delivery-on-maternal-request.

120 *People with panic or anxiety*: Rebecca Brown, "I Want a C-Section—Why Won't You Give Me One?" *Glamour*, March 5, 2020, https://www.glamour.com/story/give-me-my-elective-c-section.

120 *While research overwhelmingly supports*: Michelle J. K. Osterman, "Recent Trends in Vaginal Birth After Cesarean Delivery: United States, 2016–2018," National Center for Health Statistics Data Brief no. 359, March 2020, https://www.cdc.gov/nchs/products/databriefs/db359.htm.

121 *In 1916, Dr. Edwin Cragin*: Cassidy, *Birth*, 128.

121 *even though women who have*: Yvonne Cheng et al., "Delivery After Prior Cesarean: Maternal Morbidity and Mortality," *Clinical Perinatology* 38, no. 2 (June 2011): 297–309, https://www.ncbi.nlm.nih.gov/pmc/articles/PMC3428794.

121 *While current estimates are hard*: Morris, *Cut It Out*, 122.

121 *ACOG supports trying for a VBAC*: American College of Obstetricians and Gynecologists, "ACOG Practice Bulletin No. 205: Vaginal Birth After Cesarean Delivery," *Obstetrics & Gynecology* 133, no. 2 (February 2019): e110–e127, https://journals.lww.com/greenjournal/Abstract/2019/02000/ACOG_Practice_Bulletin_No_205_Vaginal_Birth.40.aspx.

121 *C-section rates vary widely*: Katy Backes Kozhimannil, Michael R. Law, and Beth A. Virnig, "Cesarean Delivery Rates Vary Tenfold Among US Hospitals; Reducing Variation May Address Quality and Cost Issues," *Health Affairs* 32, no. 3 (March 2013), https://www.healthaffairs.org/doi/10.1377/hlthaff.2012.1030.

121 *"Your biggest risk factor for the most"*: Kaplan, "Reducing Maternal Mortality."

121 *"Because NIH and ACOG"*: Morris, *Cut It Out*, 20.

122 *Decisions may also be affected*: Avery Plough et al., "Relationship Between Labor and Delivery Unit Management Practices and Maternal Outcomes," *Obstetrics & Gynecology* 130, no. 2 (August 2017): 358–65, https://pubmed.ncbi.nlm.nih.gov/28697107.

122 *Hospitals, like any organization*: Elizabeth Kukura, "Obstetric Violence," *Georgetown Law Journal* 106 (2018): 721–801, https://www.law.georgetown.edu/georgetown-law-journal/wp-content/uploads/sites/26/2018/06/Obstetric-Violence.pdf.

122 *In one study out of UCLA*: Rie Sakai-Bizmark et al., "Evaluation of Hospital Cesarean Delivery-Related Profits and Rates in the United States," *JAMA Network Open* 4, no. 3 (2021): e212235, https://jamanetwork.com/journals/jamanetworkopen/fullarticle/2777679.

123 *Following payment reform*: National Academies of Sciences, Engineering, and Medicine, *Birth Settings in America*, 274.

123 *Hospitals also have legal*: Carol Sakala, Y. Tony Yang, and Maureen P. Corry, *Maternity Care and Liability: Pressing Problems, Substantive Solutions* (New York: Childbirth Connection, January 2013), https://www.nationalpartnership.org/our-work/resources/health-care/maternity/maternity-care-and-liability-report.pdf.

123 *In an ACOG survey on professional*: Ibid.

123 *From a legal standpoint*: Morris, *Cut It Out*, 43.

123 *"Because all decisions around birth"*: Ibid., 57.

123 *"Pregnancy becomes an experience"*: Karkowsky, *High Risk*, 188.

124 *According to a* Listening to Mothers *survey*: Declercq et al., *Listening to Mothers III*, 34.

Chapter 12

128 *"Pregnancy makes weird vaginal secretions"*: Lenz, *Belabored*, 39.

Chapter 14

142 *Preeclampsia is one of the top three:* Kathryn R. Fingar et al., "Delivery Hospitalizations Involving Preeclampsia and Eclampsia, 2005–2014," Healthcare Cost & Utilization Project Statistical Brief, no. 222 (Rockville, MD: Agency for Healthcare Research and Quality, April 2017), https://hcup-us.ahrq.gov/reports/statbriefs/sb222-Preeclampsia-Eclampsia-Delivery-Trends.

142 *Among women diagnosed with*: Elizabeth A. Howell, "Reducing Disparities in Severe Maternal Morbidity and Mortality," *Clinical Obstetrics and Gynecology* 61, no. 2 (June 2018): 387–99, https://www.ncbi.nlm.nih.gov/pmc/articles/PMC5915910.

143 *Studies have shown that Black and Native women*: Ibid.

143 *"It's chronic stress that just"*: Nina Martin and Renee Montagne, "Nothing Protects Black Women From Dying in Pregnancy and

Childbirth," *ProPublica,* December 7, 2017, https://www.propublica.org/article/nothing-protects-black-women-from-dying-in-pregnancy-and-childbirth.

143 *As the journalist Linda Villarosa wrote in a* New York Times: Linda Villarosa, "Why America's Black Mothers and Babies Are in a Life-or-Death Crisis," *The New York Times Magazine,* April 11, 2018, https://www.nytimes.com/2018/04/11/magazine/black-mothers-babies-death-maternal-mortality.html.

143 *The physiological term for the impact*: Ryan Blitstein, "Racism's Hidden Toll," *Pacific Standard,* June 15, 2009, https://psmag.com/social-justice/racisms-hidden-toll-3643#.v5c3pmo1r.

144 *An allostatic load score aims*: Erik J. Rodriquez et al., "Allostatic Load: Importance, Markers, and Score Determination in Minority and Disparity Populations," *Journal of Urban Health* 96, Supplement 1 (March 2019): 3–11, https://www.ncbi.nlm.nih.gov/pmc/articles/PMC6430278.

144 *Even when controlling for income and education*: Arline T. Geronimus et al., "'Weathering' and Age Patterns of Allostatic Load Scores Among Blacks and Whites in the United States," *American Journal of Public Health* 96, no. 5 (May 2006): 826–33, https://www.ncbi.nlm.nih.gov/pmc/articles/PMC1470581.

144 *The risk of dying from childbirth*: Marian MacDorman et al., "Recent Increases in the U.S. Maternal Mortality Rate: Disentangling Trends from Measurement Issues," *Obstetrics & Gynecology* 128, no. 3 (2016): 1–9, https://pubmed.ncbi.nlm.nih.gov/27500333.

144 *Seven hundred to nine hundred people*: Martin and Montagne, "Nothing Protects Black Women from Dying in Pregnancy and Childbirth."

144 *Between 2003 and 2013, the US*: Luke, *Delivered by Midwives,* 4.

144 *Approximately one-third of maternal deaths*: Eugene Declercq and Laurie Zephyrin, "Maternal Mortality in the United States: A Primer," Commonwealth Fund, December 16, 2020, https://doi.org/10.26099/ta1q-mw24.

145 *The CDC estimates that rates*: Emily E. Petersen et al., "Racial

/Ethnic Disparities in Pregnancy-Related Deaths—United States, 2007–2016," *Morbidity and Mortality Weekly Report* 68, no. 35 (September 2019): 762–65, http://dx.doi.org/10.15585/mmwr.mm6835a3.

145 *In 2014, WHO, UNICEF*: World Health Organization, UNICEF, UNFPA, The World Bank, and United Nations, *Trends in Maternal Mortality: 1990 to 2013* (Geneva: Department of Reproductive Health and Research, 2014).

145 *Out of all the countries surveyed:* Center for Reproductive Rights, National Latina Institute for Reproductive Health, and SisterSong Women of Color Reproductive Justice Collective, *Reproductive Injustice: Racial and Gender Discrimination in U.S. Health Care* (Washington, DC: Center for Reproductive Rights, 2014), 12, https://cdn1.sph.harvard.edu/wp-content/uploads/sites/2413/2017/06/Reproductive-injustice.pdf.

145 *In WHO rankings, the US*: Julia Belluz, "We Finally Have a New US Maternal Mortality Estimate. It's Still Terrible," *Vox,* January 30, 2020, https://www.vox.com/2020/1/30/21113782/pregnancy-deaths-us-maternal-mortality-rate.

145 *an American woman in 1990*: Mary-Ann Etiebet, "Maternal Mortality: Reducing the Pandemic's Effect on Health Inequity," Milken Institute, August 19, 2020, https://milkeninstitute.org/article/maternal-mortality-reducing-pandemics-effect-health-inequity.

145 *Although the MMR doesn't compare*: Ibid.

145 *Black women face similar*: Martin and Montagne, "Nothing Protects Black Women from Dying in Pregnancy and Childbirth."

145 *In Chicksaw County, Mississippi*: Center for Reproductive Rights, National Latina Institute for Reproductive Health, and SisterSong Women of Color Reproductive Justice Collective, *Reproductive Injustice*, 13.

146 *The disparities have not budged*: Gopal K. Singh, *Maternal Mortality in the United States, 1935–2007: Substantial Racial/Ethnic, Socioeconomic, and Geographic Disparities Persist* (Rockville, MD: Health

Resources and Services Administration, Maternal and Child Health Bureau, 2010), https://www.pubmed.ncbi/nlm.nih.gov/pmc/articles/PMC7792749.

146 *Black and American Indian and Alaska Native*: "2021 March of Dimes Report Card," March of Dimes, November 15, 2021, https://www.marchofdimes.org/materials/March_of_Dimes_2021_Full_Report_Card_11152021_v1.pdf.

146 *each year in the US, approximately twenty-one thousand*: "Infant Health," Centers for Disease Control and Prevention, May 16, 2022, https://www.cdc.gov/nchs/fastats/infant-health.htm.

146 *As Villarosa noted in the* Times: Villarosa, "Why America's Black Mothers and Babies Are in a Life-or-Death Crisis."

146 *"It is hard to imagine"*: Kim Brooks, "America Is Blaming Pregnant Women for Their Own Deaths," *The New York Times*, November 16, 2018, https://www.nytimes.com/2018/11/16/opinion/sunday/maternal-mortality-rates.html.

147 *Black Americans are two and a half times more*: John Creamer, "Inequalities Persist Despite Decline in Poverty for All Major Race and Hispanic Origin Groups," United States Census Bureau, September 15, 2020, https://www.census.gov/library/stories/2020/09/poverty-rates-for-blacks-and-hispanics-reached-historic-lows-in-2019.htm.

147 *Despite high workforce participation*: Chandra Childers, Ariane Hegewisch, and Eve Mefferd, "Shortchanged and Underpaid: Black Women and the Pay Gap," Institute for Women's Policy Research, July 27, 2021, https://iwpr.org/iwpr-publications/fact-sheet/shortchanged-and-underpaid-black-women-and-the-pay-gap.

147 *The median white household*: Kriston McIntosh et al., "Examining the Black-White Wealth Gap," The Hamilton Project, February 26, 2020, https://www.hamiltonproject.org/blog/examining_the_black_white_wealth_gap.

147 *The more segregated the city*: Zoë Carpenter, "What's Killing

America's Black Infants?," *The Nation*, February 15, 2017, https://www.thenation.com/article/archive/whats-killing-americas-black-infants.

147 *According to the Maternal Vulnerability Index*: Sema Sgaier and Jordon Downey, "What We See in the Shameful Trends of U.S. Maternal Health," *The New York Times*, November 17, 2021, https://www.nytimes.com/interactive/2021/11/17/opinion/maternal-pregnancy-health.html.

147 *Black communities at large*: Ihab Mikati et al., "Disparities in Distribution of Particulate Matter Emission Sources by Race and Poverty Status," *American Journal of Public Health* 108 (April 2018): 480–85, https://ajph.aphapublications.org/doi/10.2105/AJPH.2017.304297.

147 *as showcased in Flint and Newark*: Kristi Pullen Fedinick, Steve Taylor, and Michele Roberts, *Watered Down Justice* (New York: National Resources Defense Council, March 27, 2020), https://www.nrdc.org/resources/watered-down-justice.

147 *Black women are also more likely*: Tiffany Onyejiaka, "Black Maternal Mortality Is Already a Crisis—Climate Change Is Making It Worse," *Glamour*, September 9, 2020, https://www.glamour.com/story/black-maternal-mortality-is-already-a-crisis-climate-change-is-making-it-worse.

147 *Heat has been linked with an increased*: Sagi Shashar et al., "Temperature and Preeclampsia: Epidemiological Evidence That Perturbation in Maternal Heat Homeostasis Affects Pregnancy Outcome," *PLoS ONE* 15, no. 5 (2020): e0232877, https://doi.org/10.1371/journal.pone.0232877.

147 *Food deserts, areas in which*: Kelly Brooks, "Research Shows Food Deserts More Abundant in Minority Neighborhoods," *Johns Hopkins Magazine*, Spring 2014, https://hub.jhu.edu/magazine/2014/spring/racial-food-deserts.

148 *Black women are more likely to be*: Martin and Montagne, "Nothing Protects Black Women from Dying in Pregnancy and Childbirth."

148 *Native American and Alaska Native:* Amnesty International, *Deadly Delivery: The Maternal Health Care Crisis in the USA* (London: Amnesty International Publications, 2010), 20.

148 *Three-quarters of Black mothers*: Elizabeth A. Howell et al., "Black-White Differences in Severe Maternal Morbidity and Site of Care," *American Journal of Obstetrics & Gynecology* 214, no. 1 (January 2016): 122.e1–122.e7, https://www.ajog.org/article/S0002-9378(15)00870-4/fulltext.

148 *In the* Birth Settings in America *report*: National Academies of Sciences, Engineering, and Medicine, *Birth Settings in America,* 115.

148 *In an analysis of two years of hospital inpatient*: Annie Waldman, "How Hospitals Are Failing Black Mothers," *ProPublica,* December 27, 2017, https://www.propublica.org/article/how-hospitals-are-failing-black-mothers.

148 *In research conducted of New York City*: Elizabeth A. Howell et al., "Site of Delivery Contribution to Black-White Severe Maternal Morbidity Disparity," *American Journal of Obstetrics & Gynecology* 215, no. 2 (August 2016): 143–52, https://pubmed.ncbi.nlm.nih.gov/27179441.

149 *In a separate study*: Howell et al., "Black-White Differences in Severe Maternal Morbidity and Site of Care," 122.e1–122.e.7.

149 *In another survey from New York City*: Lynn Freedman et al., "Disrespect and Abuse of Women of Color During Pregnancy and Childbirth" (working paper, Columbia University Mailman School of Public Health, September 2020), https://www.publichealth.columbia.edu/sites/default/files/disrespect_of_woc_during_childbirth_in_nyc_working_paper.pdf.

149 *In California, the people interviewed by*: Oparah et al., *Battling Over Birth,* 13.

149 *"If doctors and nurses give dismissive looks"*: Davis, *Reproductive Injustice,* 203.

149 *A Black woman with a college degree*: Declercq and Zephyrin, "Maternal Mortality in the United States: A Primer."

150 *In 2018, Beyoncé wrote an article*: Beyoncé, "Beyoncé in Her Own Words: Her Life, Her Body, Her Heritage," *Vogue*, August 6, 2018, https://www.vogue.com/article/beyonce-september-issue-2018.

150 *That same year, Serena Williams*: Rob Haskell, "Serena Williams on Motherhood, Marriage, and Making Her Comeback," *Vogue*, January 10, 2018, https://www.vogue.com/article/serena-williams-vogue-cover-interview-february-2018.

150 *As detailed in a* ProPublica *investigation*: Martin and Montagne, "Nothing Protects Black Women from Dying in Pregnancy and Childbirth."

150 *"There is no magic Black gene"*: Priska Neely and Julia Simon, "Reproducing Racism," *Reveal*, May 23, 2020, https://revealnews.org/episodes/reproducing-racism.

151 *"Adverse maternal health outcomes"*: "American Indian and Alaska Native Women's Maternal Health: Addressing the Crisis," National Partnership for Women & Families, October 2019, https://www.nationalpartnership.org/our-work/resources/health-care/maternity/american-indian-and-alaska.pdf.

151 *Making matters worse is the fact*: Ayla Ellison, "Why Rural Hospital Closures Hit a Record High in 2020," *Becker's Hospital Review*, March 16, 2021, https://www.beckershospitalreview.com/finance/why-rural-hospital-closures-hit-a-record-high-in-2020.html.

151 *As many as five million women*: "Nowhere to Go: Maternity Care Deserts Across the U.S.," March of Dimes, 2018, https://www.marchofdimes.org/materials/Nowhere_to_Go_Final.pdf.

151 *Mortality rates for both infants*: Danielle M. Ely, Anne K. Driscoll, and T. J. Mathews, "Infant Mortality Rates in Rural and Urban Areas in the United States, 2014," National Center for Health Statistics Data Brief, no. 285, September 2017, https://www.cdc.gov/nchs/products/databriefs/db285.htm.

152 *Following the overturning of* Roe: Amanda Jean Stevenson, Leslie Root, and Jane Menken, "The Maternal Mortality Consequences of

Losing Abortion Access," SocArXiv, June 29, 2022, https://osf.io/preprints/socarxiv/7g29k.

152 *Meanwhile, the CDC estimates*: "Pregnancy-Related Deaths: Data from Maternal Mortality Review Committees in 36 States, 2017–2019," Centers for Disease Control and Prevention, 2022, https://www.cdc.gov/reproductivehealth/maternal-mortality/erase-mm/data-mmrc.html.

152 *"These experiences collectively taught me"*: Neel Shah (@neel_shah), "These experiences collectively taught me that a bad system will beat a good person every time," Twitter, July 1, 2021, https://twitter.com/neel_shah/status/1410652104062947330.

Chapter 16

163 *Today, the term refers to a professional*: Coburn Dukehart, "Doulas: Exploring a Tradition of Support," NPR, July 14, 2011, https://www.npr.org/sections/babyproject/2011/07/14/137827923/doulas-exploring-a-tradition-of-support.

163 *The concept of the modern doula*: Sam Roberts, "Dana Raphael, Proponent of Breast-Feeding and Use of Doulas, Dies at 90," *The New York Times*, February 19, 2016, https://www.nytimes.com/2016/02/21/nyregion/dana-raphael-proponent-of-breast-feeding-and-the-use-of-doulas-dies-at-90.html.

163 *Around the same time, a neonatologist*: Karla Papagni and Ellen Buckner, "Doula Support and Attitudes of Intrapartum Nurses: A Qualitative Study from the Patient's Perspective," *Journal of Perinatal Education* 15, no. 1 (Winter 2006): 11–18, https://www.ncbi.nlm.nih.gov/pmc/articles/PMC1595283.

163 *They, too, adopted the term:* John Kennell et al., "Continuous Emotional Support During Labor in a US Hospital: A Randomized Controlled Trial," *JAMA* 265, no. 17 (1991): 2197–2201, https://jamanetwork.com/journals/jama/article-abstract/385782.

163 *In 1992, Klaus and his wife*: "DONA International History," DONA International, accessed October 19, 2021, https://www.dona.org/the-dona-advantage/about/history.

163 *A long history of judicial (and ethical) precedent*: Lisa H. Harris and Lynn Paltrow, "The Status of Pregnant Women and Fetuses in US Criminal Law," *JAMA* 289, no. 13 (2003): 1697–99, https://jamanetwork.com/journals/jama/fullarticle/196295.

164 *There are abundant examples*: Heather Ault et al., *Birth Rights: A Resource for Everyday People to Defend Human Rights during Labor and Birth* (New York: Birth Rights Bar Association and National Advocates for Pregnant Women, 2020), https://www.nationaladvocatesforpregnantwomen.org/wp-content/uploads/2020/05/BIRTH-RIGHTS-A-resource-for-everyday-people-to-defend-human-rights-during-labor-and-birth.pdf.

164 *15 percent of mothers*: Declercq et al., *Listening to Mothers III*, 36.

164 *One in six women experience*: Saraswathi Vedam et al., "The Giving Voice to Mothers Study: Inequity and Mistreatment during Pregnancy and Childbirth in the United States," *Reproductive Health* 16 (June 2019), https://doi.org/10.1186/s12978-019-0729-2.

164 *Around one in three people*: Johanna E. Soet, Gregory A. Brack, and Colleen Dilorio, "Prevalence and Predictors of Women's Experience of Psychological Trauma during Childbirth," *Birth* 30, no. 1 (March 2003): 36–46, https://pubmed.ncbi.nlm.nih.gov/12581038.

164 *The physical experience of birth*: M. H. Hollander et al., "Preventing Traumatic Childbirth Experiences: 2192 Women's Perceptions and Views," *Archives of Women's Mental Health* 20, no. 4 (2017): 515–23, https://www.ncbi.nlm.nih.gov/pmc/articles/PMC5509770/.

164 *A study from the Center for American Progress*: Shabab Ahmed Mirza and Caitlin Rooney, "Discrimination Prevents LGBTQ People from Accessing Health Care," Center for American Progress, January 18, 2018, https://www.americanprogress.org/article/discrimination-prevents-lgbtq-people-accessing-health-care.

165 *Patients sign all kinds of consent*: Karkowsky, *High Risk*, 110.

165 *In recent years, advocates in the US*: Kukura, "Obstetric Violence."

165 *"Part of what makes obstetric violence"*: Ibid.

166 *There is growing recognition of the*: National Academies of Sciences, Engineering, and Medicine, *Birth Settings in America*, 1.

166 *A review of forty-one birth practices*: Vincenzo Berghella, Jason K. Baxter, and Suneet P. Chauhan, "Evidence-Based Labor and Delivery Management," *American Journal of Obstetrics & Gynecology* 199, no. 5 (November 2008): 445–54, https://pubmed.ncbi.nlm.nih.gov/18984077.

166 *In 2017, it also released a statement*: Allison Bryant and Ann E. Borders, "Approaches to Limit Intervention During Labor and Birth," Committee Opinion, no. 766, American College of Obstreticians and Gynecologists, February 2019, https://www.acog.org/clinical/clinical-guidance/committee-opinion/articles/2019/02/approaches-to-limit-intervention-during-labor-and-birth.

166 *A Cochrane meta-analysis spanning*: Ellen D. Hodnett et al., "Continuous Support for Women During Childbirth," *Cochrane Database of Systematic Reviews* 10 (2012): CD003766, https://www.cochranelibrary.com/cdsr/doi/10.1002/14651858.CD003766.pub4/full.

167 *Other studies have shown*: National Academies of Sciences, Engineering, and Medicine, *Birth Settings in America*, 209.

167 *In one study, doula support*: Katy B. Kozhimannil et al., "Modeling the Cost-Effectiveness of Doula Care Associated with Reductions in Preterm Birth and Cesarean Delivery," *Birth* 43, no. 1 (March 2016): 20–27, https://pubmed.ncbi.nlm.nih.gov/26762249/.

Chapter 17

172 *A 2020 study from Baylor University*: K. J. Hackney et al., "Examining the Effects of Perceived Pregnancy Discrimination on Mother and Baby Health," *Journal of Applied Psychology* 106, no. 5 (2021): 774–83, https://doi.org/10.1037/apl0000788.

172 *Approximately 250,000 pregnant workers*: "The Pregnant Workers

Fairness Act," National Partnership for Women & Families, February 2021, https://www.nationalpartnership.org/our-work/resources/economic-justice/pregnancy-discrimination/fact-sheet-pwfa.pdf.

172 *Between 2010 and 2020*: Bryan Robinson, "Pregnancy Discrimination in the Workplace Affects Mother and Baby Health," *Forbes*, July 11, 2020, https://www.forbes.com/sites/bryanrobinson/2020/07/11/pregnancy-discrimination-in-the-workplace-affects-mother-and-baby-health.

172 *28.6 percent of which were filed*: "By the Numbers: Women Continue to Face Pregnancy Discrimination in the Workplace," National Partnership for Women & Families, October 2016, http://www.nationalpartnership.org/research-library/workplace-fairness/pregnancy-discrimination/by-the-numbers-women-continue-to-face-pregnancy-discrimination-in-the-workplace.pdf.

172 *People who take longer than twelve*: Pinka Chatterji and Sara Markowitz, "Family Leave After Childbirth and the Mental Health of New Mothers," *The Journal of Mental Health Policy and Economics* 15 (2012): 61–76, http://i2.cdn.turner.com/cnn/2015/images/10/28/15-061_text.pdf.

173 *Research from the Infant Studies*: Natalie Brito et al., "Paid Maternal Leave Is Associated with Infant Brain Function at 3-Months of Age," PsyArXiv, August 20, 2021, https://psyarxiv.com/t4zvn.

173 *The Family and Medical Leave Act*: M. Rossin-Slater and L. Uniat, "Paid Family Leave Policies and Population Health," Health Affairs/Robert Wood Johnson Foundation, March 1, 2019, https://www.rwjf.org/en/library/research/2019/03/paid-family-leave-policies-and-population-health.html.

173 *According to research from professors*: Michelle J. Budig, "The Fatherhood Bonus and the Motherhood Penalty: Parenthood and the Gender Gap in Pay," Third Way, September 2, 2014, https://www.thirdway.org/report/the-fatherhood-bonus-and-the-motherhood-penalty-parenthood-and-the-gender-gap-in-pay.

173 *At 20 percent, the penalty for*: Julie Kashen and Jessica Milli, "The

Build Back Better Plan Would Reduce the Motherhood Penalty," The Century Foundation, October 8, 2021, https://tcf.org/content/report/build-back-better-plan-reduce-motherhood-penalty/#easy-footnote-bottom-7.

173 *The penalty is the greatest*: Claire Cain Miller, "The Motherhood Penalty vs. the Fatherhood Bonus," *The New York Times*, September 6, 2014, https://www.nytimes.com/2014/09/07/upshot/a-child-helps-your-career-if-youre-a-man.html.

177 *"Several of our participants"*: Oparah et al., *Battling Over Birth*, 104.

178 *"expanding access to midwives and doulas"*: Nora Ellmann, "Community-Based Doulas and Midwives," Center for American Progress, April 14, 2020, https://www.americanprogress.org/article/community-based-doulas-midwives.

178 *"We have to go beyond just talking"*: Angela Doyinsola Aina, "Birth Justice in Action: Advocating for Culturally Relevant Perinatal Care for Black Mamas," American Public Health Association Conference, November 4, 2019, https://apha.confex.com/apha/2019/meetingapp.cgi/Paper/450805.

179 *When researchers from George Mason University*: Brad N. Greenwood et al., "Physician-Patient Racial Concordance and Disparities in Birthing Mortality for Newborns," *Proceedings of the National Academy of Sciences* 117, no. 35 (2020): 21194–200, https://doi.org/10.1073/pnas.1913405117.

Chapter 18

181 *That schedule, which involves a total*: Alex F. Peahl and Joel D. Howell, "The Evolution of Prenatal Care Delivery Guidelines in the United States," *American Journal of Obstetrics & Gynecology* 224, no. 4 (April 2021): 339–46, https://pubmed.ncbi.nlm.nih.gov/33316276.

181 *although there are now*: Alex F. Peahl et al., "Right-Sizing Prenatal Care to Meet Patients' Needs and Improve Maternity Care Value,"

Obstetrics & Gynecology 135, no. 5 (May 2020): 1027–37, https://pubmed.ncbi.nlm.nih.gov/32282594.

183 *For many families, Covid*: Kimiko de Freytas-Tamura, "Pregnant and Scared of 'Covid Hospitals,' They're Giving Birth at Home," *The New York Times*, April 21, 2020, https://www.nytimes.com/2020/04/21/nyregion/coronavirus-home-births.html.

183 *An analysis of CDC data*: Kalie VanDewater, "Community Births Increase During Covid-19 Pandemic—So Do Risks," *Healio*, December 23, 2021, https://www.healio.com/news/womens-health-ob-gyn/20211223/community-births-related-birth-risks-increase-during-covid19-pandemic-so-do-risks.

Chapter 19

189 *There are increased health risks*: Oster, *Expecting Better*, 7–9.

189 *According to a study from Northwestern*: Cara Murez, "Majority of Pregnant U.S. Women Were Already in Poor Health: Study," *HealthDay*, February 15, 2022, https://consumer.healthday.com/pregnancy-2656608027.html.

189 *Many studies have shown*: Zawn Villines, "What to Know About Obesity Discrimination in Healthcare," *Medical News Today*, July 26, 2021, https://www.medicalnewstoday.com/articles/obesity-discrimination-in-healthcare.

Chapter 20

201 *For all these reasons, and many others*: "What Is Postpartum Depression & Anxiety?," American Psychological Association, accessed July 29, 2021, https://www.apa.org/pi/women/resources/reports/postpartum-depression.

202 *The general consensus is that*: Amnesty International, *Deadly Delivery*, 82–83.

202 *The US is the only high-income*: Roosa Tikkanen et al., "Maternal

Mortality and Maternity Care in the United States Compared to 10 Other Developed Countries," The Commonwealth Fund, November 18, 2020, https://www.commonwealthfund.org/publications/issue-briefs/2020/nov/maternal-mortality-maternity-care-us-compared-10-countries.

202 *One study found that one*: Sharon Lerner, "The Real War on Families: Why the U.S. Needs Paid Leave Now," *In These Times*, August 18, 2015, https://inthesetimes.com/article/the-real-war-on-families.

203 *Although there is no hard scientific evidence*: Mary Marnach, "Is It Safe to Eat My Placenta?," Mayo Clinic, December 11, 2021, https://www.mayoclinic.org/healthy-lifestyle/labor-and-delivery/expert-answers/eating-the-placenta/faq-20380880.

Chapter 21

209 *A majority of new mothers*: Division of Nutrition, Physical Activity, and Obesity, National Center for Chronic Disease Prevention and Health Promotion, *Breastfeeding Report Card: United States, 2020* (Atlanta, GA: Centers for Disease Control and Prevention, August 2020), https://www.cdc.gov/breastfeeding/data/reportcard.htm.

Chapter 33

290 *After getting the surgery*: Darshali A. Vyas et al., "Challenging the Use of Race in the Vaginal Birth After Cesarean Section Calculator," *Women's Health Issues* 29, no. 3 (May–June 2019): 201–04, https://pubmed.ncbi.nlm.nih.gov/31072754.

Afterword

306 *Reproductive justice is defined*: "What Is Reproductive Justice?" SisterSong Women of Color Reproductive Justice Collective, accessed September 8, 2021, https://www.sistersong.net/reproductive-justice.

306 *"Reproductive safety and dignity"*: Ross and Solinger, *Reproductive Justice*, 360.

306 *Moreover, 60 percent of people*: Margot Sanger-Katz, Claire Cain Miller, and Quoctrung Bui, "Who Gets Abortions in America?," *The New York Times*, December 14, 2021, https://www.nytimes.com/interactive/2021/12/14/upshot/who-gets-abortions-in-america.html.

306 *"One of the things we talked"*: Zoë Beery, "What Abortion Access Looks Like in Mississippi: One Person at a Time," *The New York Times*, June 13, 2019, https://www.nytimes.com/2019/06/13/magazine/abortion-mississippi.html.

307 *An evaluation of the birth center*: Miriam Zoila Pérez, "Making Pregnancy Safer for Women of Color," *The New York Times*, February 14, 2018, https://www.nytimes.com/2018/02/14/opinion/pregnancy-safer-women-color.html.

307 *"It's a model that somewhat mitigates"*: Nina Martin, "A Larger Role for Midwives Could Improve Deficient U.S. Care for Mothers and Babies," *ProPublica*, February 22, 2018, https://www.propublica.org/article/midwives-study-maternal-neonatal-care.

308 *The startup costs for a freestanding*: Alice Callahan, "The Doctors Taking Birth Out of the Hospital," *Undark*, April 17, 2019, https://undark.org/2019/04/17/midwives-birth-centers.

308 *"The majority of birth centers"*: Rheana Murray, "What Would You Pay to Feel Safe During Childbirth?," *Today*, December 10, 2020, https://www.today.com/specials/maternal-mortality-giving-birth-at-home.

308 *That same year, Racha Tahani Lawler*: Liana Aghajanian, "Los Angeles Midwives Aim to End Racial Disparities at Birth," *Al Jazeera*, September 5, 2015, http://america.aljazeera.com/articles/2015/9/5/to-los-angeles-midwives-racial-disparities-birth.html.

308 *Dr. Nicola Pemberton, a Black*: Alice Proujansky, "Why Black Women Are Rejecting Hospitals in Search of Better Births," *The New York Times*, March 11, 2021, https://www.nytimes.com/2021/03/11

/nyregion/birth-centers-new-jersey.html; Pérez, "Making Pregnancy Safer for Women of Color."

309 *Many Native American women*: Terry Gross and Adam Cohen, "The Supreme Court Ruling That Led to 70,000 Forced Sterilizations," *Fresh Air,* NPR, March 7, 2016, https://www.npr.org/2017/03/24/521360544/the-supreme-court-ruling-that-led-to-70-000-forced-sterilizations.

309 *Gonzales is working to open*: Cecilia Nowell, "How Indigenous Women Are Taking Back the Birthing Process: 'There Is a Reclaiming Happening,'" *The Lily,* January 5, 2021, https://www.thelily.com/how-indigenous-women-are-taking-back-the-birthing-process-there-is-a-reclaiming-happening.

309 *In 2020, Stephanie Mitchell*: Stephanie Mitchell and Courtney Stallworth, "Birth Sanctuary of Gainesville," GoFundMe, June 11, 2020.

310 *In 2019, a doula named Kelsey Carroll*: Mimi Montgomery, "This Queer-Friendly Birthing and Doula Collective Is the First of Its Kind in DC," *Washingtonian,* December 13, 2019, https://www.washingtonian.com/2019/12/13/this-queer-friendly-birthing-and-doula-collective-is-the-first-of-its-kind-in-dc.

ABOUT THE AUTHOR

REBECCA GRANT is a freelance journalist based in Portland, Oregon, who covers reproductive rights, health, and justice. Her work has appeared on *This American Life* and in *New York* magazine, *Marie Claire, The Atlantic, The Guardian, Cosmopolitan, Mother Jones, The Nation,* and *VICE,* among other publications. Reporting stories around the US and the world, she has received grants and fellowships from the International Women's Media Foundation, the International Reporting Project, and Type Investigations. Rebecca studied English and art history at Cornell University and served in the Peace Corps in Thailand.

Avid Reader Press, an imprint of Simon & Schuster, is built on the idea that the most rewarding publishing has three common denominators: great books, published with intense focus, in true partnership. Thank you to the Avid Reader Press colleagues who collaborated on *Birth*, as well as to the hundreds of professionals in the Simon & Schuster advertising, audio, communications, design, ebook, finance, human resources, legal, marketing, operations, production, sales, supply chain, subsidiary rights, and warehouse departments whose invaluable support and expertise benefit every one of our titles.

Editorial
Julianna Haubner, *Editor*

Jacket Design
Alison Forner, *Senior Art Director*
Clay Smith, *Senior Designer*
Sydney Newman, *Art Associate*

Marketing
Meredith Vilarello, *Associate Publisher*
Caroline McGregor, *Marketing Manager*
Katya Buresh, *Marketing and Publishing Assistant*

Production
Allison Green, *Managing Editor*
Jessica Chin, *Manager Copyediting*
Morgan Hart, *Production Editor*
Alicia Brancato, *Production Manager*
Lexy East, *Interior Text Designer*
Cait Lamborne, *Ebook Developer*

Publicity
David Kass, *Senior Director of Publicity*
Alexandra Primiani, *Associate Director of Publicity*
Rhina Garcia, *Publicist*
Katherine Hernández, *Publicity Assistant*

Publisher
Jofie Ferrari-Adler, *VP and Publisher*

Subsidiary Rights
Paul O'Halloran, *VP and Director of Subsidiary Rights*